I0065902

Antibiotic Essentials

Antibiotic Essentials

Editor: Clancy Knightley

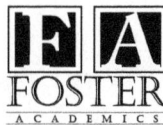

FA FOSTER
A C A D E M I C S

www.fosteracademics.com

www.fosteracademics.com

FA
FOSTER
ACADEMICS

Cataloging-in-Publication Data

Antibiotic essentials / edited by Clancy Knightley.
    p. cm.
Includes bibliographical references and index.
ISBN 978-1-63242-834-9
1. Antibiotics. 2. Antibiosis. 3. Pharmaceutical microbiology. I. Knightley, Clancy.
RM267 .A58 2019
615.792 2--dc23

© Foster Academics, 2019

Foster Academics,
118-35 Queens Blvd., Suite 400,
Forest Hills, NY 11375, USA

ISBN 978-1-63242-834-9 (Hardback)

This book contains information obtained from authentic and highly regarded sources. Copyright for all individual chapters remain with the respective authors as indicated. All chapters are published with permission under the Creative Commons Attribution License or equivalent. A wide variety of references are listed. Permission and sources are indicated; for detailed attributions, please refer to the permissions page and list of contributors. Reasonable efforts have been made to publish reliable data and information, but the authors, editors and publisher cannot assume any responsibility for the validity of all materials or the consequences of their use.

Trademark Notice: Registered trademark of products or corporate names are used only for explanation and identification without intent to infringe.

Contents

Preface

Over the recent decade, advancements and applications have progressed exponentially. This has led to the increased interest in this field and projects are being conducted to enhance knowledge. The main objective of this book is to present some of the critical challenges and provide insights into possible solutions. This book will answer the varied questions that arise in the field and also provide an increased scope for furthering studies.

Antibiotic refers to the antimicrobial substance which is active against bacteria. It plays a crucial role in fighting bacterial infections. It is used to kill or inhibit the growth of bacteria. Some antibiotics also possess the qualities of an antiprotozoal agent. Antibiotics are used in definitive therapy and empiric therapy. The interaction between some antibiotics such as tinidazole, latamoxef, furazolidone and metronidazole, with alcohol may reduce the effectiveness of antibiotics, and may cause a few side-effects. The topics included in this book on antibiotics are of utmost significance and bound to provide incredible insights to readers. It brings forth some of the most innovative concepts and elucidates the unexplored aspects of antibiotics. This book, with its detailed analyses and data will prove immensely beneficial to professionals and students involved in this area at various levels.

I hope that this book, with its visionary approach, will be a valuable addition and will promote interest among readers. Each of the authors has provided their extraordinary competence in their specific fields by providing different perspectives as they come from diverse nations and regions. I thank them for their contributions.

Editor

Non-Response to Antibiotic Treatment in Adolescents for Four Common Infections in UK Primary Care 1991–2012

Ellen Berni [1], Laura A. Scott [1], Sara Jenkins-Jones [1], Hanka De Voogd [2], Monica S. Rocha [2], Chris C. Butler [3], Christopher Ll. Morgan [1] and Craig J. Currie [1,4,*]

[1] Global Epidemiology and Medical Statistics, Pharmatelligence, Cardiff CF14 3QX, UK;
     ellen.berni@pharmatelligence.co.uk (E.B.); laura.scott@pharmatelligence.co.uk (L.A.S.);
     sara.jenkins-jones@pharmatelligence.co.uk (S.J.-J.); chris.morgan@pharmatelligence.co.uk (C.Ll.M.)
[2] Mylan Established Pharmaceuticals Division, Weesp 1381 CP, The Netherlands;
     hanka.devoogd@mylan.com (H.V.); monica.esrocha@gmail.com (M.S.R.)
[3] Nuffield Department of Primary Care Health Sciences, University of Oxford, Oxford OX2 6GG, UK;
     christopher.butler@phc.ox.ac.uk
[4] Cochrane Institute of Primary Care and Public Health, Cardiff University, The Pharma Research Centre,
     Abton House, Wedal Road, Cardiff CF14 3QX, UK
*   Correspondence: currie@cardiff.ac.uk

Academic Editor: Dan I. Andersson

Abstract: We studied non-response rates to antibiotics in the under-reported subgroup of adolescents aged 12 to 17 years old, using standardised criteria representing antibiotic treatment failure. Routine, primary care data from the UK Clinical Practice Research Datalink (CPRD) were used. Annual, non-response rates by antibiotics and by indication were determined. We identified 824,651 monotherapies in 415,468 adolescents: 368,900 (45%) episodes for upper respiratory tract infections (URTIs), 89,558 (11%) for lower respiratory tract infections (LRTIs), 286,969 (35%) for skin/soft tissue infections (SSTIs) and 79,224 (10%) for acute otitis media (AOM). The most frequently prescribed antibiotics were amoxicillin (27%), penicillin-V (24%), erythromycin (11%), flucloxacillin (11%) and oxytetracycline (6%). In 1991, the overall non-response rate was 9.3%: 11.9% for LRTIs, 9.5% for URTIs, 7.1% for SSTIs, 9.7% for AOM. In 2012, the overall non-response rate was 9.2%. Highest non-response rates were for AOM in 1991–1999 and for LRTIs in 2000–2012. Physicians generally prescribed antibiotics to adolescents according to recommendations. Evidence of antibiotic non-response was less common among adolescents during this 22-year study period compared with an all-age population, where the overall non-response rate was 12%.

Keywords: otitis media; adolescents; primary care; first line; respiratory tract infection; skin infection; treatment response; treatment failure; antibiotics

---

1. Introduction

Microbial resistance in adults and children is increasing worldwide, posing a major threat to public health [1]. Numerous strains of bacteria are becoming more difficult and time-consuming to treat [2], and now some infections cannot be treated with antibiotics [3]. Nevertheless, general practitioners (GPs) are thought to rarely report antibiotic resistance and believe that the problem is out of their control [4].

In order to address non-response to antibiotic treatment, it is essential that patterns of non-response are understood. Microbial resistance typically affects hospitalised patients, more so than in primary care settings, although antibiotics are routinely prescribed for respiratory tract infections in both primary and secondary care [5]. Considering the wide range of antibiotics available, and the different types of microbial infections, the impact of antibiotic resistance has proven difficult to characterise [6]. Extensive prescribing of antibiotics is considered to be the cause of high levels of antibiotic resistance and corresponding treatment non-response [7]. In adolescents, there is a high possibility of improper and over-prescribing of antibiotics, particularly when the prevalence of respiratory tract infections and acute otitis media (AOM) is high [8]. Children with acute respiratory tract infections treated with penicillin had reported resistance levels to be as high as 52% [9]. Nevertheless, data characterising antibiotic resistance in this younger age group are limited.

Concern regarding the effectiveness of antibiotics in adolescents has emerged. During clinical development, this age group is often studied less thoroughly than children aged 12 years and younger. Failure to respond to antibiotics does not necessarily imply a causal association with antibiotic resistance [10]. Many patients who are prescribed antibiotics in primary care are unlikely to benefit because they are suffering from viral infections. Nevertheless, information about non-response trends is important, as this may help clinicians share information with their patients about potential harm and benefits.

In our previous study [11] marking the 25th anniversary of the availability of clarithromycin, we reported that antibiotic treatment non-response rates for four common infection classes in primary care increased by 12% from 1991 to 2012. Here, given the emerging concern regarding the effectiveness of antibiotics in adolescents, our existing real-world data set was re-analysed to evaluate antibiotic non-response rates in the adolescent age group and compared these with the original study cohort, which contained patients of all ages.

2. Methods

2.1. Data Source

Data were extracted from the Clinical Practice Research Datalink (CPRD), a longitudinal anonymised research database drawn from nearly 700 primary care practices in the UK. This database contains demographic, diagnostic, treatment and referral information for approximately 8% of the UK population [12].

The data used in this study was a subgroup of the dataset from our recent study [11] and consisted of patients aged from 12 to 17 years that received prescriptions for antibiotics.

The current study received ethical approval from CPRD's Independent Scientific Advisory Committee on 31 October 2013, protocol number 13_168R.

2.2. Classification of Infection

Prescriptions for antibiotics were selected for four relevant infection classes: upper respiratory tract infections (URTIs), which included tonsillitis, laryngitis, pharyngitis and sinusitis; lower respiratory tract infections (LRTIs), including pneumonia, whooping cough and bronchitis; skin and soft tissue infections (SSTIs), including acne, abscesses, impetigo and cellulitis; and acute otitis media (AOM). These categories were the same as in our previous study [11]. The index date was set as the date of initiation of antibiotic monotherapy. Figure 1 illustrates selection of study data.

2.3. Identification of Antibiotic Treatments

Antibiotic monotherapy episodes were defined here as one or more consecutive prescriptions for a single antibiotic separated by no more than 30 days and uninterrupted by prescriptions for other antibiotic drug substances. Only first-line monotherapies, i.e. where there were no prescriptions for a different antibiotic in the 30 days prior to initiation, were included in this study. Monotherapy episodes were excluded if they began before 1991 or after 2012, or if the interval from the later of the patient's registration date and the practice's up-to-standard date to initiation was less than 365 days.

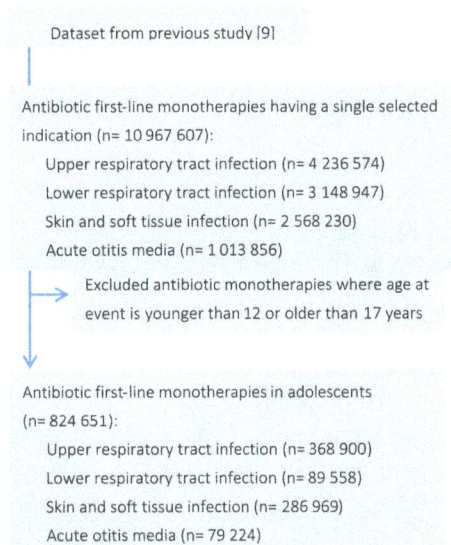

Figure 1. Data flow diagram for selection of antibiotic monotherapies in adolescents reported in the Clinical Practice Research Datalink.

2.4. Infection Rates and Antibiotic Prescription over Time

In a separate procedure (not illustrated), we measured background infection rates over time for each infection class as the proportion of all GP consultations in which the GP recorded a diagnosis of that infection in adolescents. Additionally, we determined the proportion of these infection-related consultations in which an antibiotic was prescribed. The prescription pattern of the five most commonly prescribed antibiotics over the research period in each infection is presented.

2.5. Antibiotic Treatment Non-Response Rates

For each year of the studied period, we evaluated the proportion of antibiotic monotherapies that resulted in treatment non-response. We defined antibiotic treatment non-response as the earliest occurrence of any of five events: (1) prescription of a different antibiotic within 30 days of the initial antibiotic prescription; or (2) GP record of admission to hospital with a diagnosis of infection within 30 days of initial antibiotic prescription; or (3) GP referral to an infection-related specialist service within 30 days of initial antibiotic prescription; or (4) a GP record of emergency department visit within three days of antibiotic initiation; or (5) a GP record of death with an infection-related clinical code, within 30 days of initial antibiotic prescription.

Treatment non-response rates are presented overall and for the five most frequently prescribed antibiotics within each infection class. Over the 22 years observed, the number of patients and participating practices increased, requiring treatment non-response rates to be averaged over the first five-year period (1991–1995) in order to create a more stable baseline for comparison with those in the last five-year period (2008–2012).

2.6. Statistical Analysis

Treatment non-response rates were presented as standardised ratios of observed rates to predicted rates for each year, using 1991 as the index year. Standardised ratios were adopted because of variations in antibiotic prescription patterns and age dispersion. Indexed treatment non-response rates were calculated using a matrix of infection subclass, antibiotic drug and gender; rates from 1991 were used to predict expected number of treatment non-responses, and, subsequently, to calculate the ratio.

3. Results

In this study 824,651 antibiotic monotherapies were prescribed to 415,468 adolescents. Of these, 368,900 (45%) therapies were for URTIs; 89,558 (11%) for LRTIs; 286,969 (35%) for SSTIs; and 79,224 (10%) for AOM (Figure 1).

3.1. Baseline Characteristics

The mean age of the adolescents in 1991–1995 was 14.5 years (Standard deviation (SD) 1.7 years) and in 2008–2012, 14.8 years (SD 1.7 years) (Table 1). Those with a diagnosis of AOM were younger (1991–1995: 13.9, SD 1.6 years and 2008–2012: 14.1, SD 1.7 years) and those with SSTIs slightly older (1991–1995: 15.1, SD 1.5 years and 2008–2012: 15.1, SD 1.5 years). Gender distribution was generally comparable across infection classes (1991–1995: 49.9% female; 2008–2012: 53.0% female), although URTIs were more common in females (1991–1995: 54.1%; 2008–2012: 58.7%) and LRTIs more common in males (1991–1995: 53.8%; 2008–2012: 53.1%).

Within the LRTI infection class, the proportion of co-medications increased from 1991–1995 to 2008–2012 from 2.8% to 8.0% for systemic corticosteroids, 22.3% to 29.4% for bronchodilators and 9.8% to 16.3% for inhaled corticosteroids. The proportion of co-medications in the other three infection classes remained generally constant from the first to the latter five-year period. The proportion of adolescent smokers was high (20%–27%) in the 1991–1995 period, but decreased to 5%–12% in the period 2008–2012 (Table 1).

3.2. Consultation Rates

GP consultation rates for the four infection classes, with or without antibiotic treatment, decreased over time (Figure 2). The all-cause consultation rate decreased from 466 consultations per 1000 registered patients per year in 1991 to 284 in 2012, a decrease of 39.1% ($p < 0.01$). The change in consultation rates varied by type of infection. Rates of consultations per 1000 patients per year decreased from 251 to 110 ($p < 0.01$) for URTIs, from 46 to 16 ($p < 0.01$) for AOM, and from 50 to 20 ($p < 0.01$) for LRTIs. Consultation rates for SSTI increased from 129 to 137 consultations per 1000 patients per year ($p < 0.01$).

3.3. Most Commonly Prescribed Antibiotics in Adolescents

The five most frequently prescribed antibiotics were amoxicillin (27.3%), penicillin-V (24.2%), erythromycin (11.3%), flucloxacillin (10.5%) and oxytetracycline (5.9%). Lymecycline (4.1%), co-amoxiclav (1.5%), doxycycline (1.4%) and clarithromycin (1.3%) were less frequently prescribed; the remaining antibiotics were prescribed in even lower quantities and they are reported together in a combined group termed "Others" (12.5%).

The prescription pattern of the most frequently prescribed antibiotics in each infection class, for each year between 1991 and 2012 is illustrated in Figure 3. For URTIs, penicillin-V (53.6%) was the most commonly prescribed antibiotic over the whole period. Amoxicillin was the most frequently prescribed antibiotic for the treatment of LRTIs (73.3%) and AOM (75.8%). The five most commonly prescribed antibiotics for SSTIs were flucloxacillin (30.4%), oxytetracycline (17.0%), erythromycin (15.3%), lymecycline (11.8%) and doxycycline (4.0%). In this infection class, the combined group of other antibiotics accounted for up to 21% of prescriptions.

In adolescents, skin and soft tissue infection prescriptions were more prominent than in the original, all-age study (35% vs. 23%), with therapies associated with acne comprising more than half of the antibiotic therapies in the adolescent study [11]. By contrast, antibiotic therapy for lower respiratory infection was relatively rare compared with the overall study (11% vs. 29%). Antibiotic therapies for upper respiratory infections and acute otitis media occurred in proportions comparable with the original study (45% vs. 39%, and 10% vs. 9%, respectively).

Table 1. Baseline characteristics by infection class and by early and late time period.

Baseline Characteristic	Upper Respiratory		Lower Respiratory		Skin and Soft Tissue		Acute Otitis Media		Overall	
	1991–1995	2008–2012	1991–1995	2008–2012	1991–1995	2008–2012	1991–1995	2008–2012	1991–1995	2008–2012
No of patients, n	32,150	73,528	10,063	20,259	13,768	66,937	8614	18,179	50,157	151,200
Antibiotic monotherapies, n	52,830	99,726	13,258	23,529	22,566	100,719	10,917	20,714	99,571	244,688
Male, n (%)	14,745 (45.9%)	30,354 (41.3%)	5411 (53.8%)	10,754 (53.1%)	7635 (55.5%)	33,426 (49.9%)	4309 (50.0%)	8510 (46.8%)	25,151 (50.1%)	71,113 (47.0%)
Female, n (%)	17,405 (54.1%)	43,174 (58.7%)	4652 (46.2%)	9505 (46.9%)	6133 (44.5%)	33,511 (50.1%)	4305 (50.0%)	9669 (53.2%)	25,006 (49.9%)	80,087 (53.0%)
Age, years, mean (SD)	14.4 (1.7)	14.7 (1.7)	14.4 (1.7)	14.6 (1.7)	15.1 (1.5)	15.1 (1.5)	13.9 (1.6)	14.1 (1.7)	14.5 (1.7)	14.8 (1.7)
Smoking, n (%):										
Never or not known	24,285 (46.0%)	63,936 (64.1%)	6032 (45.5%)	15,446 (65.6%)	11,216 (49.7%)	71,795 (71.3%)	4841 (44.3%)	12,127 (58.5%)	46,374 (46.6%)	163,304 (66.7%)
Ex-smoker	1575 (3.0%)	1085 (1.1%)	467 (3.5%)	277 (1.2%)	634 (2.8%)	863 (0.9%)	318 (2.9%)	120 (0.6%)	2994 (3.0%)	2345 (0.9%)
Current	12,918 (24.5%)	8646 (8.7%)	3520 (26.6%)	2645 (11.2%)	4481 (19.9%)	5044 (5.0%)	2445 (22.4%)	1085 (5.2%)	23,364 (23.5%)	17,420 (7.1%)
BMI, kg·m^{-2}, mean (SD)	21.7 (4.4)	23.0 (5.5)	21.5 (4.6)	22.8 (5.6)	21.6 (3.9)	22.9 (5.2)	21.5 (4.7)	23.3 (6.1)	21.6 (4.4)	22.9 (5.4)
Blood pressure, mmHg, mean (SD):										
Systolic	112.3 (12.3)	111.8 (12.4)	112.2 (13.0)	112.0 (12.7)	113.8 (12.4)	112.6 (12.5)	111.9 (13.6)	111.6 (12.7)	112.6 (12.6)	112.1 (12.5)
Diastolic	69.0 (8.8)	68.1 (8.7)	68.7 (8.6)	68.2 (9.1)	69.6 (8.5)	68.1 (8.6)	68.2 (8.9)	68.1 (9.1)	69.0 (8.7)	68.1 (8.7)
Co-medications, n (%):										
Systemic corticosteroid	201 (0.4%)	932 (0.9%)	370 (2.8%)	1881 (8.0%)	63 (0.3%)	348 (0.3%)	40 (0.4%)	97 (0.5%)	674 (0.6%)	3258 (1.3%)
Bronchodilator	3181 (6.0%)	7058 (7.1%)	2,951 (22.3%)	6917 (29.4%)	856 (3.8%)	3963 (3.9%)	551 (5.0%)	1138 (5.5%)	7539 (7.6%)	19,076 (7.8%)
Inhaled corticosteroid	1673 (3.2%)	4444 (4.5%)	1296 (9.8%)	3840 (16.3%)	418 (1.9%)	2560 (2.5%)	334 (3.1%)	758 (3.7%)	3721 (3.7%)	11,602 (4.7%)

n = number, SD = standard deviation.

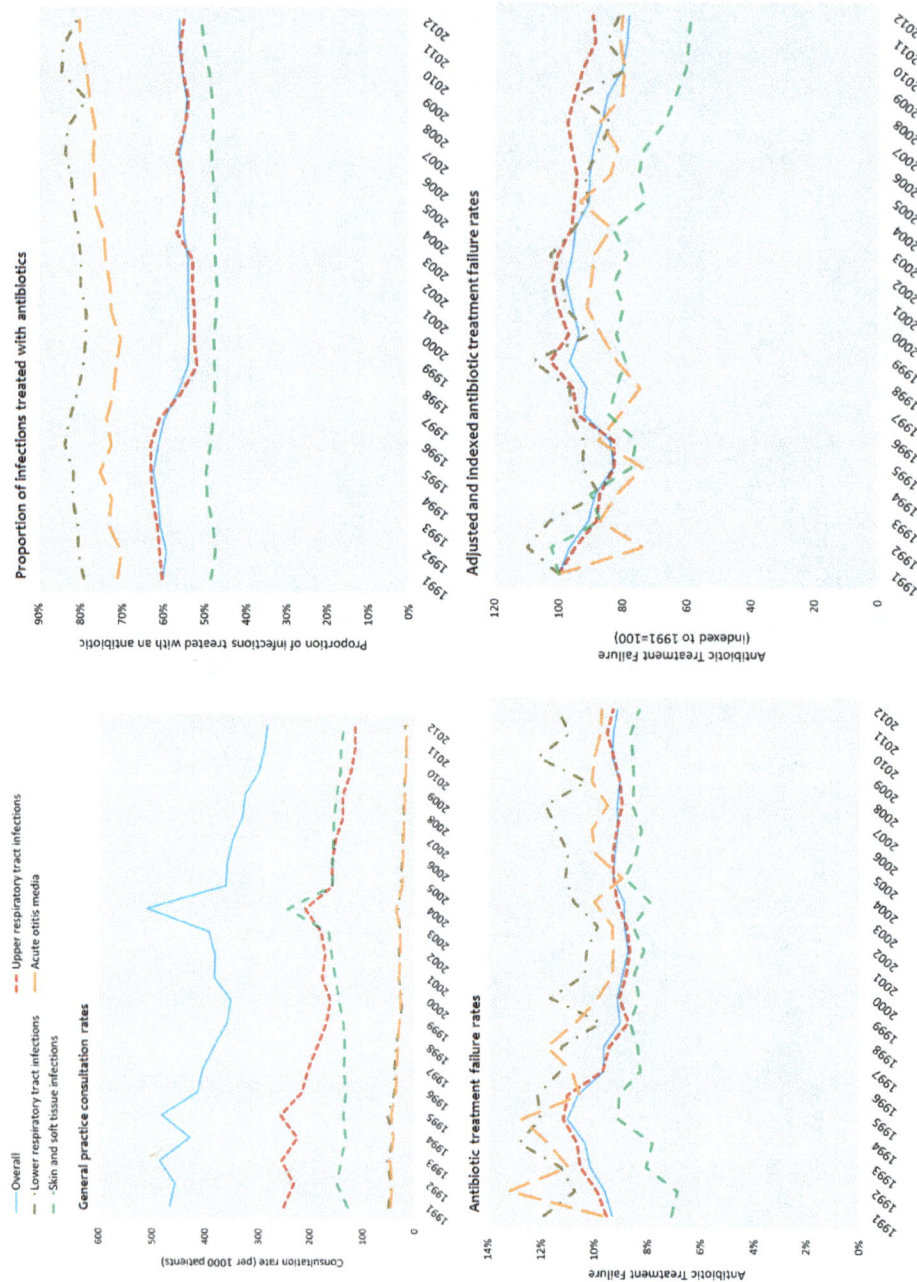

Figure 2. Consultation rates for the selected infection classes, proportion of infections in the selected classes treated with an antibiotic, antibiotic treatment non-response rates by infection class, and adjusted and indexed treatment non-response rates (indexed to 1991 = 100, and adjusted for age, sex, and type of antibiotic treatment used) observed between 1991 and 2012.

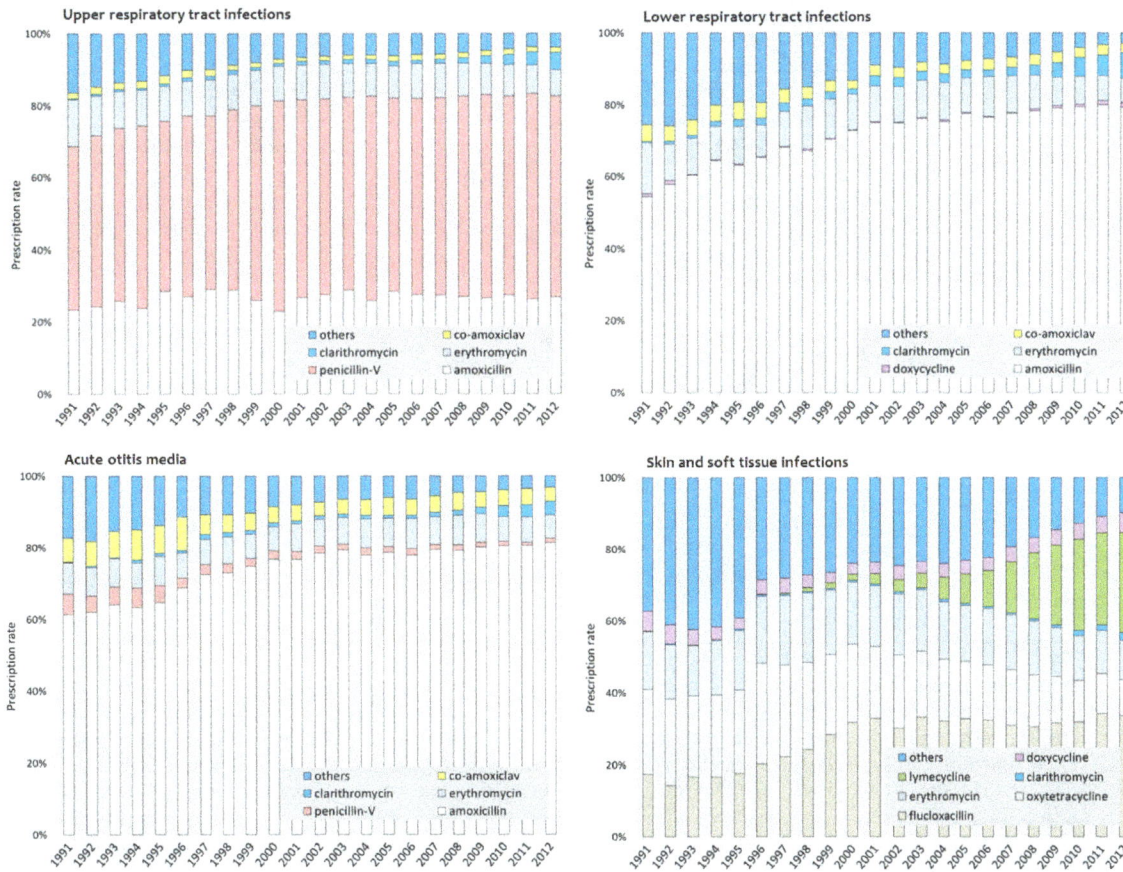

Figure 3. Five most commonly prescribed antibiotics between 1991 and 2012 by selected infection class.

A consistent prescription rate over the 22 years was generally observed in the five most frequently prescribed antibiotics for URTIs. However, antibiotics prescribed for SSTIs showed a varying pattern over time (Figure 3). For example, lymecycline showed the greatest increase in therapies since it was introduced in 1996, increasing from 0.1% to 27.9%. The proportion of oxytetracycline therapies showed the greatest decrease: from 23.6% to 10.0%.

The most frequently prescribed antibiotics in each infection class remained the same from the first five-year period to the last five-year period, albeit with changes in their ranking of relative frequency (Table 2). Penicillin-V remained the most prescribed antibiotic for the treatment of URTIs in the first and last five-year periods. For LRTIs and AOM, the most frequently prescribed antibiotic in both five-year periods was amoxicillin. In the first five-year period, oxytetracycline was the second-most-prescribed antibiotic for the treatment of SSTIs in adolescents.

Table 2. Average antibiotic therapy and treatment non-response rates (%) by infection class and by early and late time period with rank order in parentheses.

Infection Site	Antibiotic	Therapy Rates				Antibiotic Treatment Non-Response Rates			
		Average 1991–1995 % (Rank Order)		Average 2008–2012 % (Rank Order)		Average 1991–1995 % (Rank Order)		Average 2008–2012 % (Rank Order)	
URTIs	Penicillin-V	47.9	(1)	56.0	(1)	8.8%	(2)	7.4%	(1)
	Amoxicillin	25.6	(2)	26.8	(2)	9.7%	(3)	9.0%	(2)
	Others [a]	13.5	(3)	4.5	(4)	16.0%	(6)	31.3%	(6)
	Erythromycin	10.5	(4)	8.4	(3)	11.2%	(4)	9.7%	(3)
	Co-amoxiclav	2.0	(5)	1.5	(6)	12.7%	(5)	16.2%	(5)
	Clarithromycin	0.5	(6)	2.8	(5)	8.0%	(1)	10.8%	(4)

Table 2. *Cont.*

Infection Site	Antibiotic	Therapy Rates				Antibiotic Treatment Non-Response Rates			
		Average 1991–1995 % (Rank Order)		Average 2008–2012 % (Rank Order)		Average 1991–1995 % (Rank Order)		Average 2008–2012 % (Rank Order)	
LRTIs	Amoxicillin	60.9	(1)	79.1	(1)	9.6%	(2)	10.1%	(1)
	Others [b]	22.3	(2)	4.5	(4)	17.2%	(6)	37.4%	(6)
	Erythromycin	10.6	(3)	7.9	(2)	11.3%	(3)	10.7%	(2)
	Co-amoxiclav	4.5	(4)	2.9	(5)	12.6%	(4)	13.8%	(4)
	Clarithromycin	1.2	(5)	4.8	(3)	9.1%	(1)	10.7%	(3)
	Doxycycline	0.5	(6)	0.9	(6)	17.0%	(5)	16.0%	(5)
SSTIs	Others [c]	40.4	(1)	13.0	(3)	8.6%	(4)	15.9%	(7)
	Oxytetracycline	23.2	(2)	12.1	(5)	4.7%	(1)	6.3%	(2)
	Flucloxacillin	16.6	(3)	32.4	(1)	9.9%	(5)	9.0%	(4)
	Erythromycin	15.4	(4)	12.8	(4)	8.2%	(3)	9.1%	(5)
	Doxycycline	4.2	(5)	4.6	(6)	6.6%	(2)	6.7%	(3)
	Clarithromycin	0.2	(6)	1.3	(7)	18.2%	(6)	12.7%	(6)
	Lymecycline	-	-	23.8	(2)	-	-	5.1%	(1)
AOM	Amoxicillin	63.4	(1)	80.3	(1)	9.7%	(1)	8.4%	(1)
	Others [d]	15.6	(2)	4.0	(4)	16.7%	(6)	29.7%	(5)
	Erythromycin	7.9	(3)	7.5	(2)	12.8%	(3)	10.1%	(2)
	Co-amoxiclav	7.6	(4)	4.5	(3)	12.8%	(2)	13.6%	(4)
	Penicillin-V	5.0	(5)	1.2	(6)	16.2%	(4)	33.1%	(6)
	Clarithromycin	0.5	(6)	2.5	(5)	16.3%	(5)	10.7%	(3)

AOM, acute otitis media; LRTIs, lower respiratory infections; SSTIs, soft and skin tissue infections; URTIs, upper respiratory tract infections. [a] Others (URTIs): 19 antibiotics, of which the 10 most commonly prescribed were doxycycline, trimethoprim, flucloxacillin, cefalexin, lymecycline, oxytetracycline, azithromycin, cefaclor, nitrofurantoin, minocycline; [b] Others (LRTIs): 14 antibiotics (top 10: penicillin-V, cephalexin, azithromycin, trimethoprim, flucloxacillin, oxytetracycline, lymecycline, cefaclor, ciprofloxacin, cefradine); [c] Others (SSTIs): 18 antibiotics (top 10: amoxicillin, co-amoxiclav, minocycline, trimethoprim, penicillin-V, tetracycline, co-fluampicil, cephalexin, ciprofloxacin, nitrofurantoin); [d] Others (AOM): 15 antibiotics (top 10: flucloxacillin, cefalexin, trimethoprim, ciprofloxacin, doxycycline, lymecycline, oxytetracycline, cefaclor, metronidazole, co-fluampicil).

3.4. Failure to Respond to Antibiotics in Adolescents

The overall antibiotic non-response rate for the four infection classes was 9.5%, with a non-linear increase from 9.3% in 1991, peaking at 11.0% in 1995, and then declining to 9.2% in 2012. In 1991, the treatment non-response rates were 11.9% for LRTIs, 9.5% for URTIs, 7.1% for SSTIs and 9.7% for AOM. In 2012, treatment non-response rates were 11.4% for LRTIs, 9.4% for URTIs, 8.4% for SSTIs and 9.8% for AOM (Figure 2). SSTIs had the lowest treatment non-response rate in each five-year period (7.8% in 1991–1995 and 8.6% in 2008–2012). The highest treatment non-response rates were for AOM in 1991–1995 (11.7%) and for LRTIs from 2008 to 2012 (11.4%) (Table 2).

The two most frequently prescribed antibiotics for URTIs, penicillin-V and amoxicillin, both had stable non-response rates, ranging from 7% to 11% over the study period (Figure 4). Within the five most commonly prescribed antibiotics for LRTIs, amoxicillin, erythromycin and co-amoxiclav had constant treatment non-response rates of between 5% and 17% over the period (Figure 4). The five most frequently prescribed antibiotics for SSTIs had treatment non-response rates of between 4% and 13%, except for the antibiotic lymecycline, which only became available in 1996 (Figure 4).

For AOM, the treatment non-response rates of amoxicillin, erythromycin and co-amoxiclav remained stable over time (Figure 4). In contrast, for penicillin-V, treatment non-response rates increased markedly: from 16% in 1991–1995 to 33% in 2008–2012, with a rate of 40% in 2009 (Figure 4, Table 2).

3.5. Adjusted Rates of Non-Response of Antibiotic Treatment

After adjusting for antibiotic, index year and infection class, the rate of LRTI treatment non-response initially increased by 9% from 1991 to 1992 and then decreased from 1992 to 2012 by 28.3%. For SSTIs, URTIs and AOM, rates of antibiotic treatment non-response decreased from 1991 to 2012 by 40.5%, 10.2% and 19.6%, respectively. The overall adjusted treatment non-response rate decreased by 21.5% over the study period (Figure 2).

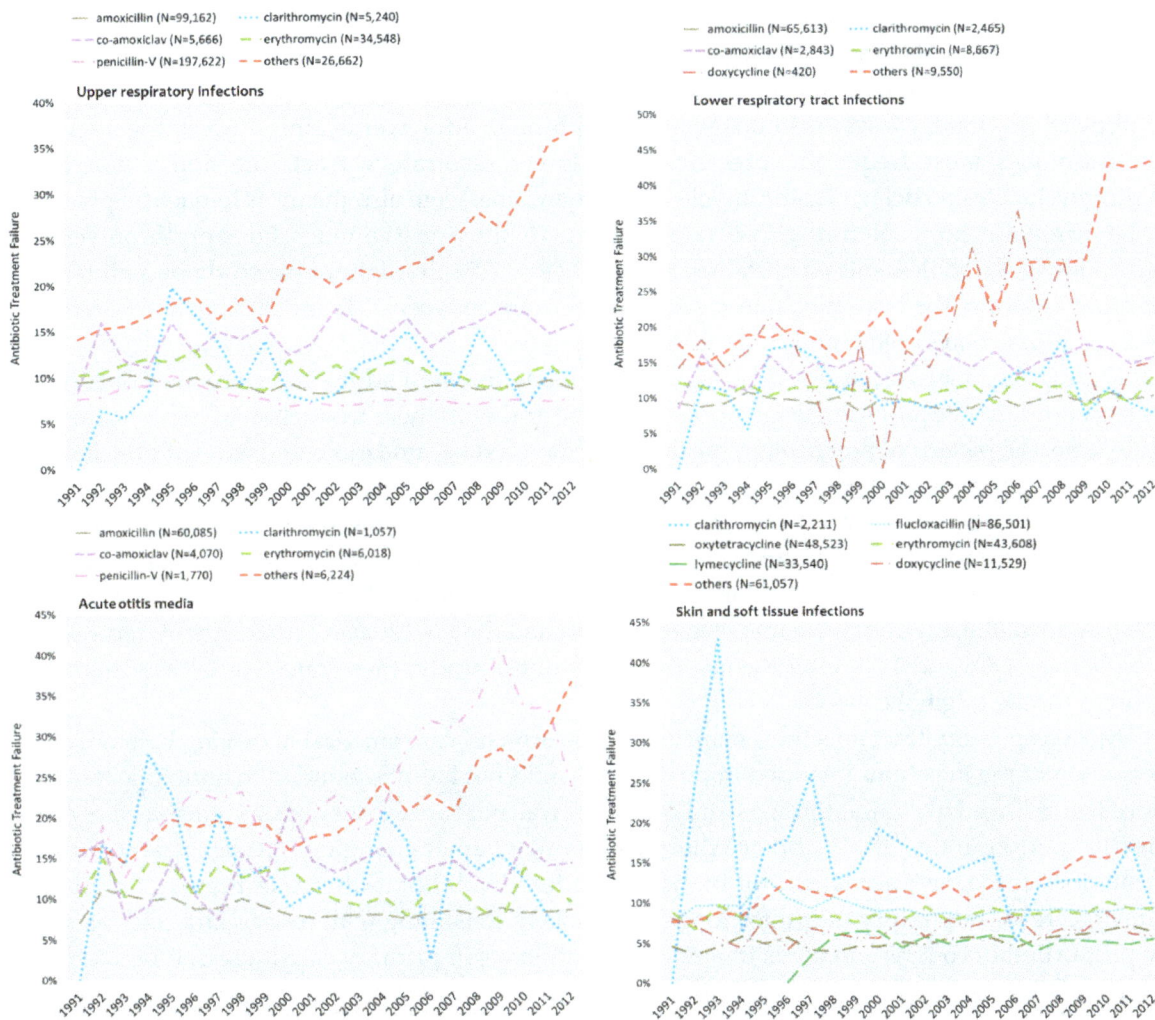

Figure 4. Antibiotic treatment non-response rates observed from 1991 to 2012 for the most commonly prescribed antibiotics in each selected infection class. "Other" antibiotics are defined in Table 2.

4. Discussion

This study examined non-response, in adolescents, to antibiotics prescribed for four common infection classes. We found that primary care physicians prescribe antibiotics to adolescents as they do for adults, rarely prescribing non-recommended compounds. In general, response to antibiotic treatment in adolescents was better than that in the all-age population.

We selected data for patients aged from 12 to 17 years from the dataset created for our original CPRD study [11] and analysed their demographic changes, consultation patterns, antibiotic treatment patterns, and treatment response rates. The proportion of adolescents in the original dataset was 7.1%, which is roughly comparable with the relative number of adolescents in the UK population over the research period [13], and the proportion of therapies prescribed to adolescents was 7.5%.

The most frequently prescribed antibiotics for upper respiratory tract infections in adolescents—penicillin-V, amoxicillin, erythromycin, co-amoxiclav and clarithromycin—were also frequent choices in the original cohort, and these are also listed in the guidelines as primary choices for bacterial infections [14]. However, antibiotics such as cefalexin, oxytetracycline, trimethoprim, cefaclor and doxycycline, which were in the top 10 for upper respiratory tract infections in the original cohort [11], were hardly prescribed to adolescents. The treatment non-response rates for penicillin and amoxicillin were below 10% in the first five years of the study period (1991–1995) and, on average, over the last five years (2008–2012). Non-response rates for the macrolides erythromycin and clarithromycin were around 10%. Co-amoxiclav and the combined "Other" antibiotics had higher and increasing treatment non-response rates. When prescribed for URTIs, penicillin and amoxicillin had lower treatment non-response rates in adolescents, compared with the original cohort.

Lower respiratory tract infections were uncommon in adolescents (only 2.6% of the infections). The antibiotics most frequently prescribed for lower respiratory tract infections: amoxicillin, erythromycin, co-amoxiclav, clarithromycin and doxycycline, were also the most frequently prescribed in the original cohort. Non-response rates for amoxicillin and the macrolides erythromycin and clarithromycin in adolescents were stable and at or below 10% throughout the study period, whilst in the original cohort, the respective non-response rates were between 15% and 20%, probably reflecting the large proportion of older and frailer patients.

During the first five years of the study period, many different antibiotics were prescribed for the treatment of skin infections in adolescence. Over time and with the introduction of lymecycline in the UK in 1996, the pattern of prescription for this infection class became more defined, with flucloxacillin and lymecycline together being prescribed in more than half of the cases.

In acute otitis media in adolescents, the top five antibiotics were amoxicillin, erythromycin, co-amoxiclav, penicillin-V and clarithromycin. In these adolescents as well as in the original study cohort, the majority of cases of AOM in the last five years of the study were treated with amoxicillin (80%). Amoxicillin, erythromycin and clarithromycin had the lowest average treatment non-response rates, between 8% and 11%, over the last five years of the study; these rates were lower than those reported for the original cohort.

Most respiratory tract infections managed in UK primary care are viral in origin, therefore a large proportion of the infections included in our study would not have responded to antibiotic treatment. Surveillance linked to clinical findings and outcomes was not carried out on a systematic basis during this time period in the UK. We do not therefore know whether changing pathogens and antibiotic sensitivities could have accounted for in the trends described. Point-of-care tests are not used in UK primary care for respiratory tract infections. The numbers consulting with coughs and colds as well as the proportion of coughs and colds treated with antibiotics in primary care increased between 2004 and 2011 [15].

5. Limitations

The adolescents formed a small subgroup of the original, all-age population and they were not excluded from the overall population values reported here. Had we compared the adolescent subgroup with the original population minus adolescent patients, the comparisons might have been more distinct. Differences observed here may therefore be somewhat underestimated but are still valid.

For infections requiring long-term antibiotic use, our algorithm may be overestimating rates of non-response because the prescription of different antibiotics in ongoing therapy would have been taken to signify non-response. Similarly, some infection episodes may have been misclassified as non-responsive because the initial therapy was followed within 30 days by the prescription of another antibiotic for a different indication.

6. Conclusions

Adolescents prescribed antibiotics are usually clinically managed as adults, and research on antibiotic non-response in this age group is scarce. In this study, we evaluated antibiotic prescription patterns and non-response rates for the treatment of four common infection classes in adolescents. Our data suggest that primary care physicians prescribe antibiotics to adolescents in line with current guidelines regarding initial prescriptions and, using our definition of antibiotic non-response, that adolescents respond generally better to these antibiotics compared with the general population as a whole. Non-response to antibiotics does not imply a causal link with antibiotic resistance, as many of the infections for which antibiotics are prescribed are viral. However, antibiotic resistance may be relevant in a minority of infections, and knowledge of non-response rates may be useful to inform discussion with patients about potential risks and benefits of antibiotic treatment for common infections.

Acknowledgments: Funding: The study was funded by Mylan (Weesp, The Netherlands). Due to the conditions of the data licence, co-authors from the funding body did not have access to the source data from the Clinical Practice Research Datalink, though they did have access to processed data. All other authors had full access to all of the data (including statistical reports and tables) in the study. All authors contributed to, read and approved the final manuscript, and all authors take responsibility for the integrity of the data and the accuracy of the data analysis. C.J.C. was the guarantor.

Author Contributions: C.J.C., E.B. and H.V. developed the study protocol. Data extraction and analysis were carried out by E.B. and S.J.-J., supervised by C.J.C. C.Ll.M. provided statistical expertise. C.C.B. advised on the interpretation of the study findings. L.A.S. and M.S.R. contributed to the writing of the manuscript.

References

1.   Bulla, A.; Hitze, K.L. Acute respiratory infections: A review. *Bull. World Health Organ.* **1978**, *56*, 481–498. [PubMed]

2.   Butler, C.C.; Hillier, S.; Roberts, Z.; Dunstan, F.; Howard, A.; Palmer, S. Antibiotic-resistant infections in primary care are symptomatic for longer and increase workload: Outcomes for patients with *E. coli* UTIs. *Br. J. Gen. Pract.* **2006**, *56*, 686–692. [PubMed]

3.   World Health Organization. *Antimicrobial Resistance: Global Report on Surveillance*; WHO Press: Geneva, Switzerland, 2014.

4.   Simpson, S.A.; Wood, F.; Butler, C.C. General practitioners' perceptions of antimicrobial resistance: A qualitative study. *J. Antimicrob. Chemother.* **2007**, *59*, 292–296. [CrossRef] [PubMed]

5.   Costelloe, C.; Metcalfe, C.; Lovering, A.; Mant, D.; Hay, A.D. Effect of antibiotic prescribing in primary care on antimicrobial resistance in individual patients: Systematic review and meta-analysis. *BMJ* **2010**, *18*, 340–2096. [CrossRef] [PubMed]

6.   Cosby, J.L.; Francis, N.; Butler, C.C. The role of evidence in the decline of antibiotic use for common respiratory infections in primary care. *Lancet Infect. Dis.* **2007**, *7*, 749–756. [CrossRef]

7.   Gonzales, R.; Malone, D.C.; Maselli, J.H.; Sande, M.A. Excessive antibiotic use for acute respiratory infections in the United States. *Clin. Infect. Dis.* **2001**, *33*, 757–762. [CrossRef] [PubMed]

8.   Grossman, Z.; del Torso, S.; Hadjipanayis, A.; van Esso, D.; Drabik, A.; Sharland, M. Antibiotic prescribing for upper respiratory infections: European primary paediatricians' knowledge, attitudes and practice. *Acta Paediatr.* **2012**, *101*, 935–940. [CrossRef] [PubMed]

9.   Kacou-N'douba, A.; Guessennd-Kouadio, N.; Kouassi-M'bengue, A.; Dosso, M. Evolution of *S. pneumoniae* antibiotic resistance in Abidjan: Update on nasopharyngeal carriage from 1997–2001. *Med. Mal. Infect.* **2004**, *34*, 83–85. [CrossRef] [PubMed]

10. Coenen, S.; Goossens, H. Antibiotic treatment failure in primary care. *BMJ* **2014**, *349*, g5970. [CrossRef] [PubMed]

11. Currie, C.J.; Berni, E.; Jenkins-Jones, S.; Poole, C.D.; Ouwens, M.; Driessen, S.; de Voogd, H.; Butler, C.C.; Morgan, C.L. Antibiotic treatment failure in four common infections in UK primary care 1991–2012: Longitudinal analysis. *BMJ* **2014**, *349*, g5493. [CrossRef] [PubMed]

12. Herrett, E.; Gallagher, A.M.; Bhaskaran, K.; Forbes, H.; Mathur, R.; van Staa, T.; Smeeth, L. Data resource profile: Clinical Practice Research Datalink (CPRD). *Int. J. Epidemiol.* **2015**, *44*, 827–836. [CrossRef] [PubMed]

13. Hagell, A.; Coleman, J.; Brooks, F. *Key Data on Adolescence 2013*; Association for Young People's Health: London, UK, 2013.

14. Public Health England. Management of Infection Guidance for Primary Care for Consultation and Local Adaptation 2015. Available online: https://www.gov.uk/government/uploads/system/uploads/attachment_data/file/455298/230415_Managing_Common_Infections_-_full_guide_with_rationale.pdf (accessed on 13 February 2016).

15. Hawker, J.I.; Smith, S.; Smith, G.E.; Morbey, R.; Johnson, A.P.; Fleming, D.M.; Shallcross, L.; Hayward, A.C. Trends in antibiotic prescribing in primary care for clinical syndromes subject to national recommendations to reduce antibiotic resistance, UK 1995–2011: Analysis of a large database of primary care consultations. *J. Antimicrob. Chemother.* **2014**, *69*, 3423–3430. [CrossRef] [PubMed]

2

Actinomycetes, an Inexhaustible Source of Naturally Occurring Antibiotics

Yōko Takahashi * and Takuji Nakashima 🆔

Kitasato Institute for Life Sciences, Kitasato University, 5-9-1 Shirokane, Minato-ku, Tokyo 108-8641, Japan; takuji@lisci.kitasato-u.ac.jp
* Correspondence: ytakaha@lisci.kitasato-u.ac.jp

Abstract: Global public health faces a desperate situation, due to the lack of effective antibiotics. Coordinated steps need to be taken, worldwide, to rectify this situation and protect the advances in modern medicine made over the last 100 years. Work at Japan's Kitasato Institute has been in the vanguard of many such advances, and work is being proactively tailored to promote the discovery of urgently needed antimicrobials. Efforts are being concentrated on actinomycetes, the proven source of most modern antibiotics. We devised a novel physicochemical screening mechanism, whereby simple physico-chemical properties, in conjunction with related detection methods, such as LC/MS, LC/UV, and polarity, could be used to identify or predict new compounds in a culture broth, simply by comparing results with existing databases. New compounds are isolated, purified, and their structure determined before being tested for any bioactivity. We used lyophilized actinomycete strains from the Kitasato Microbial Library, most more than 35 years old, and found 330 strains were producers of useful bioactive substances. We also tested organisms found in fresh samples collected in the complex environments from around plant roots, as well as from sediments of mangrove forests and oceans, resulting in the discovery of 36 novel compounds from 11 actinomycete strains. A compound, designated iminimycin, containing an iminium ion in the structure was discovered from the culture broth of *Streptomyces griseus* OS-3601, which had been stored for a long time as a streptomycin-producing strain. This represented the first iminium ion discovery in actinomycetes. Compounds with a cyclopentadecane skeleton containing 5,6-dihydro-4-hydroxyl-2-pyrone ring and tetrahydrofuran ring, designated mangromicins, were isolated from the culture broth of *Lechevalieria aerocolonigenes* K10-0216 obtained from sediment in a mangrove forest. These structures are extremely unique among natural compounds. From the same culture broth, new steroid compounds, named K10-0216 KA and KB, and other new compounds having a thiazole and a pyridine ring, named pyrizomicin A and B, were discovered. New substances can be found from actinomycetes that have been exhaustively studied. Novel compounds with different skeletons can be found from a single broth of one strain. The sought after new antibiotics will arise from continued exploitation of the actinomycetes, especially rare actinomycetes. Work on new organisms and samples should be augmented by re-examination of known actinomycetes already in storage. New research should also be carried out on the manipulation of culture media, thereby stimulating actinomycete strains to produce novel chemicals. The establishment of wide-ranging international research collaborations will facilitate and expedite the efficient and timely discovery and provision of bioactive compounds to help maintain and promote advances in global public health.

Keywords: actinomycetes; secondary metabolites; novel compounds; physicochemical screening; physical and chemical properties; structural diversity; biological activity

1. Introduction

The use of chemicals to maintain or improve human health is as old as recorded history. In recent times, the discovery and development of chemicals to kill or overcome bacteria or pathogens is regarded as one of the most significant medical achievements of the 20th century, and countless millions of human lives have been saved as a result. Natural products have been and remain the mainstay of medical treatments. Chemicals produced in nature, or compounds based on them, accounted for 65% of the 1211 small molecule drugs approved by the United States Food and Drug Administration (FDA) in the 34 years from 1981 to 2014 [1]. The wide and diverse range of microbial primary or secondary metabolites that possess potent and sometimes unique bioactivity, coupled with the enormous and as yet relatively untapped potential and promise they offer, will heavily influence and drive forward future antibiotic research, while simultaneously emphasizing the importance of prioritizing natural products discovery over the manufacturing of synthetic compounds [2].

Penicillin was first used for human treatment in 1942, and it revolutionized the treatment of bacterial infections. It has since saved hundreds of millions of lives, as well as galvanizing the search for similar antibacterial or antimicrobial chemicals. As a result of the worldwide research effort, there was a flood of new antibiotics identified throughout the 1950s and 1960s, with the approval of several distinct novel classes of efficacious antibiotics for human use. However, since that "Golden Age", the number of new antibiotics registered has steadily declined, and very few new classes of antibiotics have reached the marketplace and clinical use. In reality, scientific and economic factors will likely delay the appearance of any new antibiotics. From preclinical testing to approval for human use takes 10–15 years, and the costs involved are prohibitive [3,4]. A recent analysis suggests that, in 2014, the actual cost of driving a new compound from concept to the marketplace was in excess of $1.3 billion [5]. Furthermore, approximately 1 in 1000 potential drugs proceed to clinical trials, and then almost 90% fail in the human testing phase. For example, in the antibiotic field, the prevailing dangerous lack of new antibiotics, coupled with the loss of effectiveness of many already being widely used, threatens a return to the pre-antibiotic era, and the reversal of the gains made in global public health during the 20th century, accompanied by the potential loss of millions of lives.

The world is fast waking up to this dreadful scenario, and in 2015, the World Health Assembly endorsed the Global Action Plan on Antimicrobial Resistance [6]. This committed all member states to prepare national action plans and take proactive steps to promote the discovery, development, and sustainable exploitation of new antibiotics, especially those with novel modes of action. These commitments were reiterated by the United Nations General Assembly in 2016 [7].

So how can we find the urgently needed drugs? We firmly believe that actinomycetes will prove to be the primary source of the desperately needed biological substances over the next 2–3 decades, and this publication contains substantial evidence to support that point of view.

The actinomycetes are a heterogeneous group of Gram-positive bacteria with high guanine (G) and cytosine (C) content in their DNA. They are extremely diverse, with at least 350 genera known to date. They constitute one of the largest bacterial phyla, and are ubiquitous in aquatic and terrestrial ecosystems. Most (especially the streptomycetes are saprophytic, soil-dwelling organisms, but they are also found in fresh and salt water, and the air. They are typically present in soil at densities of 10^6 to 10^9 cells per gram of soil, with streptomycetes accounting for over 95% of all actinomycete strains isolated from soil [8]. Many species are harmless to animals and higher plants, while some are important pathogens.

The actinomycetes, particularly species from the genus *Streptomyces*, have proved to be a tremendous high-impact source of valuable chemicals. They have yielded many clinically essential antimicrobial compounds, including streptomycin, actinomycin, and streptothricin [9]. Besides streptomycin (discovered in 1944 from *Streptomyces griseus*), other examples of the success of this traditional discovery research approach are chloramphenicol (1947, *S. venezuelae*), tetracycline (1948, *S. rimosus*), erythromycin (1952, *Saccharopolyspora erythraea*), leucomycin (1952, *S. kitasatoensis*), and vancomycin (1956, *S. orientales*). Additionally, in 1963, gentamicin was discovered, isolated from *M. purpurea*, a member of the *Micromonospora*. This triggered the search for new compounds from the so-called "rare actinomycetes", which are lower frequency of isolation than members of the genus *Streptomyces* that are well isolated from soil. Compounds from the rare organisms include teicoplanin (1978, *Actinoplanes teichomyceticus*), fortimicin (1977, *M. olivoasterospora*), rosamicin (1972, *M. rosaria*), and nocardicin (1976, *Nocardia uniformis*). Incidentally, salinosporamide A, which holds promise for development of an anticancer drug, is produced by a strain of the genus *Salinispora,* a rare actinomycete isolated from a heat-treated marine sediment sample [10].

Approximately two-thirds of all known antibiotics are produced by actinomycetes, predominantly by *Streptomyces* [8]. It is believed that the actinomycetes are the source of some 61% of all microorganism-derived bioactive substances so far discovered [11], with 16% of the total originating from the "rare actinomycetes", mostly from the *Micromonosporaceae*, with additional smaller contributions from the *Pseudonocardiaceae* and *Thermomonosporaceae*. This suggests that rare actinomycetes are a valuable source of novel compounds, and that improved isolation strategies are required to increase the frequency in which they are isolated.

2. Historical Discovery of Novel Compounds from Actinomycetes by the Kitasato Ōmura-Drug Discovery Group

The Kitasato Institute has, since its inception, concentrated its investigations on soil dwelling microbes, particularly the actinomycetes, as a potential source of bioactive compounds. Up until the mid-1970s, the singular universally employed discovery process involved identifying microorganisms in soil (or other) samples, culturing them and then testing any primary or secondary metabolites or other chemicals they produced to identify predetermined bioactivity that would meet a human need.

Decades of success in our exploration of the actinomycetes is exemplified by the discovery in the Kitasato Institute by Satoshi Ōmura in the early-1970s of *Streptomyces avermectinius* (synonym *S. avermitilis*) MA-4680[T], the microbe which produces the avermectins [12,13]. The avermectin derivative, ivermectin, is perhaps the world's greatest, most effective, and safest drug for the treatment and prevention of a diverse range of human diseases and conditions [14]. The importance and significance of the discovery and development of these compounds was recognized by the 2015 Nobel Prize in Physiology or Medicine being awarded to Prof. Ōmura and Prof. William C. Campbell of Merck & Company, Inc., Kenilworth, NJ, USA, representing the industrial partner which has become essential for the discovery, development, production, marketing, and distribution process of all modern-day antibiotics. The award citation stated "William C. Campbell and Satoshi Ōmura discovered a new drug, avermectin, the derivatives of which have radically lowered the incidence of River Blindness and Lymphatic Filariasis, as well as showing efficacy against an expanding number of other parasitic diseases" [15,16]. The 2015 award was the third Nobel Prize given for discovery of an antibiotic, following those for penicillin (for Fleming, Florey, and Chain in 1945) and for streptomycin (for Waksman in 1952), the man who first coined the term "antibiotic".

The discovery of ivermectin arose because of Ōmura's unwavering belief that microorganisms are a limitless source of useful chemical compounds—"Microbes do not produce useless metabolites: we just have little knowledge of their usefulness for mankind" [17,18], and because the partnership he set up between his group and Merck scientists were looking for specific anthelmintic compounds. Although ivermectin has proved to be a multifaceted, extremely effective chemical with a wide range of impacts, the original bioactivity screening focused almost predominantly on looking for an anthelmintic. Hence, that was what was found.

In the early-1970s, Ōmura decided to introduce an innovative new approach to drug discovery, namely to simply identify novel chemicals with no fixed goal in mind, carry out preliminary assays and evaluations, catalog and store both the chemicals and the producing microorganisms, and make the chemicals available for others to assay for all variety of bioactivity, or for use as biological or chemical reagents. This novel process was referred to as physicochemical (PC) screening.

As members of the Kitasato Institute for Life Sciences' Drug Discovery Group, with Satoshi Ōmura as team leader, we have long and extensive experience in the search for novel compounds derived from microorganisms. Our cohesive integrated research program now encompasses the following three foci:

1. Isolation of microorganisms, identification, and microbial cultivation.
2. Discovery of substances from microbial metabolites.
3. Optimization of compounds by organic synthesis.

Latterly, our isolation work has been significantly refocused. We are now investigating existing but hitherto underutilized actinomycetes which exist in storage. We have also switched our attention from soil dwelling microbes to the exploration of microorganisms living in the complex environments found in the immediate vicinity of plant roots. We quickly discovered that whereas more than 90% of actinomycetes isolated from soil are *Streptomyces* strains, the rare actinomycetes dominate in strains isolated from plant roots. Currently, some 642 strains of actinomycetes have been isolated from 16 plant root locations, about 80% of which are rare. Two new genera (*Phytohabitans sufuscus* and *Rhizocola hellebori*) plus seven new species have, so far, been proposed through taxonomic study of these strains [19–21].

In our case, the discovery of useful microbial chemicals has been facilitated and accelerated by employing a two-pronged approach. Initially, using the traditional method attempting to acquire a new compound with a preconceived specific biological activity; more recently by identifying any and all novel substances by detecting and exploiting the basic physical and chemical properties and structural features of compounds. This bifurcated approach, both mechanisms of which are ongoing in Kitasato University, has led to the discovery of over 500 compounds, most of which were found using the original method [22].

In the mid-1970s, PC screening was introduced initially using Dragendorff's reagent to identify nitrogen-containing compounds (alkaloids) which would cause a simple, visible color change. Staurosporine [23] was discovered as the first indolocarbazole compound from the culture broth of *Saccharothrix aerocolonigenes* subsp. *staurosporeus* AM 2282^T [24] (renamed *Lentzea albida* in 2002 [25]) in 1977, using this method. We initially determined that the compound possessed antifungal properties, and demonstrated a hypotensive effect. Nine years after discovery, in 1986, another research group discovered that staurosporine was a nanomolar inhibitor of protein kinases, as assessed by the prevention of ATP binding to the kinase [26,27]. This interesting biological activity stimulated an explosion in exploratory research for selective protein kinase inhibitors by numerous laboratories and pharmaceutical companies worldwide, staurosporine becoming the parent compound for many of today's highly-successful anticancer agents. This example helps to illustrate that all substances produced by microbes may be of great benefit, and that they should be examined for potential use in all forms of human endeavor, especially for use in modern medicine, and that they should be made available for exhaustive testing and use by all, wherever practical and possible.

We now routinely search for novel chemicals from actinomycetes by analyzing a range of physico-chemical properties, such as LC/MS, LC/UV and polarity. It is now possible to predict whether a new substance is present by analyzing results and comparing with existing databases. This approach has so far identified some 36 novel compounds (including analogs) [28]. In this report, we describe these results, and discuss the ability of actinomycetes to produce a wide spectrum of novel chemicals, as well as draw attention to the diversity of metabolites that a single microbial strain can provide for us.

3. Novel Compounds Discovered by Physicochemical (PC) Screening of Cultured Broths of Actinomycetes

The novel compounds derived from actinomycetes discovered through our PC screening during the past eight years are displayed in Table 1. The compounds are accompanied by the name of the producing microorganism, their original source, the primary biological activity of the compound and relevant publications. The PC screening procedure was carried out as follows.

After cultivation in 10 mL of several kinds of preset media, an equivalent amount of ethanol was added, the ingredients were thoroughly mixed, the cells were then disrupted, and the ethanol extract was subjected to PC screening.

After LC/MS and LC/UV analysis, each peak recorded was compared with known data from the Dictionary of Natural Products, and our own database. A peak was predicted to be a novel substance. When this was the case, we scaled up the culture and isolated and purified the target compound using column chromatography and preparative HPLC. After obtaining the unique compound, its structure was determined by high-resolution mass spectrometry, NMR, etc. The new compounds underwent preliminary bioassays, either in-house or in established collaborative research projects with other groups.

Identification of the strains being cultured was carried out using morphological characteristics, chemical composition in cells, and phylogenetic analysis based on 16S rRNA gene sequences.

The Kitasato Ōmura-Drug Discovery Group has already discovered avermectin [14], staurosporine [23], herbimycin [29], setamycin [30], and lactacystin [31] from secondary metabolites of actinomycetes [22]. The actinomycete strains producing these compounds (as well as strains producing a variety of other chemicals) have all been catalogued, freeze-dried, and stored in the Kitasato Microbial Library (KML). In an effort to respond to the urgent global demand for new antibiotics, we have recently revived the KML strains to confirm their viability, the continuance of compound production, and the reliability of the preservation process. Survival rates and compound productivity maintenance rates have been good, but specific data in this respect will be reported elsewhere. During this work, PC screening was carried out on culture broths of 330 strains, resulting in the discovery of several new compounds (No. 1 to No. 3 in Table 1).

With respect to the three entries in question, the name of the original compound and retention period by lyophilization are stated, all three having been stored for 35 years or more. The compounds recently discovered, namely bisoxazolomycin [32], the iminimycins [33,34], and the nanaomycins [35,36], would probably not have been detected by an assay system seeking a specific bioactive property, the compounds being found as a direct result of PC screening. Discovery of the iminimycins and nanaomycins are described in detail below in Section 4.2.

With respect to new isolates (No. 4 to No. 13 in Table 1), actinomycete strains isolated from around the roots of plants (No. 4 to No. 7), sediment from mangrove forests (No. 8 to No. 10), sea sediment (No. 11), and soil samples (No. 12 & No. 13) are listed. Actinoallolides [37], hamuramicins [38], spoxazomicins [39,40], and trehangelins [41,42] were discovered from endophytic actinomycete strains, and these are classified as rare actinomycetes. The mangromicins [43–45], K10-0216 KA and KB [46], and pyrizomicins [47], which have differing core structures, were found in a culture broth of *Lechevalieria aerocolonigenes* K10-0216 isolated from sediment from mangroves. Mumiamicin [48] was found in an actinomycete strain isolated from sea sediment, while sagamilactam [49] and the dipyrimicins [50] originated in actinomycete strains from soil. In Section 5.1, we describe, in detail, the discovery of other compounds, notably the trehangelins from *Polymorphospora rubra* K07-0510 and compounds from *Lechevalieria aerocolonigenes* K10-0216.

Assays of the 36 compounds, involving collaboration with other research groups, led to the discovery of varying bioactivity, as shown in Table 1. These results help demonstrate the usefulness and cost/time effectiveness of PC screening, as well as the potential diversity of metabolites produced by a single microorganism. The outcome clearly demonstrates that, as Prof Ōmura rightly opines, "microorganisms are a treasure trove of new natural products".

Table 1. Compounds discovered by physicochemical screening of actinomycete strains (March 2018).

No.	Compound	Producing Microorganism	Source	Biological Activity	References
1	Bisoxazolomycin	*Streptomyces subflavus* subsp. *irumaensis* AM-3603	* KML Irunamycin producing strain, ** 36 years	Antibacterial	[32]
2	Iminimycin A & B	*Streptomyces griseus* OS-3601	* KML, Streptomycin producing strain, ** 43 years	Antibacterial	[33,34]
3	Nanaomycin F–H	"*Streptomyces rosa* subsp. *Notaensis*" OS-3966	* KML Nanaomycin producing strain, ** 36 years	Inhibitor of Epithelial-Mesenchymal Transition induced cells	[35,36]
4	Actinoallolide A–E	*Actinoallomurus fulvus* MK10-036	Roots of *Capsicum frutescents* in Thailand	Antitrypanosomal	[37]
		A. fulvus K09-0307	Roots of mondo grass in Saitama Pref., Japan		
5	Hamuramicin A & B	*Allostreptomyces* sp. K12-0794	Roots of fern in Hamura city, Tokyo, Japan	Antibacterial	[38]
6	Spoxazomicin A–C	*Streptosporangium oxazolinicum* K07-0460^T	Roots of orchid in Iriomote Island, Japan	Antitrypanosomal	[39,40]
7	Trehangelin A–C	*Polymorphospora rubra* K07-0510	Roots of orchid in Iriomote Island, Japan	Anti-Lipid peroxidation / Enhanced production of collagen	[41,42]
8	Mangromicin A–I	*Lechevalieria aerocolonigenes* K10-0216	Sediment from mangrove forest in Iriomote Island, Japan	Antitrypanosomal / Antioxidative	[43–45]
9	K10-0216 KA & KB	*Lechevalieria aerocolonigenes* K10-0216	Sediment from mangrove forest in Iriomote Island, Japan	Inhibitory effect on the lipid accumulation	[46]
10	Pyrizomicin A & B	*Lechevalieria aerocolonigenes* K10-0216	Sediment from mangrove forest in Iriomote Island, Japan	Antimicrobial	[47]
11	Mumiamicin	*Mumia* sp. YSP-2-79	Sea sediment, Namako Pond in Kagoshima Pref., Japan	Antibacterial / Antioxidative	[48]
12	Sagamilactam	*Actinomadura* sp. K13-0306	Soil, Kanagawa Pref., Japan	Cytotoxicity / Antitrypanosomal	[49]
13	Dipyrimicin A & B	*Amycolatopsis* sp. K16-0194	Soil, Okinawa Pref., Japan	Antibacterial	[50]

* KML: Kitasato Microbial Library, ** length of preservation by lyophilization; No. 1–3: Compounds from the KML; No. 4–13: Compounds from fresh isolates (No. 4–7; Roots of plants, No. 8–10; Sediment of mangrove forest, No. 11; Marine sediment, Nos. 12 & 13; Soil).

4. Novel Compounds Discovered from the Kitasato Microbial Library (KML)

4.1. Iminimycin A by Streptomyces griseus OS-3601, a Streptomycin Producing Strain

KML strain OS-3601 (Figure 1) was isolated from a soil sample collected at Aso, Kumamoto prefecture, Japan, in 1971, and identified as *Streptomyces griseus*, which produces streptomycin. As part of our screening of 330 preserved actinomycete strains, using four different liquid production media, a unique metabolite, predicted to be a new compound, was observed in an extract of a culture of this strain grown on defatted wheat germ medium. The metabolite was not observed following growth in the other three production media. The compound produced by strain OS-3601 showed an 242.1910 *m/z* [M + H]$^+$ and maximal absorption at 269 and 282 nm. Purification from the culture broth of strain OS-3601 yielded a new iminium compound, designated iminimycin A (Figure 1) [33], which was strongly supported by an IR absorption spectrum, indicative of the presence of an iminium ion. Several plant-derived compounds containing an iminium ion are known [51] but, to our knowledge, this is the first compound arising from an actinomycete source.

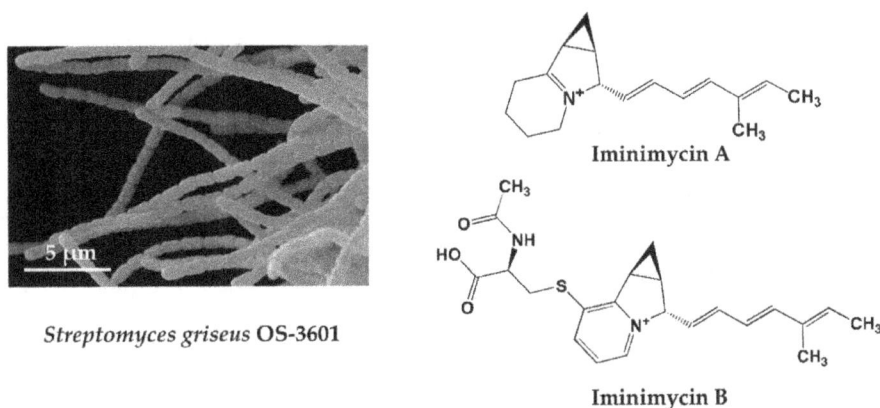

Figure 1. Scanning electron micrograph of the aerial spore chain of the streptomycin-producing strain *Streptomyces griseus* OS-3601 (**Left**) and structures of iminimycin A and B discovered from the culture broth (**Right**).

An unidentified compound with physical and chemical properties similar to iminimycin A was observed in the octadecyl silyl fraction lacking iminimycin A; the compound having an 399.1736 *m/z* [M + H]$^+$ and maximal absorption at 269 and 282 nm. Purification of this compound revealed a new indolizine alkaloid, designated iminimycin B (Figure 1) [34], that possessed *N*-acetylcysteine and pyridinium moieties, instead of the iminium moiety of iminimycin A. Iminimycin A and B both show antimicrobial activity against Gram-positive and Gram-negative bacteria. Since 1943, when Selman A. Waksman discovered streptomycin from the secondary metabolite of *Streptomyces griseus*, about 200 compounds have been reported from strains identified as *Streptomyces griseus* [9].

Among the actinomycetes, *Streptomyces griseus* is one of the organisms most frequently isolated from soil samples, and has been studied extensively. It was therefore surprising that our PC screening allowed us to find new substances from this strain, demonstrating, yet again, the unmatched ability of microorganisms, especially actinomycetes, to produce a plethora of chemicals.

One chemical component of the culture broth of strain OS-3601 was predicted to be novel from analysis of HPLC and LC/MS data gathered through PC screening. Our prediction proved true following isolation, purification, and structure determination.

Mapping of the genome of streptomycin-producing *Streptomyces griseus* has already been completed [52], and this information also indicates that production of the novel substance is predictable. So why has it not been discovered before? It is conceivable that productivity is low, or that it has been overlooked because it has been masked by the cycloheximide produced in large quantities at the same time in a lipid soluble fraction, or because the compound is inherently unstable and short-lived. We believe that prediction of the existence of new compounds can be envisaged through a combination of an enquiring mind, technological progress, and the creation and use of more sophisticated equipment. Indeed, it can be said that Prof. Ōmura's belief that "microorganisms are infinite resources" and that "microbial research has really just begun" are an accurate depiction of the current situation.

4.2. Nanaomycins F, G and H Derived from Nanaomycins A–E Produced by "Streptomyces rosa subsp. notoensis" OS-3966

Nanaomycins A, B, C, D, and E produced by "*Streptomyces rosa* subsp. *notoensis*" OS-3966 (Figure 2a,b) [53–55] were isolated from soil sampled in Nanao City, Japan. The nanaomycins contain a naphthoquinone skeleton and were found to have antimycoplasma properties. Nanaomycin A (Figure 2b) was developed as a therapeutic agent for cattle dermatophytosis in 1980 [56]. It generates semiquinone radicals by forming double bonds at positions 4a and 10a, damaging DNA in the process, consequently displaying antibacterial and antifungal activity.

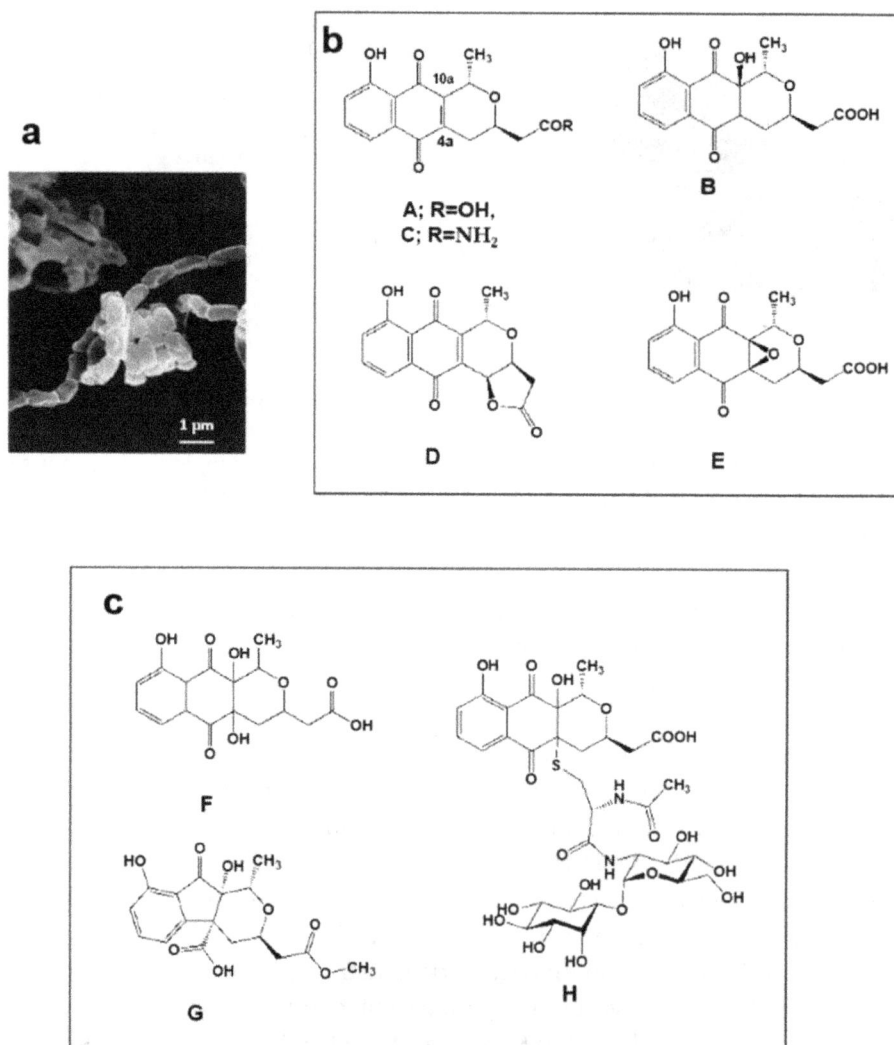

Figure 2. Nanaomycin-producing strain "*Streptomyces rosa* subsp. *notoensis*" OS-3966 and new analogs discovered by PC screening from a culture broth. (**a**) Scanning electron micrograph of aerial spore chain of "*S. rosa* subsp. *notoensis*" OS-3966 grown on agar medium; (**b**) Nanaomycins A–E discovered as antibacterial and antifungal substances during 1974–1979; (**c**) New analogs (F–H) discovered from the culture broth via PC screening.

We undertook PC screening using the culture broths of stored freeze-dried nanaomycin-producing strain OS-3966. Two new compounds appeared in the EtOH extract obtained from culturing in defatted wheat germ production medium. The first compound had 337.0917 m/z [M + H]$^+$ and maximal absorption at 231, 248 (sh), 267 (sh), and 347 nm; the second compound had 351.1075 m/z [M + H]$^+$ and maximal absorption at 225, 256 (sh), and 308 nm. Purification of these compounds revealed they were two new nanaomycin analogs. The first, which we named nanaomycin F (Figure 2c) [35], is a 4a-hydroxyl analog of nanaomycin B (Figure 2b). The second, which we named nanaomycin G (Figure 2c) [35], has a unique 1-indanone skeleton fused with a tetrahydropyran ring. During chromatographic purification of these compounds, another new compound was obtained, nanaomycin H (Figure 2c) [36]. Structure elucidation of nanaomycin H showed it to be a pyranonaphthoquinone with a mycothiol moiety. Our assays detected no antibacterial or antifungal activity in these three compounds. The reason for this seems to be that the radical-generating ability disappeared due to the reduction of the double bond of the quinone skeleton. It was found that the compounds inhibited epithelial-mesenchymal transition, inducing proliferation of mammalian cells [57]. These compounds would not have been found using an assay simply targeting bioactivity. Incidentally, the production medium of nanaomycin A to E is mainly composed of glycerol and soybean meal [53], whereas nanaomycins F, G, and H were produced on a medium containing mainly soluble starch and defatted wheat germ [35,36]. This raises the interesting possibility that simply changing the composition of culture media may allow the discovery of new compounds. These results showed to support OSMAC (one strain, many compounds) approach [58].

5. Novel Compounds Found from Fresh Isolates

5.1. Novel Substances, Trehangelins Found from Metabolites of the Plant-Derived Rare Actinomycete Polymorphospora Rubra K07-0510

Microbes isolated from plant root environments were cultured in each of four production media, with the resulting broths being subjected to PC screening. Strain K07-0510, when grown in one of the production media, yielded a peak (indicating a new compound) that was predicted based on spectrometric data.

Strain K07-0510 was isolated from the roots of an orchid collected on Iriomote Island, Okinawa, Japan. Short spore chains were formed, and spores with a smooth surface were cylindrical in shape (Figure 3). Whole-cell hydrolysates contained *meso*-DAP (diaminopimelic acid). The 16S rRNA gene sequence was determined and analyzed using the EzTaxon-e database (present name EzBioCloud) [59] to reveal a 99.9% similarity with *Polymorphospora rubra* TT97-42^T. On the basis of the morphological and cultural properties and 16S rRNA gene sequence analyses, strain K07-0510 was identified as *Polymorphospora. rubra*.

A new predicted peak showing 507.2087 m/z and maximal absorption at 216 nm was also found in the culture broth of strain K07-0510. Purification of this compound eventually identified three new compounds, which were named trehangelin A, B, C (Figure 3) [41,42]. These compounds were separated from the culture broth of strain K07-0510 by ethyl acetate extraction, followed by silica gel and ODS column chromatography, with final purification by HPLC. Eighteen liters of culture broth yielded 59 mg of trehangelin A as the major component, along with 4.4 mg and 1.3 mg of the minor components trehangelin B and C, respectively.

Structural analysis revealed that two molecules of angelic acid were bound to one molecule of trehalose. Trehangelin A, the main compound, binds angelic acid to the 3,3′ positions of trehalose, while B and C does so to the 3,2′ and 4,4′ positions, respectively. After substance isolation, preliminary bioassays were carried out, and it was found that trehangelin A and C inhibited erythrocyte hemolysis by photooxidation. Trehangelin A and C, which have symmetric structures, showed more potent inhibition than ascorbic acid. In addition, it has been found that the compounds facilitate cytoprotective action and accumulation of procollagen type I C-peptide in a cell culture assay [60], and further research is currently in progress. Our group is now close to elucidating the genetic basis of the biosynthesis of the trehangelins [42].

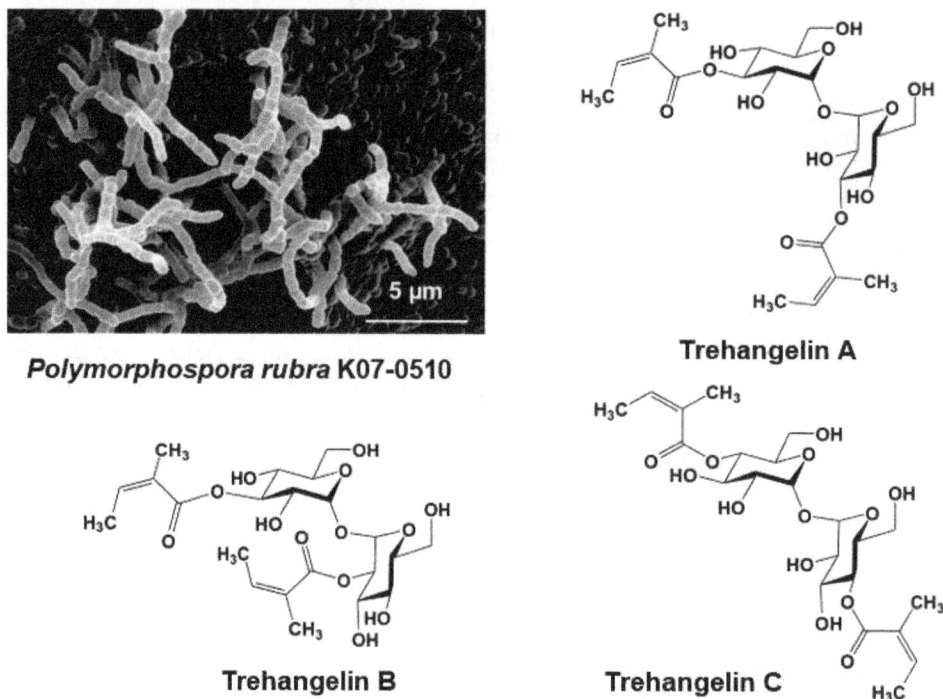

Polymorphospora rubra K07-0510

Trehangelin A

Trehangelin B

Trehangelin C

Figure 3. Scanning electron micrograph of the aerial spore chain of the trehangelin-producing strain *Polymorphospora rubra* K07-0510 and structures of trehangelin A, B, and C.

Angelic acid is known to occur in many plants, particularly chamomile, and has been used as a tonic and sedative to treat a variety of minor complaints, but reports of it being produced by microorganisms are extremely rare. It is, thus, interesting to note that a microbe in a plant root environment also produces the compound.

5.2. New Compounds Produced by Lechevalieria Aerocolonigenes K10-0216, Mangromycin A-I, K10-0216 KA & KB, and Pyrizomicin A & B

Lechevalieria aerocolonigenes K10-0216 (Figure 4a) is a rare actinomycete isolated from sediment collected in a mangrove forest in Iriomote Island, Okinawa Prefecture, Japan in 2011. In the culture broth of this strain, we found 13 new compounds.

Mangrove trees growing in brackish water are known to be a rich source of microorganisms, and many rare actinomycetes have been discovered in such environments [61]. We isolated 65 actinomycetes strains from five samples collected from a mangrove forest. Simple use of 16S rRNA gene sequences resulted in identification of 44 strains of the genus *Micromonospora*, as well as a few from the *Actinomadura* and *Verrucosispora*. The so-called rare actinomycetes accounted for 83% of organisms isolated.

Strain K10-0216 grown on an inorganic salt–starch agar medium produced sparse white aerial mycelia that formed characteristic clumps of interwoven hyphae, as shown in Figure 4a. The 16S rRNA gene sequence, which was determined and analyzed using the EzTaxon-e database [59], demonstrated a 99.8% similarity to *Lechevalieria aerocolonigenes* ISP 5034[T]. On the basis of the morphological and cultural properties and 16S rRNA gene sequence analyses, strain K10-0216 was identified as *Lechevalieria aerocolonigenes*.

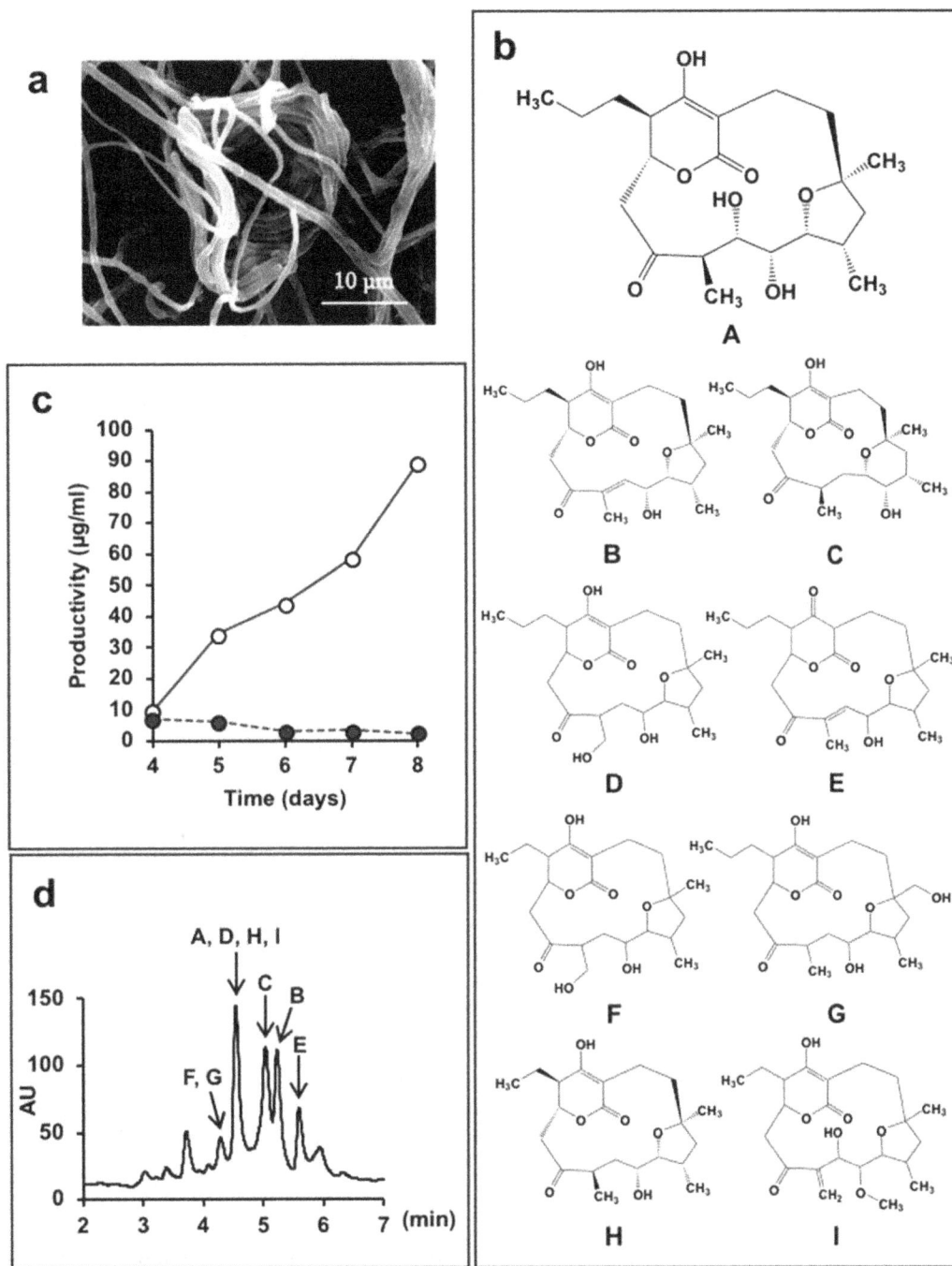

Figure 4. *Lechevalieria aerocolonigenes* K10-0216 and the mangromicins discovered from the culture broth. (a) Scanning electron micrograph of a clump of interwoven hyphae of *L. aerocolonigenes* K10-0216 grown on inorganic salt–starch agar at 27 °C for four weeks; (b) Structure of mangromicin A–I; (c) Productivity of mangromicin A. Black circle: Basic medium; soluble starch 2.0(%), defatted wheat germ 1.0, glycerol 0.5, dry yeast 0.3, CaCO$_3$ 0.5, meat extract 0.5. Open circle: Improved medium; soluble starch 5.0(%), defatted wheat germ 1.0, glycerol 0.5, dry yeast 1.0, CaCO$_3$ 0.5, meat extract 0.0. (d) HPLC analysis of the mangromicins. Chromatographic separation was undertaken using a MonoBis (3.2 × 150 mm, Kyoto Monotech Co., Ltd., Kyoto, Japan) at 40 °C. With regard to gradient elution, solvent A was water with 0.1% formic acid, and solvent B was methanol with 0.1% formic acid. The gradient elution was 0–10 min and 5–100% B. The flow rate was 0.5 mL/min, the injection volume was 5 µL, and detection occurred at 254 nm using a photodiode array detector.

We found that the culture broth contained predicted novel substances with molecular weights of 410 or 392, and maximal absorption at 251 nm or at 236 nm, respectively. We named these compounds mangromicin A and B [43]. However, these peaks were not obtained in a jar fermenter culture. A total of 500 mL Erlenmeyer flasks containing 100 mL culture medium were used to obtain the target substances that were isolated and purified. Structural analysis revealed a unique structure of a cyclopentadecane skeleton containing a 5,6-dihydro-4-hydroxyl-2-pyrone ring and a tetrahydrofuran ring (Figure 4b). Both substances displayed antitrypanosomal activity, and a patent application was filed. Subsequently, we experimented with different production media in order to obtain a large amount of the target compounds. As a result, by changing the concentration of soluble starch in the medium ingredients from 2.0% to 5.0%, and dry yeast 0.3% to 1.0%, the amount of mangromicin A increased dramatically, from 0.24 μg/mL to 88.6 μg/mL (Figure 4c). Eventually, nine analogs were obtained from 15 L of culture solution using this procedure (Figure 4b) [44,45]. The HPLC profile is shown in Figure 4d. After isolation and purification, preliminary bioassays identified DPPH radical scavenging activity and, in particular, NO scavenging was potent [44,45].

Furthermore, from the same culture broth, we also discovered four novel compounds (Figure 5). Two contained a steroid skeleton (named K10-0216 KA and KB) that inhibited lipid accumulation in 3T3-L1 adipocytes [46], while the others displayed a thiazole and a pyridine ring (named pyrizomicin A and B) that showed antibacterial activity [47].

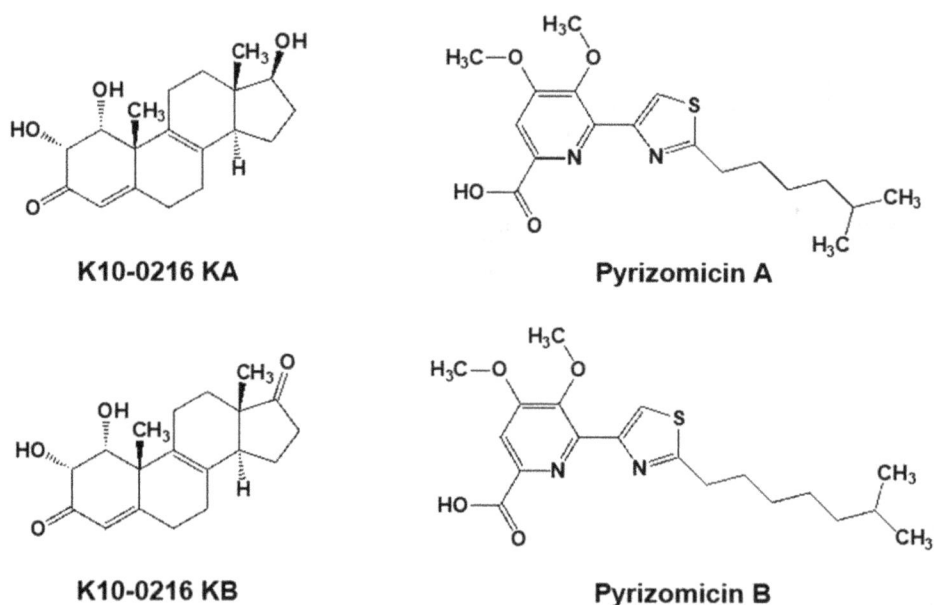

Figure 5. Two steroid compounds (K10-0216 KA and KB) and two compounds containing thiazole and pyridine (pyrizomicin A and B) from *L. aerocolonigenes* K10-0216 (Figure 4a).

As described above, 13 compounds, including three with different skeletons, were found from a single culture broth of one microorganism. This reinforces our belief that it is highly likely to be able to identify and acquire new compounds simply by changing the culture method and production medium.

6. Conclusions

This report describes compounds derived from actinomycete strains which were found via PC screening between 2011–2017 by the Kitasato Ōmura-Drug Discovery Group. Iminimycins and nanaomycins were found from culture broths of conserved KML strains, while the trehangelins from *P. rubra* K07-0510 and new compounds, mangromicins, K10-0216 KA and KB, pyrizomicin A and B, from *L. aelocolonigenes* K10-0216, originated in fresh isolates. Our results illustrate that PC screening can unearth novel compounds that are not likely to be discovered through traditional targeted bioassay systems. Genomic analysis of actinomycetes has found that more than 30 secondary metabolite biosynthetic genes may be involved in chemical production, depending on the strain. However, knowing the genetic production mechanism may not necessarily make obtaining the compound easier.

This report also shows that it is possible to obtain a novel compound from actinomycete species, such as *Streptomyces griseus*, that has already undergone long and intensive study. In addition, as in the case of *L. aerocolonigenes* K10-0216, a variety of compounds with significantly different skeletons can be obtained from a single culture broth using only one microbe strain.

Our work also demonstrates that the aptly classified "rare actinomycetes" remain a unique and, so far, relatively unexploited source of potentially useful chemicals. This is supported by work that found that strains of the genus *Actinoallomurus* (a rare actinomycete) have high secondary metabolite production capacity [62]. We also found five actinoallolide analogs [37] (shown in Table 1) produced by *A. fulvus* MK 10-036 and *A. fulvus* K 09-0307, later discovering two more new compounds together with seven known compounds from an *A. fulvus* K09-0307 broth.

Microorganisms can present us with interesting compounds with unique structures which our current scientific knowledge and expertise cannot easily predict nor easily replicate. For example, the mangromicins have unique skeletons which subsequently attracted attention in the field of organic synthesis. Organic chemists tried to devise a total synthesis of mangromicin A, and finally managed to achieve it via a complicated and lengthy 30 step process [63], whereas *L. aerocolonigenes* K10-0216 produces the compound naturally during culturing.

To illustrate the immeasurable scope for success in this respect, it has been reported that 99% of microorganisms in nature have not yet been isolated [64]. Furthermore, our results suggest that interesting compounds can be found even from *Streptomyces* strains that are thought to have been exhausted, simply by devising new identification methods or culture conditions. It is therefore essential to revisit existing actinomycetes, common and rare, and comprehensively examine them for new compounds.

Traditionally, the search for useful natural products has been advanced using approaches that focus on specific biological activity and target molecules. In this approach, there is a clearly defined goal. However, with this method alone, it is likely that many of the microorganisms isolated have been exploited and then discarded without fully utilizing their abilities. It is clearly difficult to devise a wide variety of screening systems and, certainly, almost impossible for all these systems to be operational in a single institution. Consequently, extensive, multifaceted research collaborations will need to be established to work towards full and comprehensive testing of all chemicals, be they newly isolated from existing compound libraries or from new sources. Naturally, many obstacles will need to be overcome, including protection of Intellectual Property Rights, transfer of technology, and capacity building aspects. None of these should be insurmountable, especially so if the goal of getting as many new bioactive substances in the shortest time possible is to be achieved.

We remain firm in our commitment to discover as many new compounds as possible by exploiting the ability of microorganisms, especially the actinomycetes, to produce such attractive substances. Moreover, we will continue to follow a twin-pronged approach to this task, while striving to devise other alternative screening methods, and adopt any other measures that could help expedite the research and development process.

Author Contributions: Y.T. and T.N. designed and performed the experiments, analyzed the data, and wrote the paper

Funding: This research was funded by the Institution for Fermentation, Osaka (IFO).

Acknowledgments: We deeply appreciate the guidance and support of Satoshi Ōmura (Distinguished Emeritus Kitasato Ōmura-Drug Discovery Group director, Kitasato University). And for his constant emphasis of the importance of isolation, culture and classification of microbes—to "Learn from microorganisms," and "Be grateful for microorganisms." We are grateful to all members of the Kitasato Ōmura-Drug Discovery Group, especially to Atsuko Matsumoto for management of the actinomycete strains and to Kazuro Shiomi, Toshiaki Sunazuka, Masato Iwatsuki and Kazuhiko Otoguro for structure determinations and bioassay work, and to Yuki Inahashi, Hirotaka Matsuo and Suga Takuya for their efforts in seeking new compounds by PC screening and the subsequent isolation, purification and structure determination. We would also like to extend our thanks to Toru Kimura, Rei Miyano, Yoshiyuki Kamiya, Shoko Izuta and many other researcher staff and students of the Kitasato Institute for Life Sciences for their collegiate support. We also thank Jun Nakanishi of the National Institute for Materials Science for assistance with biological activity evaluation. We would like to express our deepest gratitude to the IFO for their financial support.

References

1. Newman, D.J.; Cragg, G.M. Natural Products as sources of new drugs from 1981 to 2014. *J. Nat. Prod.* **2016**, *79*, 629–661. [CrossRef] [PubMed]

2. Bérdy, J. Thought and facts about antibiotics: Where we are now and where we are heading. *J. Antibiot.* **2012**, *65*, 385–395. [CrossRef] [PubMed]

3. Van Norman, G.A. Drugs, Devices, and the FDA: Part 1 an Overview of Approval Processes for Drugs. *JACC Basic Transl. Sci.* **2016**, *1*, 170–179. [CrossRef]

4. Morgan, S.; Grootendorst, P.; Lexchin, J.; Cunningham, C.; Greyson, D. The cost of drug development: A systematic review. *Health Policy* **2011**, *100*, 4–17. [CrossRef] [PubMed]

5. Dimasi, J.A.; Grabowski, G.H.; Hansen, R.W. Innovation in the pharmaceutical industry: New estimates of R&D costs. *J. Health Econ.* **2016**, *47*, 20–33. [PubMed]

6. World Health Organization. *Global Action Plan on Antimicrobial Resistance*; World Health Organization: Geneva, Switzerland, 2015.

7. World Health Organization. *United Nations General Assembly High-Level Meeting on Antimicrobial Resistance*; United Nations: New York, NY, USA, 2016.

8. Barka, E.A.; Vatsa, P.; Sanchez, L.; Gaveau-Vaillant, N.; Jacquard, C.; Meier-Kolthoff, J.P.; Klenk, H.P.; Clément, C.; Ouhdouch, Y.; van Wezel, G.P. Taxonomy, physiology, and natural products of Actinobacteria. *Microbiol. Mol. Biol. Rev.* **2015**, *80*, 1–43. [CrossRef] [PubMed]

9. Waksman, S.A.; Schatz, A.; Reynolds, D.M. Production of antibiotic substances by actinomycetes. *Ann. N. Y. Acad. Sci.* **2010**, *1213*, 112–124. [CrossRef] [PubMed]

10. Felling, R.H.; Buchanan, G.O.; Mincer, T.J.; Kauffman, C.A.; Jensen, P.R.; Fenical, P.R. Salinosporamide A: A highly cytotoxic proteasome inhibitor from a novel microbial source, a marine bacterium of the new genus *Salinospora*. *Angew. Chem. Int. Ed.* **2003**, *42*, 355–357. [CrossRef] [PubMed]

11. Tiwari, K.; Gupta, R.K. Rare actinomycetes: A potential storehouse for novel antibiotics. *Crit. Rev. Biotechnol.* **2012**, *32*, 108–132. [CrossRef] [PubMed]

12. Burg, R.W.; Miller, B.M.; Baker, J.; Birnbaum, E.E.; Currie, S.A.; Hartman, R.R.; Kong, Y.L.; Monaghan, R.L.; Olsen, G.; Putter, I.; et al. Avermectins, new family of potent anthelmintic agents: Producing organism and fermentation. *Antimicrob. Agents Chemother.* **1979**, *15*, 361–367. [CrossRef] [PubMed]

13. Takahashi, Y.; Matsumoto, A.; Seino, A.; Ueno, J.; Iwai, Y.; Ōmura, S. *Streptomyces avermectinius* sp. nov., an avermectin-producing strain. *Int. J. Syst. Evolut. Microbiol.* **2002**, *52*, 2163–2168.

14. Campbell, W.C.; Fisher, M.H.; Stapley, E.O.; Albers-Schönberg, G.; Jacobs, T.A. Ivermectin: A potent new antiparasitic agent. *Science* **1983**, *221*, 823–828. [CrossRef] [PubMed]

15. Crump, A.; Ōmura, S. Ivermectin, 'wonder drug' from Japan: The human use perspective. *Proc. Jpn. Acad. Ser. B Phys. Biol. Sci.* **2011**, *87*, 13–28.

16. Crump, A. Ivermectin: Enigmatic multifaceted 'wonder' drug continues to surprise and exceed expectations. *J. Antibiot.* **2017**, *70*, 495–505. [CrossRef] [PubMed]

17. The Nobel Assembly at Karolinska Institute, The Nobel Prize in Physiology or Medicine 2015. Available online: https://www.nobelprize.org/nobel_prizes/medicine/prize_awarder/ (accessed on 24 May 2018).

18. Satoshi Ōmura-Nobel Lecture: "A Splendid Gift from the Earth: The Origins and Impact of Avermectin". Nobelprize.org. Available online: http://www.nobelprize.org/nobel_prizes/medicine/laureates/2015/omura-lecture.html (accessed on 24 May 2018).

19. Takahashi, Y. Continuing fascination of exploration in natural substances from microorganisms. *Biosci. Biotechnol. Biochem.* **2017**, *81*, 6–12. [CrossRef] [PubMed]

20. Matsumoto, A.; Takahashi, Y. Endophytic actinomycetes: Promising source of novel bioactive compounds. *J. Antibiot.* **2017**, *70*, 514–519. [CrossRef] [PubMed]

21. Matsumoto, A. Potential of endophytic actinomycetes for agricultural applications. *Agric. Biotechnol.* **2018**, 2, 180–185.

22. Ōmura, S. *Splendid Gifts from Microorganisms—The Achievements of Satoshi Ōmura and Collaborators*, 5th ed.; Kitasato Institute for Life Sciences, Kitasato University: Tokyo, Japan, 2015.

23. Ōmura, S.; Iwai, Y.; Hirano, A.; Nakagawa, A.; Awaya, J.; Tsuchiya, H.; Takahashi, Y.; Masuma, R. A new alkaloid AM-2282 of *Streptomyces* origin. *J. Antibiot.* **1977**, *30*, 275–282. [CrossRef] [PubMed]

24. Takahashi, Y.; Shinose, M.; Seino, A.; Iwai, Y.; Ōmura, S. Transfer of staurosporine-producing strain *Streptomyces staurosporeus* AM-2282 to the genus *Saccharothrix* as, *Saccharothrix aerocolonigenes* (labeda 1986) subsp. *staurosporeus* subsp. nov. *Actinomycetologica* **1995**, *9*, 19–26. [CrossRef]

25. Xie, Q.; Wang, Y.; Huang, Y.; Wu, Y.; Ba, F.; Liu, Z. Description of *Lentzea flaviverrucosa* sp. nov. and transfer of the type strain of *Saccharothrix aerocolonigenes* subsp. *staurosporea* to *Lentzea albida*. *Int. J. Syst. Evolut. Microbiol.* **2002**, *52*, 1815–1820.

26. Ōmura, S.; Sasaki, Y.; Iwai, Y.; Takeshima, H. Staurosporine, a potentially important gift from a microorganism. *J. Antibiot.* **1995**, *48*, 535–548. [CrossRef] [PubMed]

27. Nakano, H.; Ōmura, S. Chemical biology of natural indolocarbazole products: 30 years since the discovery of staurosporine. *J. Antibiot.* **2009**, *62*, 17–26. [CrossRef] [PubMed]

28. Nakashima, T.; Takahashi, Y.; Ōmura, S. Search for new compounds from Kitasato microbial library by physicochemical screening. *Biochem. Pharmacol.* **2017**, *134*, 42–55. [CrossRef] [PubMed]

29. Ōmura, S.; Iwai, Y.; Takahashi, Y.; Sadakane, N.; Nakagawa, A.; Oiwa, R.; Hasegawa, Y.; Ikai, T. Herbimycin, a new antibiotic produced by a strain of *Streptomyces*. *J. Antibiot.* **1979**, *32*, 255–261. [CrossRef] [PubMed]

30. Ōmura, S.; Otoguro, K.; Nishikiori, T.; Oiwa, R.; Iwai, Y. Setamycin, a new antibiotic. *J. Antibiot.* **1981**, *34*, 1253–1256. [CrossRef] [PubMed]

31. Ōmura, S.; Fujimoto, K.; Otoguro, K.; Matsuzaki, K.; Moriguchi, R.; Tanaka, H.; Sasaki, Y. Lactacystin, a novel microbial metabolite, induces neuritogenesis of neuroblastoma cells. *J. Antibiot.* **1991**, *44*, 113–116. [CrossRef] [PubMed]

32. Koomsiri, W.; Inahashi, Y.; Kimura, T.; Shiomi, K.; Takahashi, Y.; Ōmura, S.; Thamchaipenet, A.; Nakashima, T. Bisoxazolomycin A: A new natural product from 'Streptomyces subflavus subsp. Irumaensis' AM-3603. *J. Antibiot.* **2017**, *70*, 1142–1145. [PubMed]

33. Nakashima, T.; Miyano, R.; Iwatsuki, M.; Shirahata, T.; Kimura, T.; Asami, Y.; Kobayashi, Y.; Shiomi, K.; Petersson, G.A.; Takahashi, Y.; Ōmura, S. Iminimycin A, the new iminium metabolite produced by *Streptomyces griseus* OS-3601. *J. Antibiot.* **2016**, *69*, 611–615. [CrossRef] [PubMed]

34. Nakashima, T.; Miyano, R.; Matsuo, H.; Iwatsuki, M.; Shirahata, T.; Kobayashi, Y.; Shiomi, K.; Petersson, G.A.; Takahashi, Y.; Ōmura, S. Absolute configuration of iminimycin B, the new indolizidine alkaloid from *Streptomyces griseus* OS-3601. *Tetrahedron Lett.* **2016**, *57*, 3284–3286. [CrossRef]

35. Nakashima, T.; Boonsnongcheep, P.; Kimura, T.; Iwatsuki, M.; Sato, N.; Nonaka, K.; Prathanturarug, S.; Takahashi, Y.; Ōmura, S. New compounds, nanaomycin F and G, discovered by physicochemical screening from a culture broth of *Streptomyces rosa* subsp. *notoensis* OS-3966. *J. Biosci. Bioeng.* **2015**, *120*, 596–600. [PubMed]

36. Nakashima, T.; Kimura, T.; Miyano, R.; Matsuo, H.; Hirose, T.; Kimishima, A.; Nonaka, K.; Iwatsuki, M.; Nakanishi, J.; Takahashi, Y.; et al. Nanaomycin H: A new nanaomycin analog. *J. Biosci. Bioeng.* **2017**, *123*, 765–770. [CrossRef] [PubMed]

37. Inahashi, Y.; Iwatsuki, M.; Ishiyama, A.; Matsumoto, A.; Hirose, T.; Oshita, J.; Sunazuka, T.; Watanalai, P.W.; Takahashi, Y.; Kaiser, M.; et al. Actinoallolides A-E, New anti-trypanosomal macrolides, produced by an endophytic actinomycete, *Actinoallomurus fulvus* MK10-036. *Org. Lett.* **2015**, *17*, 864–867. [CrossRef] [PubMed]

38. Suga, T.; Kimura, T.; Inahashi, Y.; Iwatsuki, M.; Nonaka, K.; Také, A.; Matsumoto, A.; Takahashi, Y.; Ōmura, S.; Nakashima, T. Hamuramicins A and B, 22-membered macrolides, produced by an endophytic actinomycete *Allostreptomyces* sp. K12-0794. *J. Antibiot.* **2018**. [CrossRef] [PubMed]

39. Inahashi, Y.; Matsumoto, A.; Ōmura, S.; Takahashi, Y. *Streptosporangium oxazolinicum* sp. nov., a novel endophytic actinomycete producing new antitrypanosomal antibiotics, spoxazomicins. *J. Antibiot.* **2011**, *64*, 297–302. [CrossRef] [PubMed]

40. Inahashi, Y.; Iwatsuki, M.; Ishiyama, A.; Namatame, M.; Nishihara-Tsukashima, A.; Matsumoto, A.; Hirose, T.; Sunazuka, T.; Yamada, H.; Otoguro, K.; et al. Spoxazomicins A-C, novel antitrypanosomal alkaloids produced by an endophytic actinomycete, *Streptosporangium oxazolinicum* K07-0460^T. *J. Antibiot.* **2011**, *64*, 303–307. [CrossRef] [PubMed]

41. Nakashima, T.; Okuyama, R.; Kamiya, Y.; Matsumoto, A.; Iwatsuki, M.; Inahashi, Y.; Yamaji, K.; Takahashi, Y.; Ōmura, S. Trehangelins A, B and C, novel photo-oxidative hemolysis inhibitors produced by an endophytic actinomycete, *Polymorphospora rubra* K07-0510. *J. Antibiot.* **2013**, *66*, 311–317. [CrossRef] [PubMed]

42. Inahashi, Y.; Shiraishi, T.; Palm, K.; Takahashi, Y.; Ōmura, S.; Kuzuyama, T.; Nakashima, T. Biosynthesis of Trehangelin in *Polymorphospora rubra* K07-0510: Identification of methabolic pathway to angelyl-CoA. *ChemBioChem* **2016**, *17*, 1442–1447. [CrossRef] [PubMed]

43. Nakashima, T.; Iwatsuki, M.; Ochiai, J.; Kamiya, Y.; Nagai, K.; Matsumoto, A.; Ishiyama, A.; Otoguro, K.; Shiomi, K.; Takahashi, Y.; et al. Mangromicins A and B: Structure and antitrypanosomal activity of two new cyclopentadecane compounds from *Lechevalieria aerocolonigenes* K10-0216. *J. Antibiot.* **2014**, *67*, 253–260. [CrossRef] [PubMed]

44. Nakashima, T.; Kamiya, Y.; Iwatsuki, M.; Takahashi, Y.; Ōmura, S. Mangromicins, six new anti-oxidative agents isolated from a culture broth of the actinomycete, *Lechevalieria aerocolonigenes* K10-0216. *J. Antibiot.* **2014**, *67*, 533–539. [CrossRef] [PubMed]

45. Nakashima, T.; Kamiya, Y.; Iwatsuki, M.; Sato, N.; Takahashi, Y.; Ōmura, S. Mangromicin C, a new analog of mangromicin. *J. Antibiot.* **2015**, *68*, 220–222. [CrossRef] [PubMed]

46. Nakashima, T.; Kamiya, Y.; Yamaji, K.; Iwatsuki, M.; Sato, N.; Takahashi, Y.; Ōmura, S. New steroidal compounds from an actinomycete strain, *Lechevalieria aerocolonigenes* K10-0216. *J. Antibiot.* **2015**, *68*, 348–350. [CrossRef] [PubMed]

47. Kimura, T.; Inahashi, Y.; Matsuo, H.; Suga, T.; Iwatsuki, M.; Shiomi, K.; Takahashi, Y.; Ōmura, S.; Nakashima, T. Pyrizomicin A and B: Structure and bioactivity of new thiazolyl pyridines from *Lechevalieria aerocolonigenes* K10-0216. *J. Antibiot.* **2018**, *71*, 606–608. [CrossRef] [PubMed]

48. Kimura, T.; Tajima, A.; Inahashi, Y.; Iwatsuki, M.; Kasai, H.; Mokudai, T.; Niwano, Y.; Shiomi, K.; Takahashi, Y.; Ōmura, S.; et al. Mumiamicin: Structure and bioactivity of a new furan fatty acid from *Mumia* sp. YSP-2-79. *J. Gen. Appl. Microbiol.* **2018**, *64*, 62–67. [CrossRef] [PubMed]

49. Kimura, T.; Iwatsuki, M.; Asami, Y.; Ishiyama, A.; Hokari, R.; Otoguro, K.; Matsumoto, A.; Sato, N.; Shiomi, K.; Takahashi, Y.; et al. Anti-trypanosoma compound, sagamilactam, a new polyene macrocyclic lactam from *Actinomadura* sp. K13-0306. *J. Antibiot.* **2016**, *69*, 818–824. [CrossRef] [PubMed]

50. Izuta, S.; Kosaka, S.; Kawai, M.; Miyano, R.; Matsuo, H.; Matsumoto, A.; Nonaka, K.; Takahashi, Y.; Ōmura, S.; Natashima, T. Dipyrimicins A and B, microbial compounds interacted with ergosterolresin, from *Amycolatopsis* sp. K16-0194. *J. Antibiot.* **2018**, *71*, 535–537. [CrossRef] [PubMed]

51. Bringmann, G.; Kajahn, I.; Reichert, M.; Pedersen, S.E.; Faber, J.H.; Gulder, T.; Brun, R.; Christensen, S.B.; Ponte-Sucre, A.; Moll, H.; et al. Ancistrocladinium A and B, the first N, C-coupled naphthyldihydroisoquinoline alkaloids, from a Congolese Ancistrocladus species. *J. Org. Chem.* **2006**, *71*, 9348–9356. [CrossRef] [PubMed]

52. Ohnishi, Y.; Ishikawa, J.; Hara, H.; Suzuki, H.; Ikenoya, M.; Ikeda, H.; Yamashita, A.; Hattori, M.; Horinouchi, S. Genome sequence of the streptomycin-producing microorganism *Streptomyces griseus* IFO 13350. *J. Bacteriol.* **2008**, *190*, 4050–4060. [CrossRef] [PubMed]

53. Ōmura, S.; Tanaka, H.; Koyama, Y.; Oiwa, R.; Katagiri, M. Nanaomycins A and B, new antibiotics produced by a strain of *Streptomyces*. *J. Antibiot.* **1974**, *27*, 363–365. [CrossRef] [PubMed]

54. Tanaka, H.; Marumo, H.; Nagai, T.; Okada, M.; Taniguchi, K. Nanaomycins, new antibiotics produced by a strain of *Streptomyces*. III. A new component, nanaomycin C, and biological activities of nanaomycin derivatives. *J. Antibiot.* **1975**, *28*, 925–930. [CrossRef] [PubMed]

55. Kasai, M.; Shirahata, K.; Ishii, S.; Mineura, K.; Marumo, H.; Tanaka, H.; Ōmura, S. Structure of nanaomycin E, a new nanaomycin. *J. Antibiot.* **1979**, *32*, 442–445. [CrossRef] [PubMed]

56. Kitaura, K.; Araki, Y.; Marumo, H. The therapeutic effect of nanaomycin A against experimental *Trichophyton mentagrophytes* infection in guinea pigs (author's transl). *Jpn. J. Antibiot.* **1980**, *33*, 728–732. [PubMed]

57. Ōmura, S.; Takahashi, Y.; Nakashima, T.; Matsumoto, A.; Nakanishi, J.; Matsuo, H. Epithelial-Mesenchymal Transition Induced Cell Proliferation Inhibitor. Patent No. PCT/JP2017/034819, 26 September 2016.

58. Bode, H.B.; Bethe, B.; Höfs, R.; Zeeck, A. Big Effects from Small Changes: Possible Ways to Explore Nature's Chemical Diversity. *ChemBioChem* **2002**, *3*, 619–627. [CrossRef]

59. Yoon, S.H.; Ha, S.M.; Kwon, S.; Lim, J.; Kim, Y.; Seo, H.; Chun, J. Introducing EzBioCloud: A taxonomically united database of 16S rRNA gene sequences and whole-genome assemblies. *Int. J. Syst. Evol. Microbiol.* **2017**, *67*, 1613–1617. [PubMed]

60. Kamiya, Y.; Enomoto, Y.; Matsukuma, S.; Nakashima, T.; Takahashi, Y.; Omura, S. Study on anti-aging effects of trehangelin, a new trehalose compound. In Proceedings of the 136th Annual Meeting of the Pharmaceutical Society of Japan, Yokohama, Japan, 26–29 March 2016; p. 137.

61. Azman, A.S.; Othman, I.; Velu, S.S.; Chan, K.G.; Lee, L.H. Mangrove rare actinobacteria: Taxonomy, natural compound, and discovery of bioactivity. *Front. Microbiol.* **2015**, *20*, 856. [CrossRef] [PubMed]

62. Pozzi, R.; Simone, M.; Mazzetti, C.; Maffioli, S.; Monciardini, P.; Cavaletti, L.; Bamonte, R.; Sosio, M.; Donadio, S. The genus *Actinoallomurus* and some of its metabolites. *J. Antibiot.* **2011**, *64*, 133–139. [CrossRef] [PubMed]

63. Takada, H.; Yamada, T.; Hirose, T.; Ishihara, T.; Nakashima, T.; Takahashi, Y.; Ōmura, S.; Sunazuka, T. Total synthesis and determination of the absolute configuration of naturally occurring mangromicin A, with potent antitrypanosomal activity. *Org. Lett.* **2017**, *19*, 230–233. [CrossRef] [PubMed]

64. Amann, R.I.; Ludwig, W.; Schleifer, K.H. Phylogenetic identification and in situ detection of individual microbial cells without cultivation. *Microbiol. Rev.* **1995**, *59*, 143–169. [PubMed]

3

LC-MS/MS Tandem Mass Spectrometry for Analysis of Phenolic Compounds and Pentacyclic Triterpenes in Antifungal Extracts of *Terminalia brownii* (Fresen)

Enass Y. A. Salih [1,3,4,*], **Pia Fyhrquist** [3], **Ashraf M. A. Abdalla** [1], **Abdelazim Y. Abdelgadir** [1], **Markku Kanninen** [4], **Marketta Sipi** [4], **Olavi Luukkanen** [4], **Mustafa K. M. Fahmi** [1,4], **Mai H. Elamin** [5] **and Hiba A. Ali** [2,†]

[1] Department of Forest Products and Industries, Faculty of Forestry, PO Box 13314, University of Khartoum, Khartoum 11111, Sudan; amahmed@uofk.edu (A.M.A.A.); ayabdelgadir@uofk.edu (A.Y.A.); mkfahmi@uofk.edu (M.K.M.F.)

[2] Commission for Biotechnology and Genetic Engineering, PO Box 2404, National Centre for Research, Khartoum, Sudan; hibaali@hotmail.com

[3] Faculty of Pharmacy, Division of Pharmaceutical Biosciences, PO Box 56, University of Helsinki, FIN-00014 Helsinki, Finland; pia.fyhrquist@helsinki.fi

[4] Viikki Tropical Resources Institute (VITRI), Department of Forest Sciences, PO Box 27, University of Helsinki, FIN-00014 Helsinki, Finland; markku.kanninen@helsinki.fi (M.K.); Marketta.Sipi@helsinki.fi (M.S.); olavi.luukkanen@helsinki.fi (O.L.)

[5] Department of Phytochemistry, Faculty of Pharmacy, PO Box 477, University of Sciences and Technology, Omdurman, Sudan; maielamin15@gmail.com

* Correspondence: enass.salih@helsinki.fi or eyabdelkareem@uofk.edu

† With this paper we would like to honor our colleague, Dr. Hiba Ali, who passed away the 29.4.2016.

Academic Editor: Leonard Amaral

Abstract: Decoctions and macerations of the stem bark and wood of *Terminalia brownii* Fresen. are used in traditional medicine for fungal infections and as fungicides on field crops and in traditional granaries in Sudan. In addition, *T. brownii* water extracts are commonly used as sprays for protecting wooden houses and furniture. Therefore, using agar disc diffusion and macrodilution methods, eight extracts of various polarities from the stem wood and bark were screened for their growth-inhibitory effects against filamentous fungi commonly causing fruit, vegetable, grain and wood decay, as well as infections in the immunocompromised host. Ethyl acetate extracts of the stem wood and bark gave the best antifungal activities, with MIC values of 250 µg/mL against *Nattrassia mangiferae* and *Fusarium verticillioides*, and 500 µg/mL against *Aspergillus niger* and *Aspergillus flavus*. Aqueous extracts gave almost as potent effects as the ethyl acetate extracts against the *Aspergillus* and *Fusarium* strains, and were slightly more active than the ethyl acetate extracts against *Nattrassia mangiferae*. Thin layer chromatography, RP-HPLC-DAD and tandem mass spectrometry (LC-MS/MS), were employed to identify the chemical constituents in the ethyl acetate fractions of the stem bark and wood. The stem bark and wood were found to have a similar qualitative composition of polyphenols and triterpenoids, but differed quantitatively from each other. The stilbene derivatives, *cis-* (**3**) and *trans-* resveratrol-3-*O*-β-galloylglucoside (**4**), were identified for the first time in *T. brownii*. Moreover, methyl-(*S*)-flavogallonate (**5**), quercetin-7-β-*O*-di-glucoside (**8**), quercetin-7-*O*-galloyl-glucoside (**10**), naringenin-4′-methoxy-7-pyranoside (**7**), 5,6-dihydroxy-3′,4′,7-tri-methoxy flavone (**12**), gallagic acid dilactone (terminalin) (**6**), a corilagin derivative (**9**) and two oleanane type triterpenoids (**1**) and (**2**) were characterized. The flavonoids, a corilagin derivative and terminalin, have not been identified before in *T. brownii*. We reported earlier on the occurrence of methyl-*S*-flavogallonate and its isomer in the roots of *T. brownii*, but this is the first report on their occurrence in the stem wood as well. Our results justify the traditional uses of macerations and decoctions of *T. brownii* stem wood and bark for crop and wood protection and demonstrate that standardized extracts could have uses for the eco-friendly control of plant pathogenic fungi in African agroforestry systems. Likewise, our results justify the traditional uses of these preparations for the treatment of skin infections caused by filamentous fungi.

Keywords: Africa; *Terminalia brownii*; antifungal stem wood and bark extracts; *Aspergillus*; *Nattrassia*; Fusarium; LC-MS/MS; flavonoids; ellagitannins; stilbenes; triterpenes

---

1. Introduction

Fungal contamination is both a pre- and a post-harvesting problem in crop production and poses a continuous and growing threat to global food crop production [1,2]. Some of the fungal species generally considered to be phytopathogens, such as *Aspergillus* spp., are also known to be increasingly significant as human pathogens, especially in the immunocompromised host [3–5].

Aspergillus niger (van Tieghem, 1867) and *Aspergillus flavus* (Link, 1809) are both human [6,7] and plant pathogens [8]. As human pathogens, especially *A. flavus*, but also *A. niger* cause aspergillosis in immunocompromised individuals [9,10]. *A. flavus* causes grain crop infections in maize (*Zea mays* L.), leading to a substantial decrease in the commercial value of maize crop due to aflatoxin contamination [11]. Moreover, *A. flavus* is often the causative agent of wood decay in timber and houses [12]. *Nattrassia mangiferae* [(Syd. and P. Syd.) B. Sutton and Dyko], previously known as *Hendersonula toruloi* Nattrass (HT) and *Dothiorella mangiferae* (Syd. and P. Syd), is a wound-invading dematiaceous (brown-pigmented) phytopathogenic fungus infecting hard wood species of *Citrus*, *Mangifera* and *Eucalyptus* and soft wood coniferous subtropical and tropical trees, causing dieback and vascular wilt diseases [13,14]. *Nattrassia mangiferae* is also a human pathogenic fungus, especially in immunocompromised individuals [15], and is even known to cause community acquired infections in rural farmer societies worldwide [13]. *Fusarium verticilloides* and some other *Fusarium* species infect maize ears (husks) causing maize ear rot disease and contaminate maize grains with fumonisin mycotoxins leading to major pre- and post-harvest losses [16]. *Fusarium* spp. mycotoxins are toxic [17,18], and fumonisin has been found to cause cancer in mammalians [19]. Another species of *Fusarium*, *F. oxysporum* is the causative agent of the "Panama disease" affecting the banana (*Musa paradisiaca*), the staple food of a large part of Africa.

Currently used fungicides are costly and toxic to the environment [20,21]. Besides, phytopathogenic and human pathogenic filamentous fungi have developed resistance to many conventional fungicides and to antibiotics [22–26]. Thus, new effective, less toxic, affordable and readily available antifungals are needed [26]. Tropical and subtropical plants are known to contain a wide range of defense compounds due to their needs for constant production of defense compounds throughout the year as well as due to the high biodiversity in rain forests, woodlands and savannahs [27]. Thus, tropical plant species used for fungal infections in African traditional medicine as well as for protection of crop plants against fungal contamination, are expected to be good sources for new antifungal compounds [28,29].

The pantropical genus of *Terminalia* (Combretaceae) contains a number of species known for their antifungal effects. Antifungal activities against *Aspergillus niger* and *A. flavus* have been reported for the Asian species, *Terminalia alata, T. arjuna, T. bellerica, T. catappa* and *T. chebula* [30,31]. Approximately 30 species of *Terminalia* occur in Africa [32]. However, despite of their frequent uses in traditional medicine for treatment of fungal infections in humans and in traditional agriculture for prevention of fungal crop plant contamination, only a small portion of these species have been studied in depth for their antifungal activity and/or antifungal compounds. Among those African *Terminalia* species investigated for their antifungal potential, either against yeasts or filamentous fungi or both, are *T. avicennoides, T. spinosa, T. sericea* and *T. nigrovenulosa* [33–36]. Ellagitannins, ellagic acid derivatives, stilbenes, lignans, flavonoids and pentacyclic triterpenes were reported from some

African species of *Terminalia*, such as *T. horrida*, *T. sericea*, *T. superba* and *T. macroptera* [33,34,37–45]. Most of these phytochemical investigations did not include antifungal screening of the characterized compounds, however.

Terminalia brownii (Fresen.) is a deciduous tree distributed throughout East African savannah regions in a wide range of temperature, rain fall and soil conditions (Figure 1) [46]. In Sudan, *T. brownii* occurs in low and high rainfall zones in Blue Nile state and El-Gadarif in the eastern part of the country and Kordofan and Darfour states in the western part of Sudan. In Sudan, *T. brownii* grows in natural forested areas such as savannah woodlands where it is listed as an endangered species due to overexploitation [47]. *T brownii* has been found to be exceptionally resistant against various pathogenic fungi that affect crops, and is frequently used in traditional agroforestry for crop plant protection [21]. Similarly to many other plant species, such as *Melianthus comosus* [48], also decoctions of various parts of *T. brownii* have traditional applications as fungicides against fungal contamination in harvested crop plants.

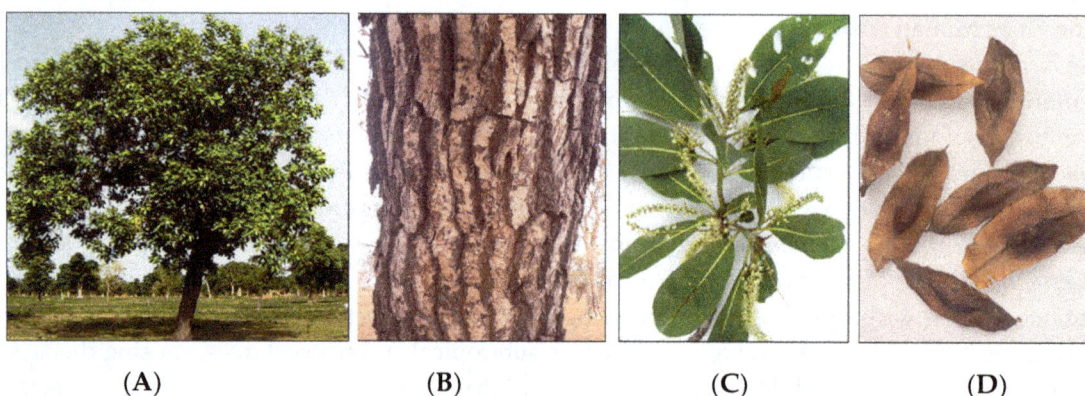

Figure 1. *Terminalia brownii.* (**A**) tree in savannah woodland; (**B**) stem bark; (**C**) flowers and leaves; (**D**) fruits. Photo: E. Y. A. Salih and Dr. H. H. Gibreel, 2006.

Terminalia brownii has been found to be a rich source of oleanane- and ursane-type pentacyclic triterpenoids, such as arjunic acid, galloyl arjunic acid, tomentosic acid, sericic acid, arjungenin, sericoside, betulinic acid, monogynol A and arjunglucoside [21,49]. In addition, a new oleanane type triterpenoid, designated as 3β,24-*O*-ethylidenyl-2α,19α-dihydroxyolean-12-en-28-oic acid, was identified in an ethyl acetate extract of the stem bark of *T. brownii* [49]. Moreover, β-sitosterol and ellagic acid derivatives have been characterized from the leaves and stem bark of *T. brownii* [21,49]. In addition, a number of unknown and known ellagitannins, including methyl-(*S*)-flavogallonate and its derivative as well as α,β-punicalagin and α,β-terchebulin have been described form the roots and the stem bark, respectively [50,51]. Moreover, a chromone derivative designated as terminalianone has been found in the stem bark of *T. brownii* [52]. However, to our knowledge, the antifungal effects of the mentioned compounds were not investigated, with the exception of arjungenin, β-sitosterol and betulinic acid [21].

Although *T. brownii* extracts are used traditionally against fungal phytopathogens and to treat human fungal infections in Sudan and in other countries of Africa, there are a limited number of reports on their in vitro antifungal activity against filamentous fungi affecting crop production and human health. Moreover, only a small number of antifungal compounds in *T. brownii* have been characterized to date [21,49], and to the best of our knowledge, no flavonoid structures have been studied in this species of *Terminalia*. Therefore, the current study was performed to verify the antifungal effects of decoctions and macerations, reported to be used for fungal infections in traditional medicine and as fungicides in traditional agriculture. In addition, extracts of various polarities made from the stem bark and wood of *T. brownii* were tested for their growth-inhibitory effects. For the screenings, significant phytopathogenic and human pathogenic opportunistic fungi of the genera *Aspergillus*, *Nattrassia* and

Fusarium were used. Thin layer chromatography (TLC) and RP-HPLC/DAD were used to study the phytochemical composition of the ethyl acetate extracts of the stem wood and bark. Tandem mass spectrometry (LC-MS/MS) was used to elucidate the molecular masses of flavonoids, triterpenes, ellagitannins and stilbenes in an antifungal stem wood extract of *T. brownii*.

2. Results

2.1. Antifungal Effects of Extracts of Terminalia brownii Stem Bark and Wood

The results of the growth inhibition of various extracts of *Terminalia brownii* stem bark and wood against *Aspergillus*, *Nattrassia* and *Fusarium* strains are shown in Table 1. When compared to the other extracts, the ethyl acetate extracts of the stem wood and bark gave the highest antifungal activity. This result is in accordance with other authors, who also reported that especially ethyl acetate extracts of the stem bark of *T. brownii* give good antifungal effects against sweet potato infecting fungi, such as *Aspergillus niger* and *Fusarium solanii* [21]. The reference antifungal used in our tests, amphotericin-B, was more growth-inhibitory than the ethyl acetate extracts, however, although the differences in potency between amphotericin-B and the ethyl acetate extracts were not big, considering that we used plant extracts instead of pure compounds present in these extracts (Table 1).

Our results demonstrate that *Nattrassia mangiferae* and *Fusarium verticilliodies* were especially sensitive to the ethyl acetate extracts of *T. brownii* stem wood and bark, giving MIC values of 250 µg/mL, whereas *Aspergillus niger* and *A. flavus* were more resistant to these extracts, demonstrating MIC values of 500 µg/mL (Table 1). We found that the obtained MIC values correlated well with the sizes of the inhibition zones produced by these ethyl acetate extracts, so that small MIC values were coupled to large diameters of the inhibition zones (Table 1). To the best of our knowledge, this is the first report on antifungal effects of *T. brownii* against *Nattrassia mangiferae*.

Interestingly, we also found that aqueous extracts of the stem bark and wood of *T. brownii* gave good growth-inhibitory effects (Table 1). Compared to the other extracts these aqueous extracts gave especially high extraction yields of 20 and 16%, respectively for bark and wood (Figure 2). Thus, our results justify the traditional application of macerations (water extracts) of the stem wood and barks of *T. brownii* for the preservation of grains and wooden house poles and for traditional medicinal treatment of fungal infections caused by *Aspergillus*, *Nattrassia* and *Fusarium*. Earlier studies have indicated that aqueous stem bark extracts of *T. brownii* are growth-inhibitory also against yeast species, such as *Candida albicans* and *Cryprococcus neoformans* and in addition the aqueous extracts were found to be less toxic than other extracts against brine shrimps [53]. Thus, standardized aqueous extracts of *T. brownii* stem wood and bark could be used to treat fungal infections and fungal contamination.

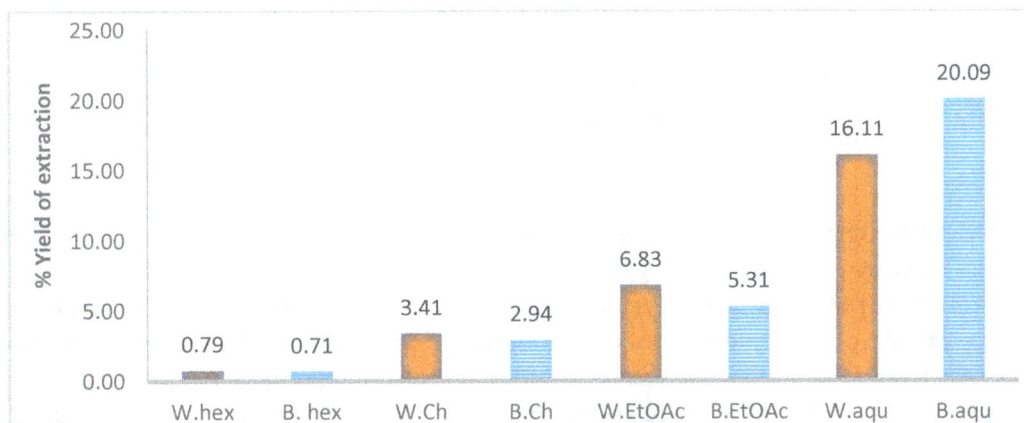

Figure 2. Percentage yield (% *w/w*) resulting from sequential extraction and liquid/liquid partition of the stem wood and stem bark of *Terminalia brownii*. W, stem wood; B, stem bark; hex, hexane extract; Ch, choloroform extract; EtOAc, ethyl acetate extract; aqu, aqueous extract.

When compared to the more polar water and ethyl acetate extracts, we found that chloroform extracts of the stem wood and bark of *T. brownii* were slightly antifungal, while the petroleum ether extracts were devoid of antifungal activity (Table 1). In contrast to our results, in an earlier investigation, it was found that an n-hexane extract of the stem bark of *Terminalia brownii* was active against another *Aspergillus* species, *A. fumigatus* [54]. Perhaps this result might indicate that different species of *Aspergillus* differ to their sensitivity to non-polar extracts of *T. brownii*, so that *A. fumigatus* is more sensitive than *A. niger* and *A. flavus*.

Table 1. Antifungal activity of stem wood and bark extracts of *T. brownii*. Results were obtained using cup well agar diffusion and agar dilution methods.

Fungal Strain	Stem Wood Extracts		Stem Bark Extracts		Amphotericin-B	
	IZ	MIC	IZ	MIC	IZ	MIC
Aspergillus niger						
Pt	NA		NA			
CHCl3	12 ± 0.9		13 ± 0.4			
EtOAc	17 ± 0.7	500	17 ± 0.8	500	35 ± 0.01	31.25
aqueous	17 ± 0.5		16.5 ± 0.4			
Aspergillus flavus						
Pt	NA		NA			
CHCl3	14 ± 0.5		14 ± 0.9			
EtOAc	18.5 ± 0.4	500	18.5 ± 0.8	500	28 ± 0.03	125
aqueous	18 ± 0.9		18 ± 0.5			
Nattrassia mangiferae						
Pt	NA		NA			
CHCl3	12 ± 0.5		12 ± 0.7			
EtOAc	19 ± 0.4	250	18.5 ± 0.4	250	30 ± 0.04	62.5
aqueous	18.5 ± 0.4		19 ± 0.4			
Fusarium verticillioides						
Pt	NA		NA			
CHCl3	13 ± 0.6		11 ± 0.9			
EtOAc	20 ± 0.4	250	19 ± 0.2	250	31 ± 0.03	62.5
aqueous	19 ± 0.3		18 ± 0.7			

For agar diffusion, extracts at the concentration 1 mg/mL were used. Diameter of inhibition zones (IZ) in mm: >18 mm: sensitive; 14–18 mm: intermediate; <14 mm: resistant [55,56]; Pt, petroleum ether extracts; CHCL3, chloroform extracts; EtOAc, ethyl acetate extracts; NA, Not active. IZ results as mean ± SEM of five measurements. MIC in µg/mL. The observed differences between the sample means of the inhibition zones (the stem bark and wood extracts) against the tested fungi did not differ significantly.

2.2. Results from the Phytochemical Screening of Antifungal Ethyl Acetate Extracts of T. brownii Stem Wood and Bark

Owing to our promising antifungal results for the ethyl acetate extracts of the stem bark and wood of *T. brownii*, and to the few existing earlier records on the activity of this species against filamentous fungi, we investigated the secondary compound composition and molecular masses as well as the fragmentation patterns of phenolic compounds and triterpenoids of these extracts.

2.2.1. TLC Results

RP-18 thin layer chromatograms of the ethyl acetate extracts of the stem wood and stem bark of *T. brownii* gave a negative reaction with Dragendorff reagent, suggesting that these extracts were devoid of alkaloids. Pink to purple colors were developed upon spraying with vanillin-H_2SO_4, which suggested the presence of triterpenoid and phenolic compounds. Spraying the TLC plates with aluminum trichloride ($AlCl_3$) and Natural Product reagent (NPR), revealed the presence of flavonoids, since color changes from quenching fluorescence to yellow, orange or blue color, typical for flavonoidal acids or other phenolic acids, could be observed at 366 nm [57].

2.2.2. HPLC-UV/DAD Results

HPLC-UV/DAD fingerprints of the ethyl acetate extracts of the stem bark and stem wood of *Terminalia brownii* are presented in Figure 3. Altogether twelve compounds with retention times between 6.8 and 25.5 min could be identified using internal standards and a computer library for standard compounds. At the wavelengths of 320 and 254 nm, which were used for detection of stilbenes and flavonoids, the wood ethyl acetate extract displayed a higher diversity of flavonoidal and stilbenoid compounds. For example, the *cis-* and *trans-*isomers of resveratrol 3-*O*-β-galloyl-glucoside (**3** and **4**) at Rt 11.1 and 13.2 min, respectively, as well as naringenin-4′-methoxy-7-pyranoside (**7**) at 15.3 min, the corilagin derivative (**9**) at Rt 18.2 min, and quercetin-7-*O*-galloyl glucoside (**10**) at Rt 18.4 min, were present in the wood extract but absent from the stem bark extract as shown in Figure 3.

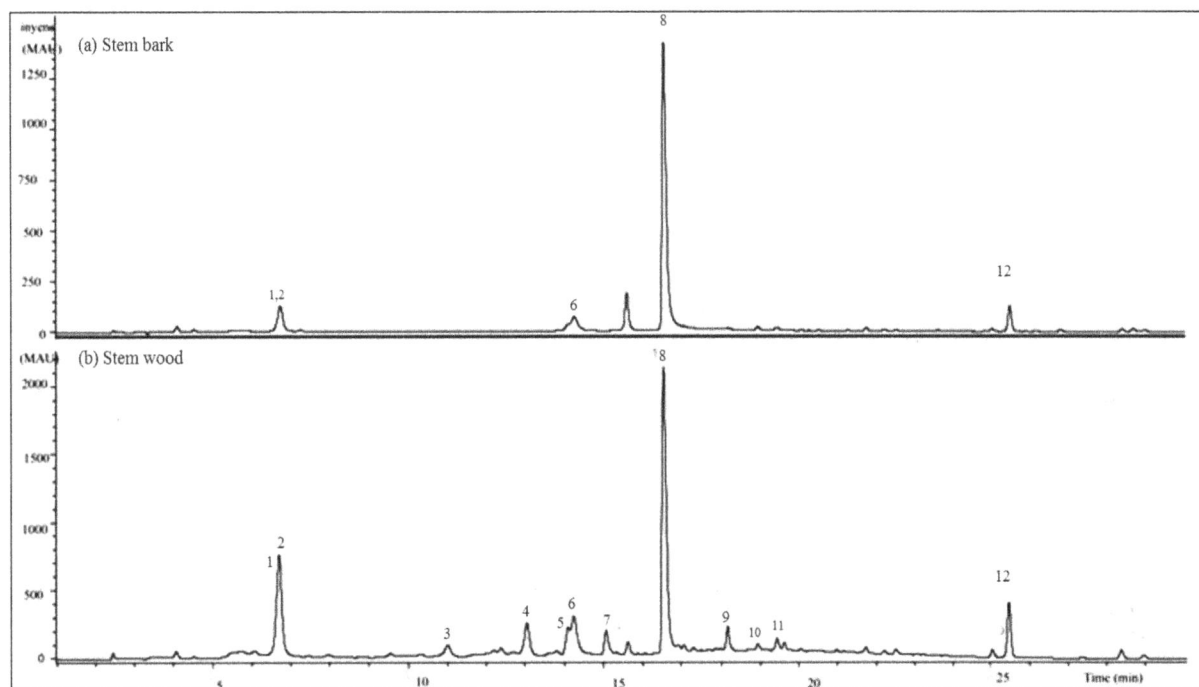

Figure 3. RP-HPLC/DAD chromatograms of ethyl acetate extracts of *T.brownii*. (**A**) stem bark and (**B**) stem wood extracts at 254 nm. (**1**) and (**2**) Oleanane type triterpenoids; (**3**) cis-resveratrol-3-*O*-β-galloyl-glucoside; (**4**) trans-resveratrol-3-*O*-β-galloyl-glucoside; (**5**) Methyl-(*S*)-flavogallonate; (**6**) Gallagic acid dilactone (Terminalin); (**7**) Naringenin-4′-methoxy-7-pyranoside; (**8**) Quercetin-7-ß-*O*-diglucoside; (**9**) Corilagin derivative; (**10**) Quercetin-7-*O*-galloyl-glucoside; (**11**) unknown ellagitannin; (**12**) 5,6-dihydroxy-3′,4′,7-trimethoxy flavone.

Because of the high number of compounds present in the wood ethyl acetate extract and due to this extract being slightly more antifungal than the stem bark, at least in terms of the sizes of the diameters of inhibition zones (Table 1), this extract was subjected to LC-MS/MS advanced analysis for identification of the major compounds.

2.2.3. LC-MS/MS Results

MS/MS combined with collision-induced dissociation (CID), has been found to enable the accurate identification of stilbenes and flavonoids in complex extracts with co-eluting peaks [58]. Therefore MS/MS was employed as the method of choice for the identification of compounds in an ethyl acetate extract of *T. brownii* stem wood. A total of twelve compounds were characterized by comparing the obtained molecular (precursor) ions and fragmentation patterns (i.e., product ions) from our LC-MS/MS data with data from the literature and with a computer library for the standard compounds

(Table 2). The MS^2, MS^3 and MS^4 ion chromatograms are presented in the supplemental part of this paper (Supplement 1).

Table 2. HPLC-DAD and MS/MS data of phenolic compounds and triterpenoids in an ethyl acetate extract of the stem wood of *T. brownii*.

Peak No	Rt (min)	[M-H] (m/z)	CID M^n Main Fragment Ions (m/z)	Identified Compound	Molecular Formula	Exact Mass (Calc.)
1	6.8	469	425, 407, 379, 353, 300, 271	oleanane type triterpenoid	-	-
2	6.8	491	447, 429, 411, 401, 385, 301	oleanane type triterpenoid	-	-
3	11.1	541	532, 425, 397, 301, 273, <u>227</u>, 199, 169	*cis*-resveratrol-3-*O*-β-galloyl-glucoside	$C_{27}H_{26}O_{12}$	542.1416
4	13.2	541	532, 424, 407, 300, 275, <u>227</u>, 199, 169	*trans*-resveratrol-3-*O*-β-galloyl-glucoside	$C_{27}H_{26}O_{12}$	542.1416
5	14.1	483	451, 433, 407, 305, 405, 377	Methyl-(*S*)-flavogallonate	$C_{22}H_{12}O_{13}$	484.0273
6	14.4	601	583, 301, 299, 271, 243, 215	Gallagic acid dilactone	$C_{28}H_{10}O_{16}$	601.9964
7	15.3	433	300, 314, 229, 271, 132	Naringenin-4′-methoxy-7-pyranoside	-	-
8	16.8	625	<u>301</u>, 284, 256, 229, 201, 185, 129	Quercetin-7-β-*O*-diglucoside	$C_{27}H_{30}O_{17}$	626.1473
9	18.2	633	481, 463, 421, 387, 305, 275, 300, 169	Corilagin derivative	-	-
10	18.4	585	<u>301</u>, 284, 257, 229, 201, 185, 153, 132	Quercetin-7-*O*-galloyl-glucoside	-	-
11	19.1	725	665, 503, 409, 441, 379, 391	Unknown ellagitannin	-	-
12	25.5	343	328, 313, 298, 285, 270, 257	5,6-dihydroxy-3′,4′,7-trimethoxy-flavone	-	-

Rt, retention time in HPLC-DAD; [M-H]$^-$ *(m/z)*, base or molecular ions at negative mode; CID M^n, Fragmentation ions resulting from collision-induced dissociation; The exact mass (calc.) according to the molecular formula of identified compounds. <u>Aglycones are underlined.</u> Peak numbers according to Figure 3.

We found that the stem wood of *T. brownii* contains two oleanane triterpenoid acids that co-eluted at 6.8 min (Figures 3 and 4). For compound (**1**) a [M-H]$^-$ molecular ion at *m/z* 469 was detected, whereas compound (**2**) gave a molecular ion of *m/z* 491. In the MS^2 chromatograms, a fragment ion at *m/z* 425 was detected for compound (**1**) and at *m/z* 447 for compound (**2**) (Table 2, Supplement 1, Slide 1). These fragment ions indicate the loss of a carboxylic acid (-COOH) group ([M-H]$^-$ for -COOH = 44) from both molecular ions. In agreement with our results, the loss of carboxylic acid at position 17 in pentacyclic triterpenoids was observed when using atmospheric pressure chemical ionization (APCI)-MS [59,60]. Moreover, we observed a fragment ion at *m/z* 407, which indicated the loss of H_2O from *m/z* 425 in compound **1**. This kind of mass spectral fragmentation pattern is typical for oleanane type triterpenes [61,62], therefore confirming that compounds 1 and 2 are oleanane type triterpenes (Figure 4A).

In our HPLC-DAD system, compounds (**3**) and (**4**) eluted at Rt 11.1 and 13.2 min, respectively (Figure 3b). Both compounds showed an identical [M-H]$^-$ molecular ion at *m/z* 541. Moreover, when subjected to MS^3, both compounds provided fragment ions of *m/z* 227 and 314 (Table 2, Supplement 1, Slide 3 and 4). The fragment ion at *m/z* 314 indicates the presence of a galloylhexose fragment [63]. A comparison with the literature showed that the fragment ion at *m/z* 227 corresponds to the resveratrol unit [44]. Therefore, compounds (**3**) and (**4**) were tentatively assigned as resveratrol-3-*O*-β-galloyl-glucoside, respectively. Due to different retention times, the compounds were proposed to be *cis*- (**3**) and *trans*- (**4**) isomers of resveratrol-3-*O*-β-galloylglucoside (Figure 4C).

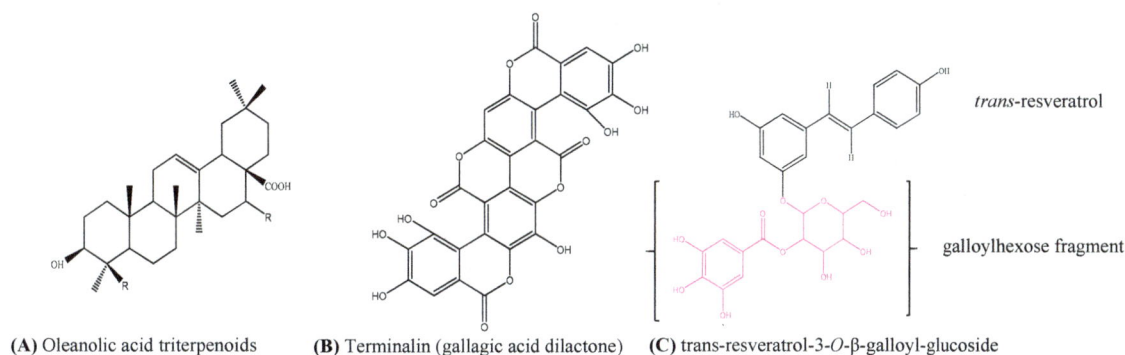

(A) Oleanolic acid triterpenoids   **(B)** Terminalin (gallagic acid dilactone)   **(C)** trans-resveratrol-3-*O*-β-galloyl-glucoside

Figure 4. Chemical structures of some of the characterized compounds in the stem wood and stem bark of *T. brownii*. (**A**) oleanane type triterpenoids (compounds **1** and **2**); (**B**) Terminalin (compound **6**) and (**C**) *trans*-resveratrol-3-*O*-β-galloyl-glucoside (compound **4**).

When subjected to MS^2, compound (**5**) at Rt 14.1 min in HPLC-DAD (Figure 3b), gave an [M-H]$^-$ molecular ion at m/z 483 (Table 2, Supplement 1, Slide 5). The loss of the two oxygen molecules {483 − 451 = 32} at MS^3, gave a fragmentation ion at m/z 433. Also, the MS^3 spectrum was devoid of the fragment of [M-H-CO$_2$]$^-$, which corresponds to a methyl ester molecule [64]. Therefore, and according to previous investigations [45,50], compound (**5**) was tentatively assigned the structure of methyl-(*S*)-flavogallonate.

Compound (**6**) at Rt 14.4 min (Figure 3b), gave a [M-H]$^-$ molecular ion at m/z 601 (Figure 3b, Table 2). When subjected to MS^3, compound (**6**) yielded the fragment ions at m/z 271 and 301, the later corresponding to free ellagic acid (Supplement 1, Slide 6). A molecular ion of m/z 601 and fragment ions at m/z 271 and 301 have been reported for gallagic acid [45]. Gallagic acid dilactone (syn. terminalin) has been reported in another species of *Terminalia*, *T. oblongata* [65]. Accordingly, compound (**6**) was tentatively assigned the structure of gallagic acid dilactone (terminalin) (Figure 4B).

Compound (**7**) at Rt 15.3 min (Figure 3b) gave an [M-H]$^-$ molecular ion at m/z 433 (Table 2). The deprotonation of [M-H]$^-$ at MS^2 resulted in a fragment ion at m/z 300, indicating the loss of one molecule of a pentose sugar ([M-H]-132) [63,66]. Moreover, MS^3 of this compound yielded the loss of an Y0 fragment at m/z 271, corresponding to the cleavage of the aglycone fragment ion of the flavanone naringenin [66–68]. In the MS^3, the [M-H]$^-$ yielded a fragment at m/z 284, therefore indicating that the methoxy group occurs at position 4′ [66] (Supplement 1, Slide 7). As flavonoids commonly occur as *O*-glycosides and *O*-glycosylation occurs at position 7 in flavanones [63,69], compound (**7**) was tentatively assigned to naringenin-4′-methoxy-7-pyranoside.

The main compound (**8**) in the HPLC chromatogram at Rt 16.8 min (Figure 3) gave a [M-H]$^-$ molecular ion at m/z 625 (Table 2). The main fragmentation product ion at m/z 301 in the MS^2 and MS^3 chromatograms indicated the loss of two glucose molecules ([M-H]$^-$-2 × 162 Da) as well the presence of a quercetin aglycone moiety corresponding to m/z 301 [68] (Supplement 1, Slide 8). Since glucose is usually β-glycosidically linked to the flavonoid aglycone and *O*-glycosidic linking is usually occurring at position 7 on the A ring of flavonoids [69], compound (**8**) was tentatively identified as quercetin-7-β-*O*-diglucoside.

Compound (**9**) at Rt 18.2 min (Figure 3b), gave a [M-H]$^-$ molecular ion at m/z 633 (Table 2). MS/MS fragmentation resulted in a loss of a fragment product ion at m/z 481, corresponding to [M-galloyl-gallic acid. Other fragment product ions resulting from MS^2 were; 463 [M-gallic acid]$^-$, 300 (hexahydroxydiphenoyl-H) and 169 corresponding to gallic acid [45,70,71] (Supplement 1, Slide 9). Consequently, compound (**9**) is suggested to be a derivative of corilagin.

Compound (**10**) at Rt 18.4 min (Figure 3b) gave a [M-H]$^-$ molecular ion at m/z 585 (Figure 3, Table 2). MS^2 fragmentation of this compound resulted in the loss of a pyranose sugar corresponding to the fragment ion at m/z 132 and a galloyl unit corresponding to a fragment ion of m/z 153. Moreover, a fragment product ion at m/z 301 {[M-H]$^-$-132-153} (Table 2), corresponding to the aglycone of quercetin, was present in the MS^2 chromatogram [68] (Supplement 1, Slide 10). Consequently, compound (**10**) was tentatively assigned to be quercetin 7-O-galloyl-glucoside.

A polyphenol (Compound **11**) with a retention time of 19.1 min in HPLC-DAD (Figure 3b) gave a molecular ion at m/z 725. In the MS^2 spectrum, the fragment ions of a hexose sugar were observed at m/z 665 and 503, indicating that the cleavage within this hexose sugar ring occurred at $_{0.3}X$ [M-H-61]$^-$ [63,69]. Moreover, the loss of two oxygen molecules was noticed at MS^3 [M-H-2 × 16]$^-$. In the spectra at MS^4, two fragments at m/z 391 and 379 were observed. These fragments resulted from the loss of one molecule of water and two methyl groups, respectively, from the fragment at m/z 409 in spectra MS^3 ([M-H]$^-$-H$_2$O-2CH$_3$]$^-$ (Supplement 1, Slide 11). Thus, compound (**11**) is suggested to be identical to an unknown ellagitannin that we have reported earlier to occur in *T. brownii* roots [50].

Compound (**12**) at Rt 25.5 min (Figure 3b), gave a [M-H]$^-$ molecular ion at m/z 343 (Table 2). MS^3 and MS^4 fragmentation of this compound resulted in the loss of three methyl groups (-CH$_3$) corresponding to product fragment ions {[M-H]$^-$ 343-328-313} (Table 2, Supplement 1, Slide 12). Moreover, in the fragment ion chromatogram resulting from MS^3, a high intensity of the product fragment ion at m/z 313 could be observed indicating the loss of a methyl group ([M-H]$^-$-15) (Table 2, Supplement 1, Slide 12). From this data, compound (**12**) was tentatively assigned as 5,6-dihydroxy-3′,4′,7-trimethoxyflavone.

3. Discussion

Pentacyclic triterpene saponins are known to complex with ergosterol and cholesterol in the fungal cell membrane, thus leading to loss of membrane integrity [72] and it has been found that triterpenoids decrease mycelial growth [73]. Accordingly, the triterpenes betulinic acid and arjungenin, isolated from ethyl acetate extracts of *T. brownii* stem bark were found to give good antifungal effects against *Aspergillus niger*, *Fusarium solanii* and *Fusarium oxysporum* with MIC values ranging from 50 to 200 μg/mL [21]. Therefore, we suggest that the two unknown oleanane-type triterpenes (**1**) and (**2**) would contribute significantly to the antifungal effects we have found for the ethyl acetate extract of the stem wood of *T. brownii* (Table 2, Figure 3).

In the genus *Terminalia*, resveratrol and its glucoside and rutinoside derivatives have been reported in *Terminalia prunioides*, *T. sericea* and *T. ferdinandiana* [44,74,75]. We reported here for the first time on the occurrence of the resveratrol derivatives, *cis*- (**3**) and *trans*-resveratrol-3-O-β-galloylglucoside (**4**) in *Terminalia brownii* stem wood. Besides, galloylglucoside derivatives of resveratrol have not been reported before in the genus *Terminalia*. Resveratrol and its derivatives are antifungal phytoalexins, protecting plants from pathogenic fungal and bacterial intrusion [76,77]. Several investigations on in vitro antifungal activities of resveratrol and its derivatives indicate good antifungal potential of this compound class [78,79]. Therefore, the good antifungal activity in the ethyl acetate extracts of *T. brownii* could partly be due to the resveratrol-galloylglucoside derivatives (**2**) and (**3**). To the best of our knowledge resveratrol-3-O-β-galloylglucoside has not been studied for its antifungal effects, which warrants further studies in this respect.

We reported here for the first time, on the occurrence of another ellagic acid derivative, gallagic acid dilactone (**6**), in the stem wood of *T. brownii*. Gallagic acid, is an analogue to ellagic acid, containing four gallic acid residues [80] and has restricted occurrence in plants. Gallagic acid and its derivatives have been found in various parts of some other *Terminalia* species such as in the leaves of *T. catappa* and *T. oblongata* [65,81] and in the fruits of *Terminalia bellerica*, *Terminalia horrida* and *T. chebula* [45]. Gallagic acid is the fully lactonized form of the gallagyl moiety in the ellagitannin punicalagin, which is common in *Terminalia* spp. [45,82]. Gallagic acid has been found to give concentration-dependent growth-inhibitory effects against *Fusarium* and *Alternaria* [83]. Thus, it is possible that gallagic acid dilactone (**6**), which we found to be present in an ethyl acetate extract of the stem wood of *T. brownii*, could be an important contributor to the antifungal effects of this extract.

Ellagitannins have been found to inhibit the growth of *Fusarium* and *Alternaria* dose-dependently [83]. Even though the genus *Terminalia* is renowned to be especially rich in ellagitannins [45] only a few studies have been performed on the antifungal effects of ellagitannins isolated from *Terminalia* species. Some of the few investigations demonstrate that ellagitannins from *Terminalia* spp. could be valuable antifungal compounds. For example, punicalagin from the leaf of *T. brachystemma* was found to give a low MIC value of 6.25 µg/mL against *Candida* strains [61]. It was found, however, that some ellagitannins were not active against filamentous fungi, although activity was demonstrated against *Candida* and *Cryptococcus neoformans* [84]. Thus, it remains to be investigated whether the ellagitannins we have found in *T. brownii* stem wood, such as methyl-*(S)*-flavogallonate (**5**), the unknown ellagitannin (**11**) and the corilagin derivative (**9**) give low MIC values against filamentous fungi such as *Aspergillus, Nattrassia* and *Fusarium* spp. among others.

Our research resulted in the characterization of the flavonoids naringenin-4′-methoxy-7-pyranoside (**7**), quercetin-7-β-*O*-diglucoside (**8**), quercetin-7-*O*-galloylglycoside (**10**) and 5,6-dihydroxy-3,4,7-trimethoxy flavone (**12**) in the ethyl acetate extracts of stem wood and bark of *Terminalia brownii*. To the best of our knowledge this is the first time these flavonoids are reported to occur in *T. brownii*. We suggest that quercetin-7-β-*O*-diglucoside (**8**), which was quantitatively the main peak in both stem bark and wood extracts of *T. brownii*, contributes significantly to the antifungal effects of these extracts. Accordingly, several authors have reported that quercetin and its derivatives give good antifungal effects against *Aspergillus* and *Fusarium* strains [85–87] and for quercetin as low MIC values as 15 µg/mL were recorded against *Aspergillus niger*, *Fusarium moniliforme* and *F. sporotrichum* [88]. Furthermore, dihydroquercetin from barley suppressed the growth of *Fusarium* spp. [89]. However, it has been demonstrated that quercetin-glycoside was not as antifungal as its aglycone [90]. In contrast to quercetin, some other flavonoids have demonstrated strong antifungal effects as glycosides. For example, naringenin pyranoside demonstrated some antifungal activity with MIC values of 1600–3200 µg/mL against *Candida albicans* and *C. krusei* [91]. Therefore, naringenin-4′-methoxy-7-pyranoside, which we have found in the stem wood of *T. brownii*, is suggested to give some antifungal activity. Moreover, it has been found that flavonoids possessing methoxy groups are especially antifungal [87]. This would apply to naringenin-4′-methoxy-7-pyranoside (**7**) and 5,6-dihydroxy-3,4,7-trimethoxy flavone (**12**) which we have found in the stem wood of *T. brownii*. These flavonoids possess one and three methoxy groups, respectively, and thus are suggested to participate in the antifungal effects of the ethyl acetate extracts of the stem wood of *T. brownii*.

4. Materials and Methods

4.1. Collection of Plant Material

The stem wood and stem bark was collected from many individuals of *Terminalia brownii* growing in natural savannah woodland, in the Blue Nile Forest, in south-eastern Sudan (Figure 1). Voucher specimen were identified by the first author, Mr. Abdelazim Yassin Abdelgadir (Ph.D), Mr. Ashraf Mohamed Ahmed Abd Alla (Ph.D., Wood Sciences) and Mr. Haytham Hashim Gibreel (Ph.D., Taxonomy) at the Faculty of Forestry, University of Khartoum, Sudan and Mr. El Sheikh Abd alla Al Sheikh (Ph.D., Taxonomy) at Soba Forest Research Center, Khartoum, Sudan (Ph.D., Taxonomy). The Voucher specimens are deposited in the herbarium at the Department of Forest Products and Industries, Faculty of Forestry, University of Khartoum, Sudan.

4.2. Extraction

Hundred (100) grams of the dried and powdered stem wood and bark were used for the extractions. Extraction was initiated with sequential extraction, beginning with petroleum ether, followed by chloroform and finally the marc was extracted using 80% methanol. The 80% methanolic extract was subjected to liquid/liquid fractionation using ethyl acetate and this fractionation resulted in aqueous and ethyl acetate fractions.

4.3. Thin Layer Chromatography (TLC)

Using micro-capillary pipettes, 5 μL of ethyl acetate extracts (5 mg/mL) of the stem bark and wood of *T. brownii* were applied on normal phase silica gel thin layer plates (Kieselgel 60 F254, aluminum backed, Merck, Darmstadt, Germany) and on reversed phase thin layer plates (RP-18 F254s, Merck, Darmstadt, Germany) to detect compounds of a wide range of polarities. Toluene: ethyl acetate: formic acid (4:5:1, *v:v:v*) was used as an eluent for NP-TLC, while methanol: water: acetic acid (6:2:2) was used for RP-TLC. The development distance was 8 cm. The plates were sprayed with Vanillin-H_2SO_4, Dragendorff reagent, aluminum chloride and Natural Products reagents to detect various compound classes such as essential oils, terpenes, phenolic compounds, alkaloids and flavonoids [57]. The plates were observed in UV-light at 254 and 366 nm. A Camaq Video documentation system was used for photographing the plates.

4.4. Solid Phase Extraction (SPE)

LC-18 reversed phase cartridges (Supelco, Sigma-Aldrich, Darmstadt, Germany) were used for solid phase extraction in order to purify and enrich flavonoids and for separation of sugars and other interfering matrix compounds. The columns were equilibrated with 100% water and elution was performed using a gradient from 100% to 50% water followed by 100% methanol.

4.5. Reversed Phase High Performance Liquid Chromatography Coupled to Diode Array Detection (HPLC-UV/DAD)

The Agilent 1100 series HPLC system was used for the HPLC runs. The system consisted of an Agilent 1100 autosampler connected to Agilent series 1200 binary pump system coupled to an Agilent series 1100 thermostatic column compartment and an Agilent series 1100 DAD detector. Separations were performed on a reversed phase column (Varian LC-18; 4.6 mm × 250 mm; ID 5 μm, USA) at 30 °C and the flow rate was 0.5 mL/min. 5 μL of samples (5 mg/mL in 80% aqueous methanol) were injected. Gradient elution was performed using solvent (A) water +1% of acetic acid to increase peak resolution. Solvent (B) 100% acetonitrile. The step gradient began with 90% A and stopped while reaching 10% B in 30 min. After this 100% B was used for 5 min followed by 10% B for 5 min. Wavelengths of 254, 320, 360 and 380 nm were used for detection. The data was compared to standard compounds and computer libraries of pure compounds.

4.6. LC-Triple Quadrupole Mass Spectrometric Analysis (LC-MS and LC-MS/MS Tandem Mass Spectrometry)

An HPLC apparatus (1100 series, Agilent, Waldbronn, Germany) connected to an electrospray ionization (ESI) triple quadruple mass spectrometer (HTC Ultra-Bruker Daltonics-Advanced Mass Spectrometry Instrumentation, Germany) was used. Gradient elution was performed using acetonitrile (MeCN) and water containing 0.005% formic acid (Solvent A) and acetonitrile and glacial acetic acid (Solvent B). A linear gradient from 4% to 33% B was employed for 35 min and was increased to 100% B for 5 min. Then 4% B was used for 5 min to re-equilibrate. Mass analysis of compounds was performed using negative ion mode. The spray voltage was set to 5000 V and the capillary temperature to +280 °C. Nitrogen was used as sheathing gas and the flow was set to 40 U. Collision-induced dissociation (CID-MSn) was applied to induce fragmentation of the molecular ions, and their fragments were analyzed using tandem mass spectrometry. Helium was used as collision gas at 0.8 m Torr. Collision energies of 15 and 30 eV were used to investigate neutral loss and product ions and scanning was performed using a mass range from 50 to 1000 *m/z*. Data from the literature, the Wiley Natural product library, and authentic samples were used for the structural identifications of phenolic compounds such as flavonoids, stilbenes and ellagic acid derivatives as well as triterpenes.

4.7. Antifungal Assays

4.7.1. Fungal Strains

Aspergillus niger ATCC 9763, *Nattrassia mangiferae* ATCC 96293, *Aspergillus flavus* ATCC 9763 and *Fusarium moniliforme* ATCC 24378 were obtained from National Research Center, Sudan. Before use, the strains were sub-cultured on Sabouraud dextrose agar (Oxoid™ CM0041B) slants, at +35 °C.

4.7.2. Agar Well Diffusion Method

A cup well agar diffusion method [55,56] with minor modifications was used. Before the test, the fungal strains were grown on petri dishes ($\varnothing$ = 9 cm) containing Sabouraud dextrose agar at +35 °C overnight [92]. The resulting fungal growth was washed with 100 mL sterile normal saline to obtain fungal suspension containing conidia, which were used for the tests. 200 µL of this fungal suspension was adjusted to 1.0×10^8 CFU/mL and mixed with 20 mL of sterile, molten Sabouraud dextrose agar which was poured into sterile petri dishes ($\varnothing$ = 9 cm). The petri dishes were left to set at room temperature. Four holes were cut in the agar using a sterile cork borer (10 mm in diameter) and each hole was filled with 100 µL of extracts (1 mg/mL in 50% methanol) and amphotericin B (Sigma-Aldrich, 1 mg/mL in 50% methanol). 100 µL of 50% methanol was used as a negative control. The extracts/antibiotics/solvents were left to diffuse into the agar in the cold room (+4 °C) for one hour. The plates were then incubated at +35 °C for 24 h. For each experiment four replicates (n = 4) were used. The diameters of the zones of inhibition (IZ) were measured in mm using a caliper and the mean of five diameters $\pm$ SD and SEM was calculated.

4.7.3. Agar Dilution Method

Minimum inhibitory concentrations were determined using a slightly modified agar macrodilution method [93]. Fungal conidial suspensions were grown for four days in Sabouraud dextrose broth at +35 °C. For the test, 1 mL of these suspensions were diluted with 0.9% (w/v) NaCl to contain 1.0×10^6 CFU/mL. 100 µL of these fungal suspensions were mixed with 10 mL molten Sabouraud dextrose agar which was pipetted into a petri dish ($\varnothing$ = 9 mm). 10 mL of twofold dilutions of plant extracts (from 500 to 31.25 µg/mL) and amphotericin B (from 500 to 15.625 µg/mL) were added to the petri dishes. Each dilution contained 500 µL of 50% methanol or hexane solutions of the plant extracts or antibiotics dissolved in 10 mL of molten Sabouraud dextrose agar. The petri dishes were incubated for 24 h at +35 °C. The MIC was taken as those concentrations that resulted in clear petri dishes showing no visible fungal growth. All tests were performed in triplicates. The solvents used for the plant extractions, 50% methanol or hexane, were used as negative controls. Hexane was used for dissolving those extracts which did not dissolve in 50% MeOH, that is very nonpolar extracts, such as those originating from hexane and petroleum ether extractions.

4.7.4. Statistical Analysis

The Student's *t*-test provided by Microsoft Excel was used for the evaluation of the statistical significance of any differences between the antifungal results of the inhibition zones (IZ) of the tested extracts.

5. Conclusions

Ethyl acetate and aqueous extracts of the stem wood and bark of *Terminalia brownii* give good antifungal effects against *Nattrassia mangiferae*, *Fusarium verticilliodes*, *Aspergillus flavus* and *Aspergillus niger*. Altogether twelve compounds were identified from an ethyl acetate extract of the stem wood of *T. brownii*. *Cis-* and *trans*-isomers of resveratrol 3-*O*-β-galloyl-glucoside were characterized for the first time in this species of *Terminalia*. Likewise, gallagic acid dilactone has not been reported previously in the stem wood of *T. brownii*. Owing to its relative chemical stability and its reported antifungal efficiency against phytopathogenic molds, gallagic acid dilactone might be an especially interesting component in standardized antifungal extracts of *T. brownii*. Also, standardized extracts of *T. brownii* stem wood, enriched with ellagitannins, could be used as natural fungicides for protecting crops and as medicines to treat fungal infections. Ellagitannins purified from these extracts, if found to be more active than the extracts, could be used for ecological crop plant protection and wood preservation, while being relatively stable and possessing less toxicity than synthetic fungicides.

Our results provide partly the justification for the uses of water-based extracts of *T. brownii* for the protection of crop plants and for wood preservation in Africa, although phytochemical analysis of these aqueous extracts would be needed. Further studies are needed on the antifungal activities of separated compounds from both the aqueous and ethyl acetate extracts as well as on various controlled combinations of these compounds. In summary, standardized extracts of *T. brownii* stem wood could be used as new, cheaper and eco-friendly fungicides for routine use in Africa instead of toxic synthetic fungicides.

Acknowledgments: The first author is grateful for the financial support for this research article by University of Khartoum, Sudan. We would also like to thank Nickoli Kuhnert and his group, School of Engineering and Science, International University, Bremen, Germany for providing LC-MS/MS research facilities.

Author Contributions: Enass Y. A. Salih, performed the data collections, extractions, antifungal analysis, and preliminary chemical identifications and wrote the draft manuscript. Hiba A. Ali, managed the study and provided support in analytical chemistry. Pia Fyhrquist has given a major contribution for the drafting of this manuscript. Other authors, Abdelazim Y. Abdelgadir, Mustafa K. M Fahmi, Mai H. Alamin and Ashraf M. Ahmed were also involved in drafting the final manuscript. All authors have thoroughly revised the paper, read and approved the final manuscript.

References

1.   Klemptner, L.R.; Sherwood, J.S.; Tugizimana, F.; Dubery, I.A.; Piater, L.A. Ergosterol, an orphan fungal microbe-associated molecular pattern (MAMP). *Mol. Plant Pathol.* **2014**, *15*, 747–761. [CrossRef] [PubMed]

2.   Anderson, P.K.; Cunningham, A.A.; Patel, N.G.; Morales, F.J.; Epstein, P.R.; Daszak, P. Emerging infectious diseases of plants: Pathogen pollution, climate change and agrotechnology drivers. *Trends Ecol. Evol.* **2004**, *19*, 535–544. [CrossRef] [PubMed]

3.   Kieren, A.M.; Thomas, P.; David, D. Aspergillosis: Pathogenesis, clinical manifestations, and therapy. *Infect. Dis. Clin. N. Am.* **2002**, *16*, 875–894.

4.   Walsh, T.J.; Anaissie, E.J.; Denning, D.W.; Herbrecht, R.; Kontoyiannis, D.P.; Marr, K.A.; Morrison, V.A.; Segal, B.H.; Steinbach, W.J.; Stevens, D.A.; et al. Treatment of Aspergillosis: Clinical Practice Guidelines of the Infectious Diseases Society of America. *Clin. Infect. Dis.* **2008**, *46*, 327–360. [CrossRef] [PubMed]

5.   Baddley, J.W. Clinical risk factors for invasive aspergillosis. *Med. Mycol.* **2011**, *49*, S7–S12. [CrossRef] [PubMed]

6.   De Aguirre, L.D.; Hurst, S.F.; Choi, J.S.; Shin, J.H.; Hinrikson, H.P.; Morrison, C.J. Rapid Differentiation of *Aspergillus* Species from Other Medically Important Opportunistic Molds and Yeasts by PCR-Enzyme Immunoassay. *J. Clin. Microbiol.* **2004**, *42*, 3495–3504. [CrossRef] [PubMed]

7.   Hadrich, I.; Makni, F.; Ayadi, A.; Ranque, S. Microsatellite Typing to Trace *Aspergillus flavus* Infections in a Hematology Unit. *J. Clin. Microbiol.* **2010**, *48*, 2396–2401. [CrossRef] [PubMed]

8.   Dagenais, T.R.T.; Keller, N.P. Pathogenesis of *Aspergillus* fumigatus in Invasive Aspergillosis. *Clin. Microbiol. Rev.* **2009**, *22*, 447–465. [CrossRef] [PubMed]

9.   U.S. Department of Health and Human Services. *Guidelines for Research Involving Recombinant DNA Molecules*; U.S. Department of Health and Human Services: Washington, DC, USA, 1986.

10. International Agency for Research on Cancer (Iarc). *IARC Monograph on the Evaluation of Carcinogenic Risk of Chemicals to Humans*; Aflatoxins; International Agency for Research on Cancer: Lyon, France, 1987; Suppl 7, pp. 83–87.

11. Fountain, J.C.; Scully, B.T.; Ni, X.; Kemerait, R.C.; Lee, R.D.; Chen, Z.Y.; Guo, B. Environmental influences on maize-*Aspergillus flavus* interactions and aflatoxin production. *Front. Microbiol.* **2014**, *5*. [CrossRef] [PubMed]

12. Gourama, H.; Bullerman, L.B. *Aspergillus flavus* and *Aspergillus parasiticus*: Aflatoxigenic Fungi of concern in Foods and Feeds. *J. Food Prot.* **1995**, *12*, 1395–1404. [CrossRef]

13. Willinger, B.; Kopetzky, G.; Harm, F.; Apfalter, P.; Makristathis, A.; Berer, A.; Bankier, A.; Winkle, S. CASE REPORTS Disseminated Infection with *Nattrassia mangiferae* in an Immunosuppressed Patient. *J. Clin. Microbiol.* **2004**, *42*, 478–480. [CrossRef] [PubMed]

14. Sigler, L.; Summerbell, R.C.; Poole, L.; Wieden, M.; Sutton, D.A.; Rinaldi, M.G.; Aguirre, M.; Estes, G.W.; Galgiani, J.N. Invasive *Nattrassia mangiferae* Infections: Case Report, Literature Review, and Therapeutic and Taxonomic Appraisal. *J. Clin. Microbiol.* **1997**, *35*, 433–440. [PubMed]

15. Frankel, D.H.; Rippon, J.W. *Hendersonula toruloidea* infection in man. Index cases in the non-endemic North American host, and a review of the literature. *Mycopathologia* **1989**, *105*, 175–186. [CrossRef] [PubMed]

16. Atanasova-Penichon, V.; Bernillon, S.; Marchegay, G.; Lornac, A.; Pinson-Gadais, L.; Ponts, N.; Zehraoui, E.; Barreau, C.; Richard-Forget, F. Bioguided Isolation, Characterization, and Biotransformation by *Fusarium verticillioides* of Maize Kernel Compounds that Inhibit Fumonisin Production. *Mol. Plant Microbe Interact.* **2014**, *27*, 1148–1158. [CrossRef] [PubMed]

17. Xing, F.; Hua, H.; Selvaraj, J.N.; Yuan, Y.; Zhao, Y.; Zhou, L.; Liu, Y. Degradation of fumonisin B1 by cinnamon essential oil. *Food Control* **2014**, *38*, 37–40. [CrossRef]

18. Dornbusch, H.J.; Buzina, W.; Summerbell, R.C.; Lass-Flörl, C.; Lackner, H.; Schwinger, W.; Sovinz, P.; Urban, C. *Fusarium verticillioides* abscess of the nasal septum in an immunosuppressed child: Case report and identification of the morphologically atypical fungal strain. *J. Clin. Microbiol.* **2005**, *43*, 1998–2001. [CrossRef] [PubMed]

19. Da Silva Bomfim, N.; Nakassugi, L.P.; Oliveira, J.F.P.; Kohiyama, C.Y.; Mossini, S.A.G.; Grespan, R.; Nerilo, S.B.; Mallmann, C.A.; Filho, B.A.A.; Machinski, M. Antifungal activity and inhibition of fumonisin production by *Rosmarinus officinalis* L. essential oil in *Fusarium verticillioides* (Sacc.) Nirenberg. *Food Chem.* **2015**, *166*, 330–336. [CrossRef] [PubMed]

20. Dias, M.C. Phytotoxicity: An Overview of the Physiological Responses of Plants Exposed to Fungicides. *Jpn. J. Bot.* **2012**, *4*. [CrossRef]

21. Opiyo, S.A.; Manguro, L.O.A.; Owuor, P.O.; Ochieng, C.O.; Ateka, E.M.; Lemmen, P. Antimicrobial Compounds from *Terminalia brownii* against Sweet Potato Pathogens. *J. Nat. Prod.* **2011**, *1*, 116–120. [CrossRef]

22. Chung, W.H.; Chung, W.C.; Ting, P.F.; Ru, C.C.; Huang, H.C.; Huang, J.W. Nature of Resistance to Methyl Benzimidazole Carbamate Fungicides in *Fusarium oxysporum* f.sp. lilii and *F. oxysporum* f.sp. gladioli in Taiwan. *J. Phytopathol.* **2009**, *157*, 742–747. [CrossRef]

23. Villa, F.; Cappitelli, F.; Cortesi, P.; Kunova, A. Fungal Biofilms: Targets for the Development of Novel Strategies in Plant Disease Management. *Front. Microbiol.* **2017**, *8*. [CrossRef] [PubMed]

24. Mazu, T.K.; Bricker, B.A.; Flores-Rozas, H.; Ablordeppey, S.Y. The Mechanistic Targets of Antifungal Agents: An Overview. *Mini Rev. Med. Chem.* **2016**, *16*, 555–578. [CrossRef] [PubMed]

25. Troskie, A.M.; de Beer, A.; Vosloo, J.A.; Jacobs, K.; Rautenbach, M. Inhibition of agronomically relevant fungal phytopathogens by tyrocidines, cyclic antimicrobial peptides isolated from *Bacillus aneurinolyticus*. *Microbiology* **2014**, *160*, 2089–2101. [CrossRef] [PubMed]

26. Martinez, J.A. Natural Fungicides obtained from Plants. In *Fungicides for Plant and Animal Diseases*; Dhanasekaran, D., Thajuddin, N., Panneerselvam, A., Eds.; InTech: Croatia, Balkans, 2012; pp. 1–28, ISBN 978-953-307-804-5. Available online: https://cdn.intechopen.com/pdfs-wm/26021.pdf (accessed on 1 May 2017).

27. Singh, A.K.; Kumar, P.; Nidhi, R.; Gade, R.M. Allelopathy—A Sustainable Alternative and Eco-Friendly Tool for Plant Disease Management. *Plant Dis. Sci.* **2012**, *7*, 127–134.

28. Rodrigues, A.M.; Theodoro, P.N.; Eparvier, V.; Basset, C.; Silva, M.R.; Beauchêne, J.; Espíndola, L.S.; Stien, D. Search for Antifungal Compounds from the Wood of Durable Tropical Trees. *J. Nat. Prod.* **2010**, *73*, 1706–1707. [CrossRef] [PubMed]

29. Gupta, S.; Dikshit, A.K. Biopesticides: An eco-friendly approach for pest control. *J. Biopestic.* **2010**, *3*, 186–188.

30. Shinde, S.L.; Wadje, S.S. Efficacy of *terminalia* bark extracts against seed-borne pathogens checked by paper disc method. *Res. J. Pharm. Biol. Chem. Sci.* **2011**, *2*, 602–607.

31. Valsaraj, R.; Pushpangadan, P.; Smitt, U.W.; Adsersen, A.; Christensen, S.; Sittie, A.; Nyman, U.; Nielsen, C.; Olsen, C.E. New Anti-HIV-1, Antimalarial, and Antifungal Compounds from *Terminalia bellerica. J. Nat. Prod.* **1997**, *60*, 739–742. [CrossRef] [PubMed]

32. Wickens, G.E. *Flora of Tropical East Africa: Combretaceae*; East African Community: Arusha, East Africa's Tanzania, 1973; p. 99.

33. Nguyen, D.-M.-C.; Seo, D.-J.; Park, R.-D.; Lee, B.-J.; Jung, W.-J. Chitosan beads combined with *Terminalia nigrovenulosa* bark enhance suppressive activity to *Fusarium solani. Ind. Crop Prod.* **2013**, *50*, 462–467. [CrossRef]

34. Samie, A.; Mashau, F. Antifungal activities of fifteen Southern African medicinal plants against five *Fusarium* species. *J. Med. Plants Res.* **2013**, *7*, 1839–1848.

35. Fabry, W.; Okemo, P.; Ansorg, R. Fungistatic and fungicidal activity of East African medicinal plants. *Mycoses* **1996**, *39*, 67–70. [CrossRef] [PubMed]

36. Baba-Moussa, F.; Akpagana, K.; Bouchet, P. Antifungal activities of seven West African Combretaceae used in traditional medicine. *J. Ethnopharmacol.* **1999**, *66*, 335–338. [CrossRef]

37. Nguyen, D.-M.-C.; Seo, D.-J.; Lee, H.B.; Kim, I.S.; Kim, K.Y.; Park, R.D.; Jung, W.J. Antifungal activity of gallic acid purified from *Terminalia nigrovenulosa* bark against *Fusarium solani. Microb. Pathog.* **2013**, *56*, 8–15. [CrossRef] [PubMed]

38. Eldeen, I.M.S.; Van Staaden, J. Antimycobacterial activity of some trees used in South African traditional medicine. *S. Afr. J. Bot.* **2007**, *73*, 248–251. [CrossRef]

39. Eldeen, I.M.S.; Elgorashi, E.E.; Mulholland, D.A.; Van Staden, J. Anolignan B: A bioactive compound from the roots of *Terminalia sericea. J. Ethnopharmacol.* **2005**, *103*, 135–138. [CrossRef] [PubMed]

40. Conrad, J.; Vogler, B.; Reeb, S.; Klaiber, I.; Roos, G.; Vasquiez, E.; Setzer, M.C.; Kraus, W. Isoterchebulin and 4,6-*O*-isoterchebuloyl-D-glucose, novel hydrolysable tannins from *Terminalia macroptera. J. Nat. Prod.* **2001**, *64*, 294–299. [CrossRef] [PubMed]

41. Conrad, J.; Vogler, B.; Klaiber, I.; Roos, G.; Walter, U.; Kraus, W. Two triterpene esters from *Terminalia macroptera* bark. *Phytochemistry* **1998**, *48*, 647–650. [CrossRef]

42. Silva, O.; Duarte, A.; Pimentel, M.; Viegas, S.; Barroso, H.; Machado, J.; Pires, I.; Cabrita, J.; Gomes, E. Antimicrobial activity of *Terminalia macroptera* root. *J. Ethnopharmacol.* **1997**, *57*, 203–207. [CrossRef]

43. Kuete, V.; Tabopda, T.K.; Ngameni, B.; Nana, F.; Tshikalange, T.E.; Ngadjui, B.T. Antimycobacterial, antibacterial and antifungal activities of *Terminalia superba* (Combretaceae). *S. Afr. J. Bot.* **2010**, *76*, 125–131. [CrossRef]

44. Joseph, C.C.; Moshi, M.J.; Innocent, E.; Nkunya, M.H.H. Isolation of a stilbene glycoside and other constituents of *Terminalia sericeae. Afr. J. Tradit. Complement. Altern. Med.* **2007**, *4*, 383–386. [CrossRef] [PubMed]

45. Pfundstein, B.; El Desouky, S.K.; Hull, W.E.; Haubner, R.; Erben, G.; Owen, R.W. Polyphenolic compounds in the fruits of Egyptian medicinal plants (*Terminalia bellerica, Terminalia chebula* and *Terminalia horrida*): Characterization, quantitation and determination of antioxidant capacities. *Phytochemistry* **2010**, *71*, 1132–1148. [CrossRef] [PubMed]

46. Schmidt, L.H. *Terminalia brownii* Fresen. *Seed Leafl.* **2010**, *148*, 363–374.

47. Mosango, D.M. Terminalia brownii. In *Plant Resources of Tropical Africa 11(2): Medicinal plants 2*; Schmelzer, G.H., Gurib-Fakim, A., Eds.; PROTA Foundation: Wageningen, The Netherlands, 2013; pp. 245–248.

48. Shuping, D.S.S.; Eloff, J.N. The use of plants to protect plants and food against fungal pathogens: A review. *Afr. J. Tradit. Complement. (Ajtcam)* **2017**, *14*, 120–127. [CrossRef] [PubMed]

49. Machumi, F.; Midiwo, J.O.O.; Jacob, M.R.; Khan, S.I.; Tekwani, B.L.; Zhang, H.; Walker, L.A.; Muhaamed, L. Phytochemical, antimicrobial and antiplasmodial investigation of *Terminalia brownii. J. Nat. Prod. Commun.* **2013**, *8*, 761–764.

50. Salih, E.Y.A.; Kanninen, M.; Sipi, M.; Luukkanen, O.; Hiltunen, R.; Vuorela, H.; Julkunen-Tiitto, R.; Fyhrquist, P. Tannins, flavonoids and stilbenes in extracts of African savanna woodland trees *Terminalia brownii, Terminalia laxiflora* and *Anogeissus leiocarpus* showing promising antibacterial potential. *S. Afr. J. Bot.* **2017**, *108*, 370–386. [CrossRef]

51. Yamauchi, K.; Mitsunaga, T.; Muddathir, A.M. Screening for melanogenesis-controlled agents using Sudanese medicinal plants and identification of active compounds in the methanol extract of *Terminalia brownii*. *J. Wood Sci.* **2016**, *62*, 285–293. [CrossRef]

52. Negishi, H.; Maoka, T.; Njelekela, M.; Yasui, N.; Juman, S.; Mtabaji, J.; Miki, T.; Nara, Y.; Yamori, Y.; Ikeda, K. New chromone derivative terminalianone from African plant *Terminalia brownii* Fresen (Combretaceae) in Tanzania. *J. Asian Nat. Prod. Res.* **2011**, *13*, 281–283. [CrossRef] [PubMed]

53. Mbwambo, Z.H.; Moshi, M.J.; Masimba, P.J.; Kapingu, M.C.; Nondo, R.S. Antimicrobial activity and brine shrimp toxicity of extracts of *Terminalia brownii* roots and stem. *BMC Complement. Altern. Med.* **2007**, *7*, 1–5. [CrossRef] [PubMed]

54. Masoko, P.; Picard, J.; Eloff, J.N. Antifungal activities of six South African *Terminalia* Species (Combretaceae). *J. Ethnopharmacol.* **2005**, *99*, 301–308. [CrossRef] [PubMed]

55. Elegami, A.A.; El-Nima, E.I.; El Tohami, M.S.; Muddathir, A.K. Antimicrobial activity of some species of the family Combretaceae. *Phytother. Res.* **2002**, *16*, 555–561. [CrossRef] [PubMed]

56. Kavanagh, F. *Analytical Microbiology*, 2nd ed.; Academic Press: New York, NY, USA, 1972; p. 11.

57. Wagner, H.; Bladt, S. *Plant Drug Analysis: A Thin Layer Chromatography Atlas*, 2nd ed.; Springer: New York, NY, USA, 1996; 320p.

58. Stecher, G.; Huck, C.; Popp, M.; Bonn, G.K. Determination of flavonoids and stilbenes in red wine and related biological products by HPLC and HPLC–ESI–MS–MS. *J. Anal. Chem.* **2001**, *371*, 73–80. [CrossRef]

59. Otto, A.; Simoneit, B.R.; Wilde, V.; Kuntzmann, L.; Pűttmann, W. Terpenoids Composition of three fossil resins from Cretaceae and tertiary Conifers. *Rev. Palaeobatony Palynol.* **2002**, *120*, 203–215. [CrossRef]

60. Van der Doelen, G.A.; van den Berg, K.J.; Boon, J.J.; Shibayama, N.; De La Rie, E.R.; Genuit, W.J.L. Analysis of fresh triterpenoid resin and aged triterpenoid varnishes by HPLC. APCI.MS/MS. *J. Chromatogr. A* **1998**, *809*, 21–37. [CrossRef]

61. Liu, M.; Katerere, D.R.; Gray, A.I.; Seidel, V. Phytochemical and antifungal studies on *Terminalia mollis* and *Terminalia brachystemma*. *Fitoterapia* **2009**, *80*, 369–373. [CrossRef] [PubMed]

62. Xia, B.; Bai, L.; Li, X.; Xiong, J.; Xu, P.; Xue, M. Structural analysis of metabolites of asiatic acid and its analogue madecassic acid in zebrafish using LC/IT-MSn. *Molecules* **2015**, *20*, 3001–3019. [CrossRef] [PubMed]

63. Pinheiro, P.F.; Justino, G.C. Structural analysis of flavonoids and related compounds-a review of spectroscopic applications. In *Phytochemicals—A Global Perspective of Their Role in Nutrition and Health*; InTech: Croatia, Balkans, 2012; pp. 1–26.

64. Marzouk, M.S.; El-Toumy, S.A.; Moharram, F.A. Pharmacologically active ellagitannins from *Terminalia myriocarpa*. *Planta Med.* **2002**, *68*, 523–527. [CrossRef] [PubMed]

65. Oeirichs, P.B.; Pearce, C.M.; Zhu, J.; Filippich, L.J. Isolation and structure determination of terminalin A toxic condense tannin from *Terminalia oblongata*. *Nat. Toxins* **1994**, *2*, 144–150. [CrossRef]

66. Canedo, E.M.; Fill, T.P.; Pereira-Filho, E.R.; Rodrigues-Filho, E. Enzymatic Potential of *Mucor inaequisporus* for Naringin Biotransformation, Accessed by Fractional Factorial Design and Mass Spectrometry Analysis. *J. Anal. Bioanal. Tech.* **2014**, *S6*. [CrossRef]

67. Lee, M.K.; Bok, S.H.; Jeong, T.S.; Moon, S.S.; Lee, S.E.; Park, Y.B.; Choi, M.S. Supplementation of naringenin and it is synthetics derivatives altars antioxidant enzyme activities of erythrocyte and liver high cholesterol-fed rats. *Bioorg. Med. Chem.* **2002**, *10*, 2239–2244. [CrossRef]

68. Fabre, N.; Rustan, I.; de Hoffmann, E.; Quetin-Leclercq, J. Determination of Flavone, Flavonol, and Flavanone Aglycones by Negative Ion Liquid Chromatography Electrospray Ion Trap Mass Spectrometry. *J. Am. Soc. Mass Spectrom.* **2001**, *12*, 707–715. [CrossRef]

69. Cuyckens, F.; Claeys, M. Mass spectrometry in the structural analysis of flavonoids. *J. Mass Spectrom.* **2004**, *39*, 1–15. [CrossRef] [PubMed]

70. Nuengchamnong, N.; Ingkaninan, K. An on-line LC-MS/DPPH approach towards the quality control of antioxidative ingredients in Sahastara. *Songklanakarin J. Sci. Technol.* **2017**, *39*, 123–129. [CrossRef]

71. Xiao, H.-T.; Tsang, S.-W.; Qin, H.-Y.; Choi, F.F.; Yang, Z.-J.; Han, Q.-B.; Chen, H.-B.; Xu, H.-X.; Shen, H.; Lu, A.-P.; et al. A bioactivity-guided study on the anti-diarrheal activity of *Polygonum chinense* Linn. *J. Ethnopharmacol.* **2013**, *149*, 499–505. [CrossRef] [PubMed]

72. Morrissey, J.P.; Osbourn, A.E. Fungal resistance to plant antibiotics as a mechanism of pathogenesis. *Microbiol. Mol. Biol. Rev.* **1999**, *63*, 708–724. [PubMed]

73. Smaili, A.; Mazoir, N.; Aicha Rifai, L.; Koussa, T.; Makroum, K.; Benharref, A.; Faize, L.; Alburquerque, N.; Burgos, L.; Belfaiza, M.; et al. Antimicrobial Activity of two Semisynthetic Triterpene Derivatives from *Euphorbia officinarum* Latex against Fungal and Bacterial Phytopathogens. *Nat. Prod. Commun.* **2017**, *12*, 331–336.

74. Sirdaarta, J.; Matthews, B.; Cock, I.E. Kakadu plum fruit extracts inhibit growth of the bacterial triggers of rheumatoid arthritis: Identification of stilbene and tannin components. *J. Funct. Food* **2015**, *17*, 610–620. [CrossRef]

75. Cock, I.E.; van Vuuren, S.F. Anti-*Proteus* activity of some South African medicinal plants: Their potential for the prevention of rheumatoid arthritis. *Inflammopharmacology* **2014**, *22*, 23–36. [CrossRef] [PubMed]

76. Sebastià, N.; Montoro, A.; León, Z.; Soriano, J.M. Searching *trans*-resveratrol in fruits and vegetables: A preliminary screening. *J. Food Sci. Technol.* **2017**, *54*, 842–845. [CrossRef] [PubMed]

77. Zainal, N.; Chang, C.-P.; Cheng, Y.-L.; Wu, Y.-W.; Anderson, R.; Wan, S.-W.; Chen, C.-L.; Ho, T.-S.; AbuBakar, S.; Lin, Y.S. Resveratrol treatment reveals a novel role for HMGB1 in regulation of the type 1 interferon response in dengue virus infection. *Sci. Rep. UK* **2017**, *7*, 42998. [CrossRef] [PubMed]

78. Caruso, F.; Mendoza, L.; Castro, P.; Cotoras, M.; Aguirre, M.; Matsuhiro, B.; Isaacs, M.; Rossi, M.; Viglianti, A.; Antonioletti, R. Antifungal Activity of Resveratrol against *Botrytiscinerea* Is Improved Using 2-Furyl Derivatives. *PLoS ONE* **2011**, *6*, 1–10. [CrossRef] [PubMed]

79. Jung, H.J.; Hwang, I.A.; Sung, W.S.; Kang, H.; Kang, B.S.; Seu, Y.B.; Lee, D.G. Fungicidal effect of resveratrol on human infectious fungi. *Arch. Pharm. Res.* **2005**, *28*, 557–560. [CrossRef] [PubMed]

80. Crozier, A.; Jaganath, I.B.; Clifford, M.N. Phenols, Polyphenols and Tannins: An Overview. In *Plant Secondary Metabolites: Occurrence, Structure and Role in the Human Diet*, 1st ed.; Crozier, A., Clifford, M.N., Ahihara, H., Eds.; Blackwell Publishing: Oxford, UK, 2006; pp. 1–25.

81. Silva, L.P.; de Angelis, C.D.; Bonamin, F.; Kushima, H.; Mininel, F.J.; dos Santos, L.C.; Delella, F.K.; Felisbino, S.L.; Vilegas, W.; da Rocha, L.R.M.; et al. *Terminalia catappa* L.: A medicinal plant from the Caribbean pharmacopeia with anti-*Helicobacter pylori* and antiulcer action in experimental rodent models. *J. Ethnopharmacol.* **2015**, *159*, 285–295. [CrossRef] [PubMed]

82. Cerdá, B.; Cerón, J.J.; Tomás-Barberán, F.A.; Espín, J.C. Repeated oral administration of high doses of the pomegranate ellagitannin punicalagin to rats for 37 days is not toxic. *J. Agric. Food Chem.* **2003**, *51*, 3493–3501. [CrossRef] [PubMed]

83. Glazer, I.; Masaphy, S.; Marciano, P.; Bar-Ilan, I.; Holland, D.; Kerem, Z.; Amir, R. Partial identification of antifungal compounds from *Punica granatum* peel extracts. *J. Agric. Food Chem.* **2012**, *60*, 4841–4848. [CrossRef] [PubMed]

84. Latté, K.P.; Kolodziej, H. Antifungal effects of hydrolysable tannins and related compounds on dermatophyte, mould fungi and yeasts. *Z. Naturforsch.* **2000**, *55c*, 467–472.

85. Alves, C.T.; Ferreira, I.C.; Barros, L.; Silva, S.; Azeredo, J.; Henriques, M. Antifungal activity of phenolic compounds identified in flowers from North Eastern Portugal against *Candida* species. *Future Microbiol.* **2014**, *9*, 139–146. [CrossRef] [PubMed]

86. Tempesti, T.C.; Alvarez, M.G.; de Arau'jo, M.F.; Ju'nior, F.E.; de Carvalho, M.G.; Durantini, E.N. Antifungal activity of a novel quercetin derivative bearing a trifluoromethyl group on *Candida albicans*. *Med. Chem. Res.* **2012**, *21*, 2217–2222. [CrossRef]

87. Weidenbörner, M.; Hindorf, H.; Jha, H.C.; Tsotsonos, P. Antifungal activity of flavonoids against storage fungi of the genus *Aspergillus*. *Phytochemistry* **1990**, *29*, 1103–1105. [CrossRef]

88. Céspedes, C.L.; Salazar, J.R.; Ariza-Castolo, A.; Yamaguchi, L.; Avila, J.G.; Aqueveque, P.; Kubo, I.; Alarcón, J. Biopesticides from plants: *Calceolaria integrifolia* sl. *Environ. Res.* **2014**, *132*, 391–406. [CrossRef] [PubMed]

89. Mierziak, J.; Kostyn, K.; Kulma, A. Flavonoids as important molecules of plant interactions with the environment. *Molecules* **2014**, *19*, 16240–16265. [CrossRef] [PubMed]

90. Liu, H.; Mou, Y.; Zhao, J.; Wang, J.; Zhou, L.; Wang, M.; Wang, D.; Han, J.; Yu, Z.; Yang, F. Flavonoids from *Halostachys caspica* and Their Antimicrobial and Antioxidant Activities. *Molecules* **2010**, *15*, 7933–7945. [CrossRef] [PubMed]

91. Orhan, D.D.; Özçelik, B.; Özgen, S.; Ergun, F. Antibacterial, antifungal, and antiviral activities of some flavonoids. *Microbiol. Res.* **2010**, *165*, 496–504. [CrossRef] [PubMed]

92. Tokarzewski, S.; Ziółkowska, G.; Nowakiewicz, A. Susceptibility testing of *Aspergillus niger* strains isolated from poultry to antifungal drugs-a comparative study of the disk diffusion, broth microdilution (M 38-A) and Etest® methods. *Pol. J. Vet. Sci.* **2012**, *15*, 125–133. [CrossRef] [PubMed]
93. Guarro, J.; Soler, L.; Rinaldi, M.G. Pathogenicity and antifungal susceptibility of *Chaetomium* species. *EUR J. Clin. Microbiol.* **1995**, *14*, 613–618. [CrossRef]

4

Reevaluation of the Acute Cystitis Symptom Score, a Self-Reporting Questionnaire: Development, Diagnosis and Differential Diagnosis

Jakhongir F. Alidjanov [1,2] (iD)**, Kurt G. Naber** [3,*,†]**, Ulugbek A. Abdufattaev** [1]**, Adrian Pilatz** [2] **and Florian M. E. Wagenlehner** [2]

[1]   The Republican Specialized Center of Urology, 100109 Tashkent, Uzbekistan;
       jakhonghir@hotmail.com (J.F.A.); abdufattaev@gmail.com (U.A.A.)
[2]   Clinic of Urology, Paediatric Urology and Andrology, Justus-Liebig-University, 35392 Giessen, Germany;
       pilatz@t-online.de (A.P.); Florian.Wagenlehner@chiru.med.uni-giessen.de (F.M.E.W.)
[3]   Department of Urology, School of Medicine, Technical University of Munich, D-80333 Munich, Germany
*   Correspondence: kurt@nabers.de
†   Current address: Karl-Bickleder-Str. 44c, 94315 Straubing, Germany.

Abstract: This study aimed to reevaluate the Acute Cystitis Symptom Score (ACSS). The ACSS is a simple and standardized self-reporting questionnaire for the diagnosis of acute uncomplicated cystitis (AC) assessing typical and differential symptoms, quality of life, and possible changes after therapy in female patients with AC. This paper includes literature research, development and evaluation of the ACSS, an 18-item self-reporting questionnaire including (a) six questions about "typical" symptoms of AC, (b) four questions regarding differential diagnoses, (c) three questions on quality of life, and (d) five questions on additional conditions that may affect therapy. The ACSS was evaluated in 228 women (mean age 31.49 ± 11.71 years) in the Russian and Uzbek languages. Measurements of reliability, validity, predictive ability, and responsiveness were performed. Cronbach's alpha for ACSS was 0.89, split-half reliability was 0.76 and 0.79 for first and second halves, and the correlation between them was 0.87. Mann-Whitney U test revealed a significant difference in scores of the "typical" symptoms between patients and controls (10.50 vs. 2.07, $p < 0.001$). The optimal threshold score was 6 points, with a 94% sensitivity and 90% specificity to predict AC. The "typical" symptom score decreased significantly when comparing before and after therapy (10.4 and 2.5, $p < 0.001$). The reevaluated Russian and Uzbek ACSS are accurate enough and can be recommended for clinical studies and practice for initial diagnosis and monitoring the process of the treatment of AC in women. Evaluation in German, UK English, and Hungarian languages was also performed and in other languages evaluation of the ACSS is in progress.

Keywords: cystitis; female; quality of life; urinary tract infection; symptom score; questionnaire

1. Introduction

Urinary tract infections (UTIs) are common, with an estimated annual global incidence of at least 250 million, with the vast majority (84%) of visits related to female patients presenting with acute uncomplicated cystitis (AC) [1–3]. Although AC is a benign condition, recurrent episodes are associated with a reduction in quality of life, a negative impact on everyday activity and working ability, disturbances in sexual life and psychosexual disorders [4–6]. In the recent years, several studies have shown specific risk factors for recurrent AC [7,8], and large studies revealed its microbial etiology. Clinical tests for diagnosing AC vary widely, depending on comorbidities and different treatment strategies [9–11].

Several studies and current guidelines do not consider urinalysis or microbiologic investigation necessary but rely on patients' complaints only, even though telephone conversation [12–14]. Various urinary symptoms have been used to assess the diagnosis and severity of AC in women. Diaries, questionnaires, and symptom scores used in these studies were mainly adapted from other tools. Only a few publications devoted to the studies regarding the development of the questionnaires, evaluating the severity of symptoms of the AC and their interference with activities [15,16]. However, up to today, no single, unified, valid, and specific questionnaire existed for diagnosis, differential diagnosis, assessment of symptoms' severity, and quality of life that is also available to monitor treatment efficacy [4,15–17]. We have recently presented a new self-reporting questionnaire—ACSS—for diagnosis, differential diagnosis, and patient-reported outcome in female patients with AUC, assessing typical and differential symptoms, quality of life, and possible changes after therapy [18,19].

Since the first 58 subjects who filled in the precursor version of the ACSS (USQOLAT) [20], which differed in a few aspects from the current version of the ACSS, were included in the former validation, a reevaluation of the current Uzbek and Russian versions of the ACSS was performed excluding these patients. Now, the present study includes only the results of the final 228 subjects (107 patients with AC and 121 controls without AC) who filled in the current versions of the Uzbek or Russian ACSS (Supplementary Figures S1 and S2).

2. Development and Evaluation Process of the Acute Cystitis Symptom Score (ACSS) Questionnaire

Regarding the purpose of the development of the ACSS questionnaire, PubMed's medical subject headings (MeSH) service was used for the literature search. Different combinations of such MeSH terms as "urinary tract infections", "cystitis", and "signs and symptoms" were used for the identification of the key clinical symptoms/signs of AC. The literature search was limited to the publications in the English language. Thereafter, different versions of multiple choice questions regarding the presence and severity of symptoms were developed in Uzbek and Russian languages, and furtherly were revised and commented by Russian-speaking, Uzbek-speaking, and bilingual (speaking both in Uzbek and Russian languages) female staff of the hospital. Although the Uzbek language is the official state language in Uzbekistan, Russian is the second common language and remains in widespread use (https://en.wikipedia.org/wiki/Uzbekistan), with the majority of the population speaking both languages.

Following the approval of the Institutional Review Board (Clinical ethics committee) of the Republican Specialized Center of Urology/JSC "Republican Specialized Center of Urology" (RSCU) (Akilov FA, Mukhtarov ShT, Khvan AL: No. 429/23) in September 2009, preliminary versions of the questionnaire were tested as described earlier with females from different social areas, with different levels of education, nationalities, and age after informed consent was obtained prior to enrollment of the participants [18]. Based on their comments and requests, a multidimensional scaling analysis was performed, and the most appropriate versions of questions and answers were chosen by the research team for the development of the preliminary questionnaire titled as "Urinary Symptoms and Quality of Life Assessment Tool (USQOLAT)." The reliability analysis, performed on the first 58 subjects (32 patients with AC and 26 controls without AC), showed a mean Cronbach's alpha of 0.84, a Split-half reliability of 0.82, and a Spearman-Brown prophecy of 0.9 [20].

From the preliminary (precursor) version (USQOLAT), the current ACSS was further updated as follows: (i) the scores for question 1 (frequency of urination) were related to the number of urinations per 24 h, (ii) the symptoms were clearly divided into "typical" and "differential" symptoms, and (iii) five questions on additional conditions were added.

3. Current Acute Cystitis Symptom Score Questionnaire (ACSS)

The current so-called ACSS is now an 18-item self-reporting questionnaire including (a) six items (questions) about "typical" symptoms of AC, (b) four items regarding differential diagnoses,

(c) three items on quality of life, and (d) five items on additional conditions that may affect therapy (Supplementary Figures S1 and S2).

Part A of the ACSS is filled in at the first office visit, prior to treatment. Part A of the ACSS includes four subscales (domains): Typical, Differential, Quality of Life, and Additional. Part B of the questionnaire, which also includes the previously mentioned for domains of the Part A and "Dynamics" domain, in addition, is completed at a follow-up visit, e.g., after treatment [21].

4. Procedures for the Validation and Methods of the Statistical Analysis

4.1. Study Population

The Uzbek and Russian versions of the ACSS questionnaire (Supplementary Figures S1 and S2) were applied in 228 women (187 Uzbek and 41 Russian versions of the ACSS) presenting with and without symptoms of AC at the outpatient clinic of the RSCU. All participants signed written informed consent before filling out the questionnaire. Data obtained from filled-in paper-form questionnaires were then recorded into the electronic database, using PC software specially developed for the purpose of recording, storing and processing inputted data (e-USQOLAT).

The clinical diagnosis of AC was established by the physicians of the RSCU based on subject's complaints that are typical for UTI (acute onset, dysuria, urgency, the sensation of pain/discomfort above the pubic area, etc.) and the results of the laboratory tests. Respondents for whom the AC was ruled out were included in the control group, regardless of the total score obtained from the ACSS questionnaire or the presence or absence of other urological pathology.

4.2. Clinical Procedures

All patients were to undergo routine diagnostic procedures such as renal and bladder ultrasound, microscopy of centrifuged mid-stream urine sediment using a Goryaev's chamber (hemocytometer) and urine culture. Urinalysis was performed according to Nechiporenko [22] with taken reference normal values of white blood cells (WBC) for females ≤ 2000/mL. Microscopic bacteriuria was registered as negative or positive. Any amount of bacteria was regarded as positive [23]. For the urine culture, a bacteriuria of $\geq 10^4$ colony forming units (CFU) per mL was considered positive. Other clinical and/or instrumental investigations and tests were performed when indicated. All required data, including patients' answers, their age, ethnicity, employment status, place of residence, number of previous episodes of AC within the last year, duration of current episode, and results of laboratory tests, were recorded into the electronic database.

4.3. Validation Methods and Statistical Tests

4.3.1. Testing Variables for Normality

The distributions of all the data obtained were tested visually (Q-Q Plots, histograms) and numerically (Shapiro-Wilk test). Parametric or non-parametric statistical tests were then performed in dependence of normality of distributions.

4.3.2. Descriptive Statistics

Ordinary statistical parameters (mean, standard deviations, standard error etc.) were used for the description of patients' demographics and characteristics.

4.3.3. Validity and Reliability

Validity and reliability of the questionnaire were estimated calculating internal consistency by Cronbach's alpha, split-half, and Spearman-Brown prophecy [24]. Spearman's rank correlation coefficient was used for assessing relations between results of subjective self-assessment (answers marked on the questionnaire) and objective lower UTI symptoms (pyuria, hematuria, and bacteriuria).

4.3.4. The Process of Distribution into the Groups

For revealing true negative and true positive, false-negative, and false-positive results, two members of the research team were chosen. One of them (JFA) had access to case histories and results of patient's clinical and laboratory investigations but was blinded to the results of the questionnaire. The second member (UAA) was blinded to all results of patient's investigations apart from the ACSS test results and final diagnosis of the urologist. Based on information available to them individually, they have made independent diagnostic decisions whether the respondent has AC or not. Their decisions were documented and then compared by the final decision maker (FAA, see "Acknowledgements"). In cases when their opinions coincided true-negative (both of them decided that the patient did not have AC) or true-positive (both of them decided that patient did have AC), diagnoses were marked. All disagreements were discussed with the project supervisor and final decision was achieved by consensus. Using this algorithm, patients were divided into two groups (patients with AC and controls without).

4.3.5. Predictive Ability and Responsiveness

Two-by-two (2×2) contingency tables were used for physician's diagnosis taken as an outcome and binominal variable (positive/negative) taken as an exposure. To determine the predictive ability of the test, sensitivity and specificity were calculated. Odds ratios and absolute risk differences were also calculated.

Nonparametric Wilcoxon's signed rank test was used for comparative analysis of variables for related samples, and parametric paired t-test was used for a reassessment of statistical significance [25,26].

The nonparametric Mann-Whitney test was used for comparing different variables between patients and controls. Wilcoxon signed rank test was used for comparing symptom severity before and after therapy in patients admitted for subsequent visits and assessing the responsiveness of the questionnaire.

Means and 95% confidence intervals (CI) were calculated. A p-value less than or equal to 0.05 was considered statistically significant. Substantive significance (effect size) was estimated by the modified correlation coefficient (r) proposed by Rosenthal and Rosnow using the Z-value retrieved from Wilcoxon's signed-rank test.

The Statistical Package for the Social Sciences (IBM SPSS Statistics for Windows, Version 22.0. IBM Corp., Armonk, NY, USA) was used for statistical analysis and graphical presentations of the results.

5. Results

5.1. Development of ACSS Questionnaire

The literature search resulted in 56 articles covering the period from 1971 to 2012. Of those, 4 articles were selected as a basis for the items of the questionnaire [27–30]. The following main symptoms of women diagnosed with AC were identified: frequent voiding of small volumes, urgency, painful urination, feeling of incomplete bladder emptying after voiding, suprapubic discomfort and hematuria. These six symptoms were combined into the first domain of the questionnaire and labeled as "Typical". Symptoms regarding other genitourinary problems (e.g., flank pain, vaginal/urethral discharge, fever, etc.) were selected for the second domain labeled as "Differential". In the third domain, questions concerning the impact on quality of life were included and labeled as "Qol". Finally, five questions regarding additional health conditions (menstruation, premenstrual and menopausal syndrome, pregnancy, diabetes mellitus) were labeled as "Additional". For each question in the "Typical", "Differential", and "Qol" domains, a 4-point Likert-type scale assessing severity of each symptom ranged from 0 (no symptom) to 3 (severe) was introduced, while questions in the "Additional" domain contained only dichotomously fashioned "yes/no" questions. This procedure resulted in an 18 item self-reporting questionnaire for AC.

5.2. Study Population: Characteristics of Patients and Controls

Among 228 women, 107 (46.9%), with mean age 30.02 ± 10.35 y.o., had physician-diagnosed AC. Of the 107 patients, urinalysis was performed for 106 (99.1%). Of those 106, 100 (94.3%) had pyuria (>2000 WBC/mL) and 75 (70.8%) had microscopic bacteriuria. Urine culture was performed for only 64 (59.8%) of all urine samples. Of them, 39/64 (60.9%) were culture-positive (CFU $\geq 10^4$/mL). The average duration of the episode at the time of the visit was 6.04 ± 4.37 days. All patients received appropriate treatment according to Uzbek national urological guidelines (standards), and a subsequent test-of-cure visit was recommended after its completion. Forty-eight of 107 patients (44.9%) came for a follow-up investigation after the treatment period and were asked to fill in the Part B of the questionnaire for further monitoring.

The control group consisted of 121 female patients (mean age 32.79 ± 12.69 years) without ($n = 88$) or with ($n = 33$) urologic pathologies (other than lower UTIs). There were no significant differences between patients and controls in terms of nationality, employment, age, pregnancy, and place of residence ($p > 0.05$).

5.3. ACSS Analysis in Subjects with AC and Controls at Visit 1

5.3.1. Validity and Reliability

As the separately analyzed results of the Russian and Uzbek versions of the questionnaire published earlier did not differ significantly, a "combined" analysis for both versions was performed. Internal consistency and reliability of the ACSS were considered as good. Cronbach's alpha for the entire questionnaire was 0.88, split-half reliability was 0.76 and 0.79 for both halves, Guttman split-half was 0.93, correlation (rho) between first and second halves was 0.87, and Spearman-Brown prophecy coefficient was 0.93.

Cronbach's alpha for "Typical" domain (combination of the six most typical symptoms of AC) was 0.89, split-half reliability resulted in 0.82 and 0.76 for both halves, Guttman split-half was 0.92, and the correlation between first and second half was 0.85. Mean inter-item correlation of the domain was 0.55, the interclass correlation for average measures was 0.89 (95% CI: 0.87–0.91).

The same tests performed for the "Differential" domain (five questions) showed the following results: Cronbach's alpha 0.53, split-half reliability 0.35 and 0.21 for both halves, respectively, and Guttman split-half 0.57 and the interclass correlation coefficient was 0.53 (95% CI: 0.44–0.61).

The results of the reliability tests of the "QoL" domain (three questions regarding symptoms with negative influence on usual lifestyle) were excellent. In particular, Cronbach's alpha was 0.91 average inter-item correlation was 0.76, the interclass correlation coefficient was 0.92 (95% CI: 0.90–0.93) and Spearman-Brown prophecy coefficient was 0.91.

Since items of the "Additional" domain had a dichotomous view, they were not included in this analysis.

5.3.2. Discriminative Ability

Discriminative ability of the "Typical" domain was evaluated using Receiver-Operating-Characteristic (ROC) curve analysis (Figure 1). Changes in predictive ability of the questionnaire depending on scores in "Typical" domain showed that the most appropriate cut-off summary score for the "Typical" domain was equal to 6 (Table 1). Among 107 women with confirmed AC, 99 (92.5%) had a summary score of 6 and higher (true-positive result), and only 8 women (7.5%) with approved AC had a score less than 6 (false-negative result). Among the group of 121 women who did not have AC, the false-positive result was noted in 13 cases (10.7%) (false-positive value), and the true-negative result (<6) was reported for 108 women (89.3%). These results were similar to those published earlier, when the first 58 patients having filled in the precursor version, USQOLAT, were also included in the analysis (Table 2). A scatter plot chart according to a summary score of the "Typical" domain at visit 1 including 228 subjects (107 patients with AC, 121 controls without AC) is given in Figure 2.

Table 1. Changes in the predictive ability of the ACSS including 228 women (107 with AC and 121 without AC) depending on the summary scores obtained in the "Typical" domain at visit 1. The most appropriate discriminative summary score for the "Typical" domain was equal to 6.

Score ≥	TP Result	TN Result	FP Result	FN Result	Sensitivity	Specificity	Pos. Predictive Value	Neg. Predictive Value	Pos. Likelihood Ratio	Neg. Likelihood Ratio	Relative Risk	Risk Difference	Diagnostic Odds Ratio	Diagnostic Effectiveness
0	107	0	121	0	100.0%	0.0%	46.9%	NA	1.0	NA	NA	NA	NA	46.9%
1	107	34	87	0	100.0%	28.1%	55.2%	100.0%	1.4	0.0	NA	55.2%	NA	61.8%
2	107	79	42	0	100.0%	65.3%	71.8%	100.0%	2.9	0.0	NA	71.8%	NA	81.6%
3	106	85	36	1	99.1%	70.2%	74.6%	98.8%	3.3	0.0	64.2	73.5%	250.3	83.8%
4	104	96	25	3	97.2%	79.3%	80.6%	97.0%	4.7	0.0	26.6	77.6%	133.1	87.7%
5	100	101	20	7	93.5%	83.5%	83.3%	93.5%	5.7	0.1	12.9	76.9%	72.1	88.2%
6	99	108	13	8	92.5%	89.3%	88.4%	93.1%	8.6	0.1	12.8	81.5%	102.8	90.8%
7	96	110	11	11	89.7%	90.9%	89.7%	90.9%	9.9	0.1	9.9	80.6%	87.3	90.4%
8	86	113	8	21	80.4%	93.4%	91.5%	84.3%	12.2	0.2	5.8	75.8%	57.8	87.3%
9	78	116	5	29	72.9%	95.9%	94.0%	80.0%	17.6	0.3	4.7	74.0%	62.4	85.1%
10	65	119	2	42	60.7%	98.3%	97.0%	73.9%	36.8	0.4	3.7	70.9%	92.1	80.7%
11	53	120	1	54	49.5%	99.2%	98.1%	69.0%	59.9	0.5	3.2	67.1%	117.8	75.9%
12	42	121	0	65	39.3%	100.0%	100.0%	65.1%	NA	0.6	2.9	65.1%	NA	71.5%
13	30	121	0	77	28.0%	100.0%	100.0%	61.1%	NA	0.7	2.6	61.1%	NA	66.2%
14	19	121	0	88	17.8%	100.0%	100.0%	57.9%	NA	0.8	2.4	57.9%	NA	61.4%
15	16	121	0	91	15.0%	100.0%	100.0%	57.1%	NA	0.9	2.3	57.1%	NA	60.1%
16	8	121	0	99	7.5%	100.0%	100.0%	55.0%	NA	0.9	2.2	55.0%	NA	56.6%
17	5	121	0	102	4.7%	100.0%	100.0%	54.3%	NA	1.0	2.2	54.3%	NA	55.3%
18	3	121	0	104	2.8%	100.0%	100.0%	53.8%	NA	1.0	2.2	53.8%	NA	54.4%

TP = true-positive; TN = true-negative; FP = false-positive; FN = false-negative.

Table 2. Predictive ability of the current ACSS including 228 women (107 with AC and 121 without AC) using for diagnostics of AC a summary score of 6 or higher obtained in the "Typical" domain at visit 1 as compared with the study published earlier [19] including in addition 58 women (total 286), in whom the precursor questionnaire, USQOLAT, was applied.

Questionaire	ACSS	ACSS + USQOLAT
Women total (*n*)	228	286
Women with AC	107	139
Women without AC	121	147
Sensitivity	92.5%	93.5%
Specificity	89.3%	89.8%
True-positive (*n*, %)	99 (92.5%)	138 (99.2%)
True-negative (*n*, %)	108 (89.3%)	132 (89.8%)
False-positive (*n*, %)	13 (10.7%)	15 (10.2%)
False-negative (*n*, %)	8 (7.5%)	9 (6.5%)
Positive predictive value	88.4%	89.7%
Negative predictive value	93.1%	93.6%
Positive likelihood ratio	8.6	9.2
Negative likelihood ratio	0.1	0.1
Relative risk	12.8	14.0
Risk difference	81.5%	83.3%
Diagnostic Odds ratio	102.8	127.1
Diagnostic effectiveness	90.8%	91.6%

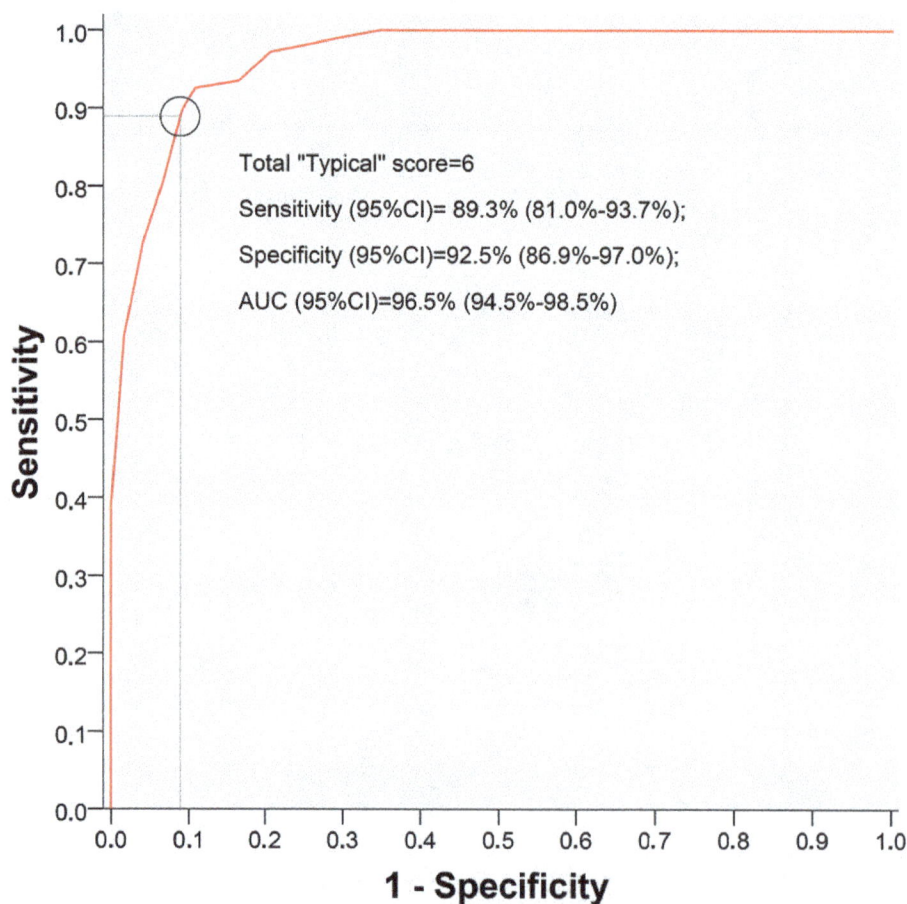

Total "Typical" score=6

Sensitivity (95%CI)= 89.3% (81.0%-93.7%);

Specificity (95%CI)=92.5% (86.9%-97.0%);

AUC (95%CI)=96.5% (94.5%-98.5%)

Figure 1. Receiver-Operating-Characteristic (ROC) curve analysis of the "Typical" domain of the Acute Cystitis Symptom Score (ACSS) at the first visit with results from 228 subjects (107 patients with acute uncomplicated cystitis (AC), 121 controls without AC).

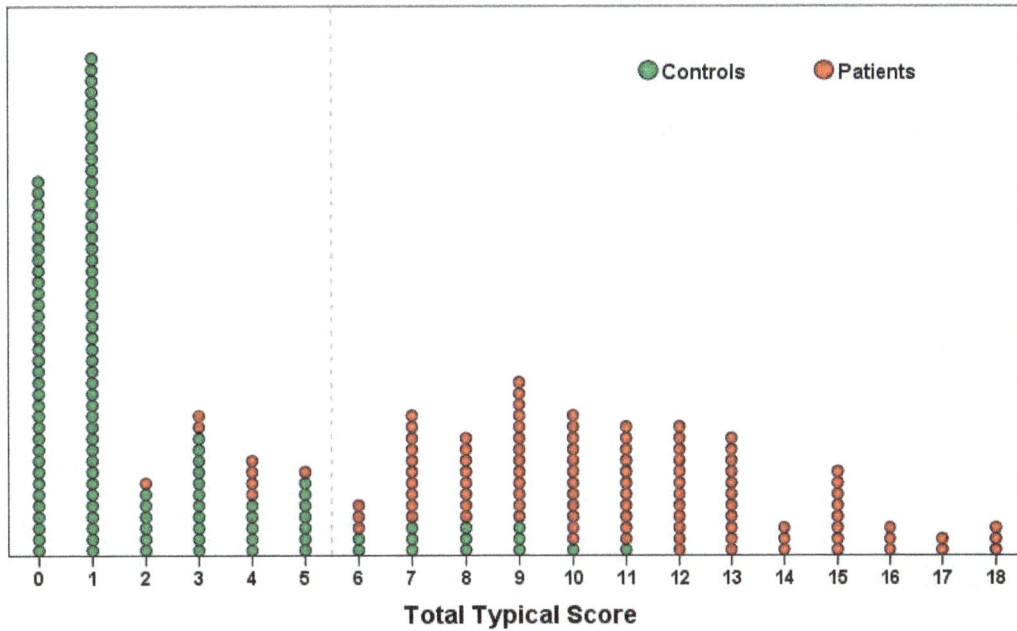

Figure 2. Distribution of 228 subjects (107 patients with AC, 121 controls without AC) according to a summary score of the "Typical" domain of the ACSS at the first visit.

5.3.3. Predictive Ability and Responsiveness

Using a summary score of the "Typical" domain of 6 as discriminative, assessment of sensitivity and specificity resulted in values around 90% (92.5% and 89.3%, respectively) (Table 2). The positive likelihood ratio was as high as 8.6 and negative likelihood ratio was low enough (0.1). The absolute risk difference was 81.5%, and values of the odds ratio and relative risk for the AC group were 102.8 and 12.8, respectively (Table 3).

Differences in scores between the group of patients with AC compared to those without AC were significant ($p < 0.0001$) in items of "Typical" and "QoL" domains. Scores in items of the "Differential" domain did not differ significantly between groups except for questions regarding "vaginal discharge" and "urethral discharge" (Table 4).

For the group of patients at the time of the first visit, the most common symptom was urgency: 86 (80.37%) patients rated the intensity of this symptom as "moderate" and "severe" (46 and 40 patients, respectively). Painful urination was recognized as the second most common symptom, with 84 (78.50%) patients suffering correspondingly rating this symptom as moderate (43 patients) or severe (41 patients) (Table 5).

Table 3. Estimation of risks depending on "cut-off" value in "Typical" domain of ACSS at visit 1.

	'Typical' Score ≥ 6	'Typical' Score < 6
Number of subjects	112	116
Risk of having AC	0.88	0.07
Risk of not having AC	0.12	0.93
Odds of having AC	7.62	0.07
Odds against having AC	0.13	13.5
Absolute risk difference	81.5%	
Odds ratio	102.81	

Table 4. Differences in scores of the ACSS between patients with AC (*n* = 107) and controls without AC (*n* = 121) at visit 1.

Item/Domain	Mann-Whitney U	Patients (*n* = 107)		Controls (*n* = 121)		*p*-Value
		Mean	SD	Mean	SD	
Frequency	1720.50	2.05	0.85	0.71	0.68	0.000
Urgency	1364.50	2.07	0.95	0.28	0.70	0.000
Painful urination	1066.50	2.09	0.91	0.24	0.66	0.000
Incomplete bladder emptying	1329.50	1.87	0.81	0.36	0.74	0.000
Suprapubic discomfort	1761.50	1.77	0.90	0.39	0.78	0.000
Hematuria	4155.00	0.66	0.90	0.09	0.37	0.000
Total "Typical" score	458.50	10.50	3.49	2.07	2.55	0.000
Flank pain	6097.00	1.32	1.01	1.40	0.97	0.428
Vaginal discharge	5539.00	0.49	0.79	0.26	0.60	0.013
Urethral discharge	5573.00	0.27	0.61	0.09	0.39	0.002
Feeling of chill/fever	5774.50	0.27	0.62	0.14	0.49	0.018
Hyperthermia (measured) *	5883.00	0.27 [a]	0.59	0.17 [b]	0.53	0.058
Total "Differential" score	5630.50	2.35	1.84	1.90	1.51	0.082
General dyscomfort	2923.00	2.06	0.66	1.18	0.86	0.000
Impairment of everyday activity	2541.00	1.87	0.67	0.91	0.84	0.000
Impairment of social activity	2863.50	1.75	0.75	0.84	0.83	0.000
Total "QoL" score	2396.50	5.67	1.80	2.93	2.34	0.000

* Hyperthermia (measured): [a] *n* = 90; [b] *n* = 94.

Table 5. The number of patients with AC (*n* = 107) with symptoms of severity "moderate" (score 2) and "severe" (score 3) in "Typical" and "Differential" domain of the ACSS at visit 1.

Domain	Symptom	'Moderate'	'Severe'	Total	Percentage
Typical	Urgency	46	40	86	80.4%
	Painful urination	43	41	84	78.5%
	Frequency	45	36	81	75.7%
	Incomplete bladder emptying	47	25	72	67.3%
	Suprapubic discomfort	40	25	65	60.7%
	Hematuria	16	15	31	29.0%
Differential	Flank pain	32	15	47	43.9%
	Vaginal discharge	11	3	14	13.1%
	Feeling of chill/fever	4	2	6	5.6%
	Hyperthermia	5	1	6	5.6%
	Urethral discharge	3	2	5	4.7%

Table 6 represents the distributions of scores of the typical symptoms in the groups of patients and controls. Note, blood in urine is only seen in patients with acute hemorrhagic cystitis, a specific form of cystitis, which is not the case in the majority of the patients with AC.

Table 6. Distribution of scores in Typical Symptoms of ACSS in women without AC (Controls) and in those with AC (Patients).

Symptom/Severity	Controls (*n* = 121)	Patients (*n* = 107)
Frequency		
No (4 or less times per day)	41.32%	4.67%
Yes, mild (5–6 times/day)	46.28%	19.63%
Yes, moderate (7–8 times/day)	12.40%	42.06%
Yes, severe (9–10 or more times/day)	0.00%	33.64%

Table 6. *Cont.*

Symptom/Severity	Controls (*n* = 121)	Patients (*n* = 107)
Urgency		
No	81.82%	11.21%
Yes, mild	12.40%	8.41%
Yes, moderate	1.65%	42.99%
Yes, severe	4.13%	37.38%
Painful urination		
No	85.95%	7.48%
Yes, mild	6.61%	14.02%
Yes, moderate	4.96%	40.19%
Yes, severe	2.48%	38.32%
Incomplete bladder emptying		
No	77.69%	3.74%
Yes, mild	11.57%	28.97%
Yes, moderate	8.26%	43.93%
Yes, severe	2.48%	23.36%
Suprapubic pain		
No	76.86%	7.48%
Yes, mild	9.92%	31.78%
Yes, moderate	10.74%	37.38%
Yes, severe	2.48%	23.36%
Visible blood in the urine		
No	93.39%	57.94%
Yes, mild	4.13%	22.43%
Yes, moderate	2.48%	14.95%
Yes, severe	0.00%	4.67%

Table 7 shows total typical scores in patients and controls and in their corresponding subgroups: pregnant women, women ≤50 years of age and not pregnant, and women ≥51 years of age. The discrimination between patients and controls is in the subgroups as good as in the total group. Therefore, the ACSS is a reliable diagnostic tool for premenopausal, non-pregnant women, pregnant women, and postmenopausal women.

Table 7. Differences (Mann-Whitney test) in total "Typical" scores of the ACSS between patients with AUC (*n* = 107) and controls without AUC (*n* = 121), substratified in pregnant women, women 50 years of age and younger, and women 51 years of age and older. N: number; SD: standard deviation; CI: confidence interval.

	Patients with AUC				Controls without AUC				*p*-Value *
	"Typical" Scores				"Typical "Scores				
Respondents	*N*	mean	SD	95% CI	*N*	mean	SD	95% CI	
Pregnant women	21	9.29	4.11	7.41–11.16	20	2.55	3.03	1.13–3.97	4.00×10^{-6}
≤50 years, not pregnant	79	10.73	3.32	9.99–11.48	87	2.05	2.45	1.52–2.57	2.51×10^{-26}
≥51 years	7	11.57	2.82	8.96–14.18	14	1.50	2.50	0.05–2.95	3.40×10^{-05}
Total	107	10.50	3.49	9.84–11.17	121	2.07	2.55	1.61–2.53	4.07×10^{-34}

* *p* values in the table are given in scientific (exponential) notation and are lower than 0.0001 for all cases.

5.4. ACSS Analysis in Subjects with AC and Controls at Follow-Up Visit

Of the total 107 patients with AC, 48 had subsequently a "test-of-cure" visit after 5.08 ± 2.71 days of therapy. Differences between scores obtained at the first and subsequent visits are shown in Table 8. The total "typical" symptom score decreased significantly when comparing the two visits (10.4 and 2.5, $p < 0.001$). A more detailed analysis will be discussed in part II [21].

Table 8. Differences in scores between first and follow-up visit (*n* = 48).

Scores in Different Domains of the ACSS	First Visit		Subsequent Visit		Mean Difference [a]	*p*-Value [b]
	Mean	SD	Mean	SD		
Total "Typical" score	10.8	3.2	2.5	3.2	8.3	<0.0001
Total "Differential" score	2.2 [a]	1.6	0.8 [a]	1.2	1.4	<0.0001
Total "QoL" score	5.7	1.7	1.5	2.2	4.2	<0.0001

[a] Based on the sum of scores of 46 patients with non-missing values. [b] *p*-values are generated by Wilcoxon Signed Rank Test.

6. Discussion

The consulting physicians diagnosed AC according to their clinical practice and based on the results of laboratory investigations. Besides the typical history and symptoms, urinalysis was performed in 99.1% patients (only 1 missing data) with positive pyuria in 94.5% of cases. Although microscopic bacteriuria and positive urine culture was only found in 75/106 (70.8%) and 39/64 (60.9%) of patients, respectively, it should be noted that only cases with a bacteriuria of at least 10^5 CFU/mL found in microscopy [23] and at least 10^4 CFU/mL in urine culture, could be considered as positive in the clinical practice.

In contrast, Stamm et al. had already shown that the traditional diagnostic criterion, $\geq 10^5$ CFU/mL of midstream urine, has a very high degree of diagnostic specificity (99%) but a very low level of sensitivity (51%) [31]. That means that this threshold of urine culture may identify only 51% of symptomatic women with lower UTI whose bladder urine (obtained by suprapubic aspiration or by catheter) contains coliforms. The authors found the best diagnostic criterion to be $\geq 10^2$ CFU/mL (sensitivity, 95%; specificity, 85%) and suggested that clinicians and microbiologists should alter their approach to the diagnosis and treatment of women with acute symptomatic coliform infection of the lower urinary tract.

Hooton et al., however, confirmed in a more recent study that colony counts of *E. coli* as low as even 10^1 to 10^2 CFU/mL in midstream urine were sensitive and specific for the presence of *E. coli* in catheter urine in symptomatic women [32]. Although using such low counts as a threshold, still no uropathogens could be cultured neither from catheter nor midstream urine in 22% of patients with typical symptoms of AC. It follows, that for diagnosing AC the symptomatology has become more decisive than any urinary bacterial count.

The results of our investigation demonstrate that the ACSS is a reliable, valid, and easy-to-use questionnaire, which may help to diagnose AC in women in primary healthcare settings and to assess treatment efficacy. The ACSS is a reliable diagnostic tool for patients and physicians, not only in premenopausal, non-pregnant women but also in pregnant women and in postmenopausal women. It can be self-administered and completed in a short time by respondents or surveyees. Questions and versions of answers are easy to understand and may be used for epidemiological surveys and/or drug studies.

The current version of the ACSS was tested in 228 women visiting urologist's office for different reasons. The Uzbek, as well as the Russian versions, are clear and understandable for women of any age, educational level, and employment status. Our study demonstrated high reliability and validity of the questionnaire. The items of ACSS have excellent internal consistency and validity.

The results of the present study, including only the 228 women to whom the current ACSS was applied, did not show clinically relevant diagnostic differences to the study published earlier [19], which included an additional 58 women, to whom the precursor questionnaire, USQOLAT, was administered (Table 1).

Health-related quality of life is gaining increasing importance, combining characteristics of physical, psychological, emotional, and social human functioning based on subjective perception [33–35]. The assessment of the quality of life is usually performed by patient self-reporting and may be much more useful even if it mismatches the physician's view. Although standard medical and biological parameters are often basic criteria of treatment efficacy, they cannot reflect the patient's feeling of well-being and performance of everyday activities. Therefore, indeed the self-assessment may be the most informative index of the patient's status of health in many cases [36]. In this context, symptom scores and questionnaires are valuable tools. In urology, international validated questionnaires such as the IPSS (International Prostate Symptom Score) and the NIH-CPSI (National Institutes of Health Chronic Prostatitis Symptom Index) are broadly used for various conditions [37,38].

Until recently, there was no generally accepted questionnaire for AC available for combined assessment of severity of symptoms and impact on quality of life. Our study aimed to develop a highly sensitive and specific as well as simple patient self-reporting questionnaire assessing the symptoms of AC and their impact on quality of life, differentiating AC from other urogynecological disorders with similar symptomatology, and assessing treatment efficacy.

In previous studies on UTIs, numerous different diaries, symptoms questionnaires and scales for separately assessing "bladder symptoms" and health-related quality of life were used separately [4,15,16,27,28,39–41]. Some researchers assessed general conditions and wellbeing of patients rather than urinary symptoms [17,29]. Others have used "self-made" questionnaires or algorithmic schemes for assessing symptoms in patients with pre-diagnosed AC before and after treatment [12,13,39]. The symptom score used in the study of Bleidorn et al. [27] contained questions regarding only three key symptoms of AC (dysuria, frequency, and lower abdominal pain), while the ACSS contains also questions about other key symptoms of AC (urgency, incomplete bladder emptying and hematuria). However, the ACSS is not the first questionnaire in the area of UTIs. Earlier, two other questionnaires—the UTI Symptoms Assessment (UTISA) and the Activity Impairment Assessment (AIA)—were published [15,16]. While the UTISA evaluates the severity of lower UTI, the AIA investigates the impact on impaired activity. Unfortunately, important statistical information like sensitivity, specificity, responsiveness and discriminative abilities have not been reported for both. The ACSS was developed and validated considering these parameters. It also contains questions to differentiate AC from other commonly community-acquired urological and gynecological diseases ("Differential" domain) and items for conditions that may affect therapy ("Additional" domain) and therefore requiring broader and more thorough investigation. These additional items may add more accuracy and be useful for epidemiological surveys.

The discriminative ability of "Typical" domain of the questionnaire may allow easier distinguishment of the patients with AC from those without it. During our analysis, we have found statistically significant correlations between scores of the questionnaire and results of urinalyses. High levels of sensitivity and specificity in combination with excellent discriminative ability and responsiveness make this questionnaire very useful for diagnosing AC in women and assessment of treatment efficacy. The ACSS also evaluates the severity of symptoms and their influence on the quality of life and may assist to differentiate AC from other urological disorders with the help of the "Differential" domain. Complicating and affecting factors may be revealed by the analysis of the "Additional" domain. A special domain assessing dynamics evaluates treatment efficacy. These distinctive features are the main advantages of the ACSS compared to other existing UTI symptom scores [12,13,15,16,39].

Our study has limitations that should be acknowledged. First, the questionnaire was limited to Uzbek- and Russian-speaking women. Second, the study was performed in a single center, and only 48% of all patients with AC returned for a follow-up visit to test responsiveness. Nevertheless, the reevaluation of the questionnaire was performed in a large number of patients and controls. Results of the validation of the ACSS in German and UK English languages were published recently [42,43] and is planned or ongoing in other languages.

7. Conclusions

The Uzbek and the Russian ACSS was reevaluated—excluding 58 patients having filled in also the precursor version, USQOLAT—to assess the severity of symptoms in women with AC and their impact on quality of life as well as to differentiate from other urogenital disorders with the possibility to monitor treatment efficacy. The ACSS questionnaire was validated in 228 women with and without AC and demonstrated good values of reliability, validity, predictive ability, and responsiveness. This facilitates its use in the primary healthcare setting as well as in clinical studies. For a broader use validation of the ACSS in other languages will be necessary.

8. Patents

Copyright and Translations of the ACSS in Other Languages

The ACSS is copyrighted by the Certificate of Deposit of Intellectual Property in Fundamental Library of Academy of Sciences of the Republic of Uzbekistan, Tashkent (Registration number 2463; 26 August 2015) and the Certificate of the International Online Copyright Office, European Depository, Berlin, Germany (Nr. EU-01-000764; 21 October 2015). The Rightholders are Jakhongir Fatikhovich Alidjanov (Uzbekistan), Ozoda Takhirovna Alidjanova (Uzbekistan), Adrian Martin Erich Pilatz (Germany), Kurt Guenther Naber (Germany), Florian Martin Erich Wagenlehner (Germany).

http://avtor-web.com/index.php?option=com_desposition&task=display_desp_det&id=2612&lang=ru (assessed on 13 January 2018);

http://interoco.com/all-materials/work-of-science/1013-1951954939.html (assessed on 13 January 2018)

The e-USQOLAT is copyrighted by the Authorship Certificate of the International Online Copyright Office, European Depository, Berlin, Germany (Nr. EC-01-001179; 18 May 2017) 19.

http://inter.interoco.com/copyright-depository/computer-programs/1438-2017-05-18-10-59-16.html?path=computer-programs (assessed on 13 January 2018).

Translations of the ACSS in other languages are available on the website: http://www.acss.world/downloads.html.

Acknowledgments: The authors would like to express their special gratitude to Dmitrii L. Aroustamov (former director of RSCU) for initiating this study. We thank all the participants of the study for their contribution. Research team acknowledges the staff of the RSCU, Farkhad A. Akilov and Saidamin A. Makhsudov, for their priceless help with study population and during the decision-making process. J.F. Alidjanov received a 1-year Clinical/Lab Scholarship grant of the European Urological Scholarship Programme (EUSP) of the European Association of Urology (EAU).

Author Contributions: J.F.A. and K.G.N. conceived and designed the study; J.F.A. and U.A.A. recruited respondents and inputted the data; J.F.A., U.A.A. and K.G.N. analyzed the data; F.M.E.W., J.F.A. and A.P. contributed analysis tools; K.G.N., J.F.A. and F.M.E.W. wrote the manuscript.

References

1. Foxman, B.; Brown, P. Epidemiology of urinary tract infections: Transmission and risk factors, incidence, and costs. *Infect. Dis. Clin. N. Am.* **2003**, *17*, 227–241. [CrossRef]
2. Ronald, A.R.; Nicolle, L.E.; Stamm, E.; Krieger, J.; Warren, J.; Schaeffer, A.; Naber, K.G.; Hooton, T.M.; Johnson, J.; Chambers, S.; et al. Urinary tract infection in adults: Research priorities and strategies. *Int. J. Antimicrob. Agents* **2001**, *17*, 343–348. [CrossRef]
3. Schappert, S.M.; Rechtsteiner, E.A. Ambulatory medical care utilization estimates for 2007. *Vital Health Stat.* **2011**, *13*, 1–38.
4. Colgan, R.; Keating, K.; Dougouih, M. Survey of symptom burden in women with uncomplicated urinary tract infections. *Clin. Drug Investig.* **2004**, *24*, 55–60. [CrossRef] [PubMed]

5. Ernst, E.J.; Ernst, M.E.; Hoehns, J.D.; Bergus, G.R. Women's quality of life is decreased by acute cystitis and antibiotic adverse effects associated with treatment. *Health Qual. Life Outcomes* **2005**, *3*, 45. [CrossRef] [PubMed]

6. Foxman, B.; Gillespie, B.; Koopman, J.; Zhang, L.; Palin, K.; Tallman, P.; Marsh, J.V.; Spear, S.; Sobel, J.D.; Marty, M.J.; et al. Risk factors for second urinary tract infection among college women. *Am. J. Epidemiol.* **2000**, *151*, 1194–1205. [CrossRef] [PubMed]

7. Scholes, D.; Hooton, T.M.; Roberts, P.L.; Stapleton, A.E.; Gupta, K.; Stamm, W.E. Risk factors for recurrent urinary tract infection in young women. *J. Inf. Dis.* **2000**, *182*, 1177–1182. [CrossRef] [PubMed]

8. Zincir, H.; Kaya Erten, Z.; Ozkan, F.; Sevig, U.; Baser, M.; Elmali, F. Prevalence of urinary tract infections and its risk factors in elementary school students. *Urol. Int.* **2012**, *88*, 194–197. [CrossRef] [PubMed]

9. Berg, A.O. Variations among family physicians' management strategies for lower urinary tract infection in women: A report from the washington family physicians collaborative research network. *J. Am. Board Fam. Pract.* **1991**, *4*, 327–330. [PubMed]

10. Wigton, R.S.; Longenecker, J.C.; Bryan, T.J.; Parenti, C.; Flach, S.D.; Tape, T.G. Variation by specialty in the treatment of urinary tract infection in women. *J. Gen. Intern. Med.* **1999**, *14*, 491–494. [CrossRef] [PubMed]

11. Yamamichi, F.; Shigemura, K.; Matsumoto, M.; Nakano, Y.; Tanaka, K.; Arakawa, S.; Fujisawa, M. Relationship between urinary tract infection categorization and pathogens' antimicrobial susceptibilities. *Urol. Int.* **2012**, *88*, 198–208. [CrossRef] [PubMed]

12. Bent, S.; Nallamothu, B.K.; Simel, D.L.; Fihn, S.D.; Saint, S. Does this woman have an acute uncomplicated urinary tract infection? *JAMA* **2002**, *287*, 2701–2710. [CrossRef] [PubMed]

13. Bent, S.; Saint, S. The optimal use of diagnostic testing in women with acute uncomplicated cystitis. *Am. J. Med.* **2002**, *113* (Suppl. 1A), 20S–28S. [CrossRef]

14. Schauberger, C.W.; Merkitch, K.W.; Prell, A.M. Acute cystitis in women: Experience with a telephone-based algorithm. *WMJ* **2007**, *106*, 326–329. [PubMed]

15. Clayson, D.; Wild, D.; Doll, H.; Keating, K.; Gondek, K. Validation of a patient-administered questionnaire to measure the severity and bothersomeness of lower urinary tract symptoms in uncomplicated urinary tract infection (UTI): The UTI Symptom Assessment questionnaire. *BJU Int.* **2005**, *96*, 350–359. [CrossRef] [PubMed]

16. Wild, D.J.; Clayson, D.J.; Keating, K.; Gondek, K. Validation of a patient-administered questionnaire to measure the activity impairment experienced by women with uncomplicated urinary tract infection: The Activity Impairment Assessment (AIA). *Health Qual. Life Outcomes* **2005**, *3*, 42. [CrossRef] [PubMed]

17. Barry, H.C.; Ebell, M.H.; Hickner, J. Evaluation of suspected urinary tract infection in ambulatory women: A cost-utility analysis of office-based strategies. *J. Fam. Pract.* **1997**, *44*, 49–60. [CrossRef] [PubMed]

18. Alidjanov, J.F.; Abdufattaev, U.A.; Makhsudov, S.A.; Pilatz, A.; Akilov, F.A.; Naber, K.G.; Wagenlehner, F.M. New self-reporting questionnaire to assess urinary tract infections and differential diagnosis: Acute cystitis symptom score. *Urol. Int.* **2014**, *92*, 230–236. [CrossRef] [PubMed]

19. Alidjanov, J.F.; Abdufattaev, U.A.; Makhsudov, S.A.; Pilatz, A.; Akilov, F.A.; Naber, K.G.; Wagenlehner, F.M. The Acute Cystitis Symptom Score for Patient- Reported Outcome assessment. *Urol. Int.* **2016**, *97*, 402–409. [CrossRef] [PubMed]

20. Akilov, F.A.; Naber, K.G.; Rakhmonov, O.M.; Alidjanov, J.F.; Abdufattaev, U.A. Development and validation of self-administered questionnaire to assess severity of acute cystitis symptoms and their influence to quality of life: Urinary Symptoms and Quality of Life Assessment Tool *(USQOLAT)*. In *Collected Articles of the Congress "Current Problems of Theoretical and Practical Medicine"*; The Research Center of Urology named after B.U. Dzharbussynov: Almaty, Kazakhstan, 2011; pp. 8–9, ISBN 978-601-80076-2-0.

21. Alidjanov, J.F.; Abdufattaev, U.A.; Pilatz, A.; Naber, K.G.; Wagenlehner, F.M. Reevaluation of the Acute Cystitis Symptom Score, a Self-reporting Questionnaire for Patient-Reported Outcome Assessment (Part II); (in preparation)

22. Nechiporenko, A.Z. Leukocyte and erythrocyte counts in 1 mL of urine. *Lab. Delo* **1969**, *2*, 121. (In Russian) [PubMed]

23. Simerville, J.A.; Maxted, W.C.; Pahira, J.J. Urinalysis: A comprehensive review. *Am. Fam. Phys.* **2005**, *71*, 1153–1162.

24. Cronbach, L.J. Test "reliability": Its meaning and determination. *Psychometrika* **1947**, *12*, 1–16. [CrossRef] [PubMed]

25.   Wilcoxon, F. Individual comparisons by ranking methods. *Biom. Bull.* **1945**, *1*, 80–83. [CrossRef]

26.   Student. The probable error of a mean. *Biometrika* **1908**, *6*, 1–25.

27.   Bleidorn, J.; Gagyor, I.; Kochen, M.M.; Wegscheider, K.; Hummers-Pradier, E. Symptomatic treatment (ibuprofen) or antibiotics (ciprofloxacin) for uncomplicated urinary tract infection?—Results of a randomized controlled pilot trial. *BMC Med.* **2010**, *8*, 30. [CrossRef] [PubMed]

28.   Ferry, S.A.; Holm, S.E.; Stenlund, H.; Lundholm, R.; Monsen, T.J. The natural course of uncomplicated lower urinary tract infection in women illustrated by a randomized placebo controlled study. *Scand. J. Infect. Dis.* **2004**, *36*, 296–301. [CrossRef] [PubMed]

29.   Malterud, K.; Baerheim, A. Peeing barbed wire. Symptom experiences in women with lower urinary tract infection. *Scand. J. Prim. Health Care* **1999**, *17*, 49–53. [PubMed]

30.   Savaris, R.F.; Teixeira, L.M.; Torres, T.G. Bladder tenderness as a physical sign for diagnosing cystitis in women. *Int. J. Gynaecol. Obstet.* **2006**, *93*, 256–257. [CrossRef] [PubMed]

31.   Stamm, W.E.; Counts, G.W.; Running, K.R.; Fihn, S.; Turck, M.; Holmes, K.K. Diagnosis of coliform infection in acutely dysuric women. *N. Engl. J. Med.* **1982**, *307*, 463–468. [CrossRef] [PubMed]

32.   Hooton, T.M.; Roberts, P.L.; Cox, M.E.; Stapleton, A.E. Voided midstream urine culture and acute cystitis in premenopausal women. *N. Engl. J. Med.* **2013**, *369*, 1883–1891. [CrossRef] [PubMed]

33.   Novick, A.A.; Ionova, T.I.; Kaind, P. *Conception of Life Quality Research in Medicine*; Elby: Saint-Petersburg, Russia, 1999. (In Russian)

34.   Spilker, B. *Quality of Life and Pharmacoeconomics in Clinical Trials*, 2nd ed.; Lippincott-Raven: Philadelphia, PA, USA, 1996.

35.   Staquet, M.J. *Quality of Life Assessment in Clinical Trials: Methods and Practice*; Oxford University Press: Oxford, UK; New York, NY, USA, 1998.

36.   Staquet, M.; Berzon, R.; Osoba, D.; Machin, D. Guidelines for reporting results of quality of life assessments in clinical trials. *Qual. Life Res.* **1996**, *5*, 496–502. [CrossRef] [PubMed]

37.   Barry, M.J.; Fowler, F.J.; O'Leary, M.P.; Bruskewitz, R.C.; Holtgrewe, H.L.; Mebust, W.K.; Cockett, A.T. The American Urological Association symptom index for benign prostatic hyperplasia. The measurement committee of the American Urological Association. *J. Urol.* **1992**, *148*, 1549–1557. [CrossRef]

38.   Litwin, M.S.; McNaughton-Collins, M.; Fowler, F.J., Jr.; Nickel, J.C.; Calhoun, E.A.; Pontari, M.A.; Alexander, R.B.; Farrar, J.T.; O'Leary, M.P. The National Institutes of Health Chronic Prostatitis Symptom Index: Development and validation of a new outcome measure. Chronic prostatitis collaborative research network. *J. Urol.* **1999**, *162*, 369–375. [CrossRef]

39.   Baerheim, A.; Digranes, A.; Jureen, R.; Malterud, K. Generalized symptoms in adult women with acute uncomplicated lower urinary tract infection: An observational study. *MedGenMed* **2003**, *5*, 1. Available online: https://www.medscape.com/viewarticle/457337 (accessed on 10 January 2018). [PubMed]

40.   Ellis, A.K.; Verma, S. Quality of life in women with urinary tract infections: Is benign disease a misnomer? *J. Am. Board Fam. Pract.* **2000**, *13*, 392–397. [CrossRef] [PubMed]

41.   Little, P.; Merriman, R.; Turner, S.; Rumsby, K.; Warner, G.; Lowes, J.A.; Smith, H.; Hawke, C.; Leydon, G.; Mullee, M.; et al. Presentation, pattern, and natural course of severe symptoms, and role of antibiotics and antibiotic resistance among patients presenting with suspected uncomplicated urinary tract infection in primary care: Observational study. *BMJ* **2010**. [CrossRef] [PubMed]

42.   Alidjanov, J.F.; Pilatz, A.; Abdufattaev, U.A.; Wiltink, J.; Weidner, W.; Naber, K.G.; Wagenlehner, F. German validation of the Acute Cystitis Symptom Score. *Urologe A* **2015**, *54*, 1269–1276. (In German) [CrossRef] [PubMed]

43.   Alidjanov, J.F.; Lima, H.A.; Pilatz, A.; Pickard, R.; Naber, K.G.; Safaev, Y.U.; Wagenlehner, F.M. Preliminary Clinical Validation of the UK English Version of the Acute Cystitis Symptom Score in UK English-speaking female population of Newcastle, Great Britain. *JOJ Urol. Nephrol.* **2017**, *1*, 555561. [CrossRef]

5

Complementation Studies of Bacteriophage λ O Amber Mutants by Allelic Forms of O Expressed from Plasmid, and O-P Interaction Phenotypes

Sidney Hayes * [ID], Karthic Rajamanickam and Connie Hayes

Department of Microbiology and Immunology, College of Medicine, University of Saskatchewan, Saskatoon, SK S7N 5E5, Canada; kar029@mail.usask.ca (K.R.); clh127@outlook.com (C.H.)
* Correspondence: sidney.hayes@usask.ca

Abstract: λ genes O and P are required for replication initiation from the bacteriophage λ origin site, *ori*λ, located within gene *O*. Questions have persisted for years about whether O-defects can indeed be complemented *in trans*. We show the effect of original null mutations in O and the influence of four origin mutations (three are in-frame deletions and one is a point mutation) on complementation. This is the first demonstration that O proteins with internal deletions can complement for O activity, and that expression of the N-terminal portion of gene P can completely prevent O complementation. We show that *O-P* co-expression can limit the lethal effect of P on cell growth. We explore the influence of the contiguous small RNA OOP on O complementation and P-lethality.

Keywords: bacteriophage lambda (λ); bi-directional replication initiation from *ori*λ; O and P initiator proteins; *ori*λ interaction site; O complementation by *ori*λ-defective alleles; influence of O:P interactions on cell growth and O activity

1. Introduction

Bacteriophage λ prophage is maintained within the chromosome of *Escherichia coli* cells by its CI repressor protein, which prevents the transcription of λ genes positioned leftward and rightward from promoters *pL* and *pR* that straddle *cI* (Figure 1A). CI binds to operator sites that overlap these promoters. Upon inactivation of CI, the derepressed prophage genes *N-int* are expressed from *pL*, and genes *cro-cII-O-P-Q* are expressed from *pR*. Transcription initiated from *pR* requires gpN activity to proceed effectively past the rho-dependent t_{R1} termination site positioned between *cro* and *cII* (reviewed in [1–4]).

The mechanism for bi-directional initiation of λ DNA replication involves a complex interaction of phage proteins gpO and gpP (designated herein as O and P) with *E. coli* host DNA replication proteins. In brief, O acts to bind the replicator site, *ori*λ, or origin for replication initiation that is situated midway within the *O* sequence [5,6]. The P protein recruits DnaB, the major replicative helicase for unwinding double-stranded DNA, bringing it to *ori*λ-bound O to form a DnaB:P:O:*ori*λ preprimosomal complex. P can commandeer DnaB away from its cellular equivalent, DnaC [7]. Since the interaction of P with DnaB inactivates the helicase activity of DnaB, the dissociation of P bound to DnaB in the preprimosomal complex is required to restore DnaB activity, which involves *E. coli* heat shock proteins DnaK, DnaJ, and GrpE [8,9]. By inhibiting transcription from *pR*, CI blocks a *cis* requirement for replication initiation described as transcriptional activation, explaining why providing O and P from a superinfecting heteroimmune phage will not stimulate replication initiation from an integrated resident *imm*λ prophage [10,11]. This requirement for *pR* transcription can be suppressed by *ri*^{C} (replicative-inhibition constitutive) mutations which lie outside of *ori*λ [12,13].

The excision of a λ prophage from the host chromosome between B.P′ and P.B′ sites (Figure 1A) is dependent upon λ genes *int* and *xis* (reviewed in [1,4,14]. Their expression requires that gpN antiterminate transcription at t_L terminator signals positioned between *pL-N* and ahead of *xis*. The PDS selection (refer to Abbreviations, Unique λ Terminology) for cell survivors of λ *N cI* ([Ts], temperature sensitive) prophage, named for its inventor [15], takes advantage of the induced prophage being unable to excise from the chromosome or lyse its host cell. In addition, the *N* null mutation reduces late λ gene expression and cell lysis, which depend on N for transcriptional antitermination at several t_R sites upstream of the late genes. Examinations for *E. coli* cell survival using the PDS selection led to the suggestion that mutations preventing the initiation of λ replication suppress cell killing [15–21].

The induction lethality phenotype for non-excisable prophage was termed Replicative Killing [18]. Accordingly, starting cells with de-repressible, but non-excisable prophage, as in Figure 1A,B, are termed RK$^+$ (Replicative Killing competent) cells and the selected survivor cells that form CFU at 42 °C were named Replicative Killing defective (RK$^-$) mutants (Figure 1C–G). The concept evolved that the starting cells possess the capacity for λ replication initiation upon prophage induction, whereas the survivor clones do not. The results of these early studies were reviewed [22]. Only a few mutations conferring the RK$^-$ phenotype for survivor CFU derived from the PDS selection or those from the N$^+$ λ fragment strains (an example is shown in Figure 1) have been characterized by DNA sequence analysis. Most all the RK$^-$ mutants were obtained before the possibility for PCR amplification of a mutated region of the chromosome, which enables direct sequence determination of the RK$^-$ mutation. Hence, those RK$^-$ mutations that have been characterized depended mainly upon genetic analysis using phage mapping and complementation.

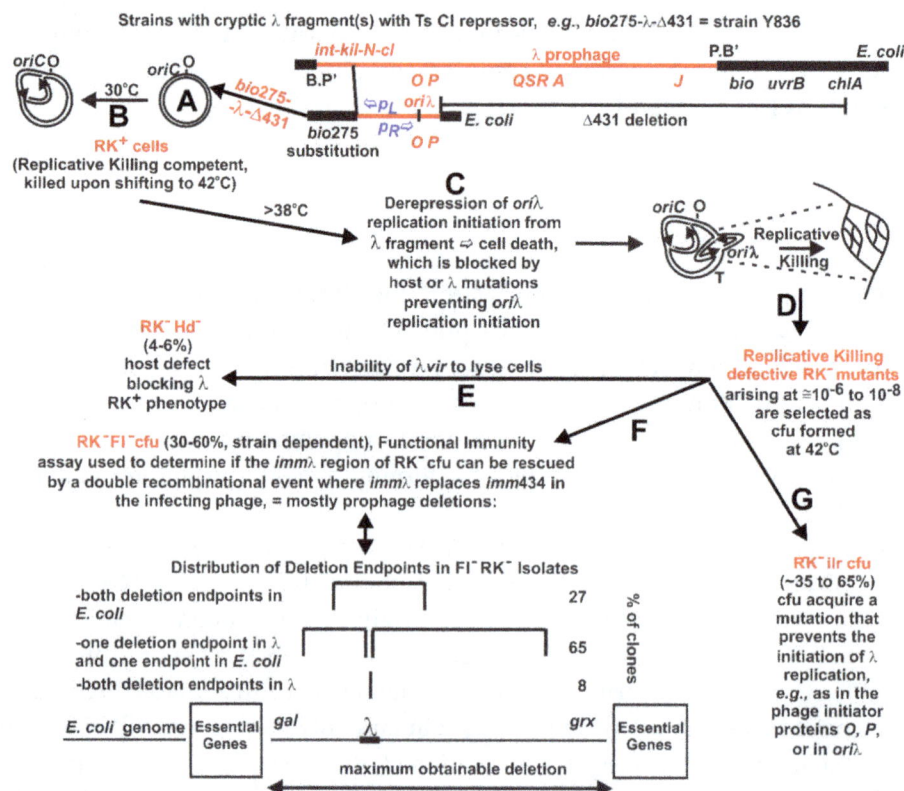

Figure 1. Replicative Killing, RK$^+$ phenotype and selection for RK$^-$ mutants. (**A**) Defective prophage strains were made where the *int-kil* or *int-ral* genes of λ were substituted with the *bio*275 or *bio*10 regions of specialized transducing phage to remove a phenotype termed "killing to the left", dependent on *kil* [23]. The starting cells included the *chlA* deletion Δ434 that removed all of the late genes, i.e., cell lysis, head and tail for λ [11]. These constructs include (i) an active *imm*λ region with gene *cI*[Ts]857

encoding a repressor that blocks transcription from promoters *pL* and *pR* along with the *cro* repressor just right of *pR*, and (ii) the *rep*λ region that includes genes *O* and *P* and the *ori*λ target for replication initiation from the λ genome. The genome for strain Y836, shown, has the *bio*+ operon to the left of the λ fragment and Δ431deletion to the right; (**B**) As long as strain Y836 maintains CI repressor activity the cells can grow normally without gene expression from the repressed λ fragment; (**C**) When the cells are shifted to growth conditions where the CI[Ts] repressor loses its ability to block transcription from *pL* and *pR* the remaining λ genes become derepressed, the phage replication initiation genes *O* and *P* are expressed and rounds of replication initiation arise from *ori*λ. The λ replication forks extend bidirectionally into the adjacent regions of the *E. coli* genome, likely colliding with *E. coli* replication forks. The event is highly lethal to the cell because the λ fragment has no mechanism for excision from the genome and was termed Replicative Killing [18]; (**D**) When cells with a conditionally repressible defective λ prophage are shifted from growth at 30 °C to 42 °C the Replicative Killing, RK+, phenotype is triggered, resulting in cell death. Rare mutations that suppress the loss of λ replication control are selected as RK− clones capable of colony formation at 42 °C. These survivor CFU have lost the capacity for λ replication. This strategy is based on the PDS selection [15], where an intact prophage is made *N*-defective, so that expression of *int-xis* and late/cell lysis gene expression is limited without *N*-antitermination of *pL* and *pR* transcription upon prophage induction. There are many possibilities for RK− mutants; (**E**) Cells acquiring defects in host genes participating λ replication are termed RK− Hd−. For example, the GrpD55 mutation in *dnaB* is of this type, though not isolated as shown [24,25]; (**F**) A marker rescue recombination assay is used to determine if the *imm*λ regions genes and target sites remain functional (i.e., FI+) when substituted for the *imm*434 region of a hybrid phage. The FI assay scores for the activity of the *pR* promoter, but in practice it is a good indication of whether the λ fragment in Y836 cells was partially or fully deleted. An example of the deletion endpoints of RK− FI− mutants from Y836 is shown [26–28]; (**G**) It was found that brief pretreatment RK+ of cells held at 30 °C with a mutagenic substance, prior to shifting them to 42 °C increases the frequency of RK− mutants. This assay, termed the RK Mutatest, proved very sensitive due to the rather large target potential for RK− mutants [29–31].

Genetic mapping of RK− mutations within *O* or *P* requires that both *O* and *P* initiator gene products can complement and function *in trans*. When a cell is infected with two phages, one defective in *O* and the other in *P*, complementation is observed suggesting that the products of these genes are diffusible [32]. However, Rao and Rodgers [33] were unable to demonstrate that cells carrying a ColE1 plasmid expressing *O*+ could complement, i.e., support the efficient plating of an infecting λ*imm*21 *O*am29 phage, even though the plasmid copy number varied between 50 copies at 32 °C and 260 copies at 42 °C. However, they could demonstrate *trans* complementation for phages with amber mutations in *N* or *P* by plasmids that can express these genes. Kleckner [34] suggested that *O* might act *in cis* or be poorly complemented under *N* defective conditions, and other experiments suggesting that O functions in *cis* were reported in [22]. These findings throw into question whether it is possible to designate using a phage complementation assay whether an induced RK− mutant has an *O*+ or *O*− phenotype. Alternatively, these divergent observations suggest that the ability of *O* to complement is more complex than initially assumed. A complicating problem in addressing this historical issue is that the mutant λ phages used in these early complementation assays were never subjected to DNA sequence analysis, so that in many cases their designations depend only upon unreported phage mapping studies, without accompanying proof of mutational site determination.

In this report, we examine the sequences of some early *O* mutations provided by A. Campbell from his original collection [35], and phages we have acquired over the years from laboratories that have participated in studies on *O*. We have cloned out *O* alleles from the chromosomes of RK− mutants and inserted them into a plasmid where the expression of the allele is regulated by CI[Ts], and is repressed in cells growing at 30 °C, or can be slightly to fully induced at growth temperatures between 37 °C and 42 °C. Each of these alleles was examined for their ability to complement the growth of a λ *O* amber mutant(s) *in trans*. We have explored the influence of O:P interactions on cell growth and toxicity, since the expression of *P* by itself, using the same system, is highly toxic [25,36]. These studies reveal that some alleles of *O* with internal deletions can complement as well or better than *O*[+] and that the co-expression of *O-P*, or of *O* with portions of the N-terminal end of *P*, prevents an ability of *O* to complement *in trans*.

2. Results

2.1. Taking Stock of O Mutations in Phage and Prophage Collections

DNA sequence characterization of *O* mutations in phage and prophage collections available to us is summarized, Table 1. Campbell (AC) described and mapped *O*am mutations 8, 29 and 125 [35]. Furth genetically mapped *O*am mutations and ordered them (N- to C-terminal) 905, 29, 1005, 8, 125, 205 by marker rescue using six prophage strains, each with a deletion designated as extending into *O* [37,40]. The original AC prophage in strain R573 representing *O*am125 included two missense mutations in addition to an amber mutation at 39511 bpλ. These three mutations were carried on a phage (our lysate #1024, Table 1) from LT designated MMS254. In contrast, isolate #1023 for *O*am29 designated LT-MMS99 included a silent mutation in addition to the amber mutation at 39511. Of relevance, four phage lysates (designated as carrying *O*am8 or *O*am29 mutations) that were obtained from researchers were found WT for λ genes *cII-O-P* through base 40712 in orf *ninB*, but they did include a nonsense mutation somewhere in λ since they grew well on a *supE* host but not on a *sup*[o] host. These results can explain why the initial assignment of an *O*[+] phenotype to some RK[−] ilr mutants proved incorrect (Figure 2).

Table 1. Collection of sequenced phage mutants in O and P.

Collection Isolate	Mutated Base in λ, Mutation(s), Comment, Strain Source [a]
Phage lysates (#)	
Mutations in *O*	
λ*cI*857 *O*am905 (#1022)	38797 G to T GAG to TAG), LT; 37 AA at N-terminal of *O*
λ [Ts] *O*am29 (#51)	38914 G to T (GAG to TAG), λ induced from AC 1966 slant R473, sc1,2; 76 AA from N-terminal of *O*
λ*cI*857 *O*am317 (#52)	39166 G to T (GAG to TAG), LT; 160 AA at N-terminal of *O*
λ *O*am8 (#50)	39301 A to T (AAG to TAG), λ induced from AC 1966 slant R377, sc1,2; 205 AA at N-terminal of *O*
λ*cI*857 *O*am8 (#1025)	39301 A to T (AAG to TAG), LT
λ*cI*857 *O*am205 (#586, 630)	39570, C to G, (TAC to TAG), WD; 294 AA from N-terminal of *O*
Mutations in *P*	
λ*imm*434*cI* Pam3 (#664)	39786 (CAG to TAG), WD
λ*cI*[+]*prm*116 Pam902 (#719,722)	39894 (CAG to TAG), GG
Host [b] (prophage), strain #	
C600(λ[Ts] *O*am29) #1170	38914 G to T (GAG to TAG) AC 1966 slant R473 (both sc's)
C600(λ *O*am8) #Y1169	39301 A to T (AAG to TAG), AC 1966 slant R377 (both sc's)
C600(λ Nam7 *cI*857[Ind] *O*am8) #Y239	39301 G to T (GAG to TAG), WD
M72 *su*[+] (λ Nam7 *cI*857 r95) #Y85 [c]	12 bpΔ λ bases 39123–39134, WD
M72 *su*[+] (λ Nam7 *cI*857 r96) #Y84 [c]	15 bpΔ λ bases 39139–39153, WD
M72 *su*[+] (λ Nam7 *cI*857 r98) #Y88	24 bpΔ λ bases 39096–39119, WD
594(λ Nam7 *cI*857 ti12) #188	39122 C to A (ACA to AAA), WD
Aberrant designations or with additional mutations, as received (lysate or strain #)	
λ*cI*857 *O*am8 (#16)	has nonsense mutation, but WT for *cII-O-P*-40712 in *ninB*; WS
λ*imm*434 *O*am8 (#656)	has nonsense mutation, but WT for *cII-O-P*-40712 in *ninB*; WD
λ*cI*857 *O*am8 (#518)	no mutation in *O*; 39786 in *P*, (CAG to TAG), same as Pam3; WS
λ*cI*857 *O*am29 (#582)	has nonsense mutation, WT for *cII-O-P*-40712 in *ninB*; WS
λ*cI*857 *O*am29 (#1023)	38914 G to T (GAG to TAG); 38713 T to C (TTC to TCC); LT-MMS99
λ*cI*857 *O*am125 (#1024)	39511 C to T (CAG to TAG); 39182 C to T (TCC to TTC); and 39510 A to T (CAA to CAT); LT-MMS254
594(λ*cI*857 *O*am8) #Y49, Y52	38914 G to T (GAG to TAG), really is *O*am29; WS
C600(λ *O*am125) #1171	39182 C to T (TCC to TTC); and 39510 A to T (CAA to CAT); and 39511 C to T (CAG to TAG), AC 1966 slant R573

[a] Known strain sources: AC, A. Campbell; LT, L. Thomason; GG, G. Gussin, WD, W. Dove; WS, W. Szybalski. Furth [37] reported the original sources of the *O*am mutations as: 8, 29 and 125 from [35], 905 from P. Toothman and I. Herskowitz, 1005 from I. Herskowitz, and 205 [38]. "AA" = amino acid(s). [b] Host C600 is *SupE*; The Pm[−] hosts 594 and M72 are *sup*[o]. [c] Transcription from *pL* and *pR*, the lack of replication arising from *ori*λ, and the absence of any increase in phage titer following prophage induction were reported for these strains in [39].

2.2. Replicative Killing Selection and Mutants

The selection of RK⁻ mutants with defects in λ replication initiation were categorized (Figure 1) as follows: RK⁻ clones designated Hd⁻ (host defects), representing about 4% to 6% of selected spontaneous RK⁻ clones [22], are not lysed by λ*vir*. These mutants are arbitrarily considered to have an altered host gene whose product participates in vegetative λ growth, or a λ-fragment mutation whose effect is to complement negatively for the growth of λ*vir*. The RK⁻ clones that are lysed by λ*vir*, retain the *imm*λ phenotype at 30 °C, and were FI⁺, were designated RK⁻ ilr (initiation of λ replication defective). The FI, or functional immunity assay [11,41], represents a stab of an RK⁻ CFU to a lawn of cells lysogenized with λ*imm*434T to which is added free λ*imm*434*cI*. If *imm*λ double recombinant phage can be generated (indicated by a lysis area forming around the RK⁻ clone stabbed to the overlay plate), this is taken to indicate that the *imm*λ region encoding *o*L/*p*L -*cI*- *o*R/*p*R is functional both in the RK⁻ mutant and in the *imm*λ recombinant. The RK⁻ FI⁻ Imm⁻ isolates mainly have had large deletions (>10 Kb) [26–28]. In an examination of the spontaneous RK⁻ mutants/mutations arising from four RK⁺ N⁺ selector strains, 256/650 RK⁻ isolates were the RK⁻ ilr type [22].

Figure 2 shows eight sequences for RK⁻ ilr mutants falling within *O-P* that were derived from induced *N*⁺ prophage, along with mutants derived from induced *N*⁻ prophage, including ori-95, -96, -98 obtained by Rambach [20] and ti12 from the Dove laboratory [18]). The sequences for ori95 and ori98 were not previously reported [42]. The ori96 mutation was a 15 bp deletion of λ bases 39139–39153 (not 39138–39152 as reported [42]). Mutation ori98 removed the entire iteron-ITN4 region, and ori95 and ori96 each deleted part of the High-AT rich region within *O*. Except for ilr541c, which included a stop codon that eliminated translation of the last 35 codons of *O*, the remaining RK⁻ ilr *O* mutations (Figure 2) represented small deletions within *O* or insertions that could exert a polar effect on downstream *P* expression. Each of the ilr mutants were initially scored as being *O*⁺, which clearly was not proved correct by sequence analysis. None of the ilr mutations had in-frame deletions within *O* as with those obtained in Rambach's λ *N*⁻ selection.

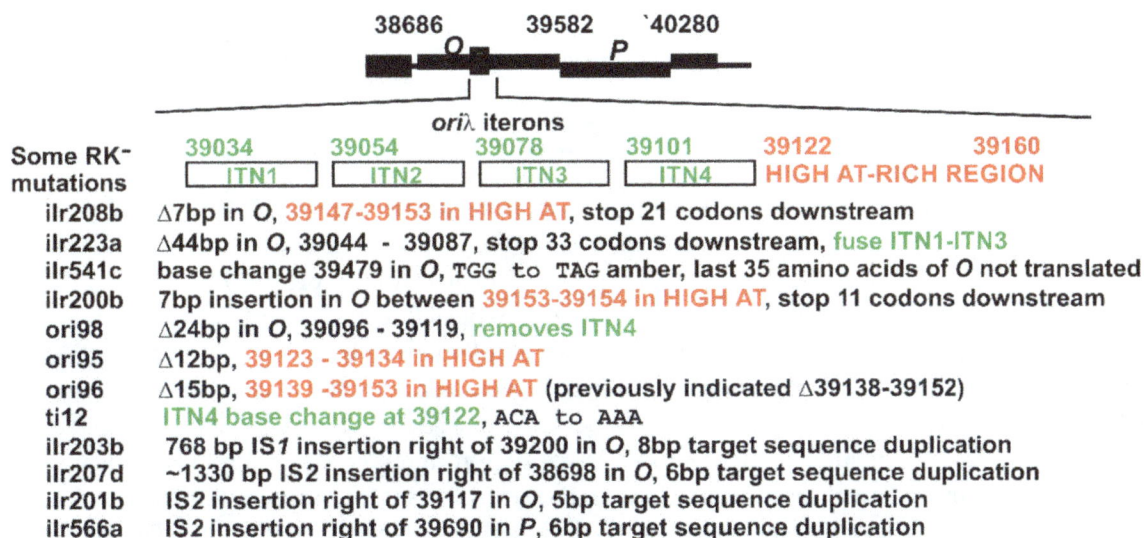

Figure 2. RK⁻ ilr mutations characterized within λ genes *O-P*. The minimal *ori*λ size was suggested to include a HIGH-AT-rich region to the right of four iteron sequences, ITN's1-4 [43,44], which each contain an 18 bp inverted repeat of hyphenated symmetry, joined by adenine residues that can cause *ori*λ to assume a bent structure [45]. The mutants shown designated ori95, ori96 and ori98 were obtained from WD from prophage with *r*-mutants *r-95*, *r-96*, and *r-98*. Note that Denniston-Thompson, et al., [46] sequenced the *r*-mutants *r-99*, *r-96* and *r93* which represent Δ12 bp (39120–39131), Δ15 bp (39138–39152) and Δ24 bp (39092–39115) [42]. Our sequence localization for ori96 (*r96*) differs by one bp from that assigned in [42].

2.3. Complementation for O Activity in Trans

The wild type *O* protein is 299 amino acids (AA) [43]. Alleles of *O* were cloned into an expression plasmid, Figure 3. Each allele was from an RK⁻ mutant for which complementation analysis had suggested was *O*⁺.

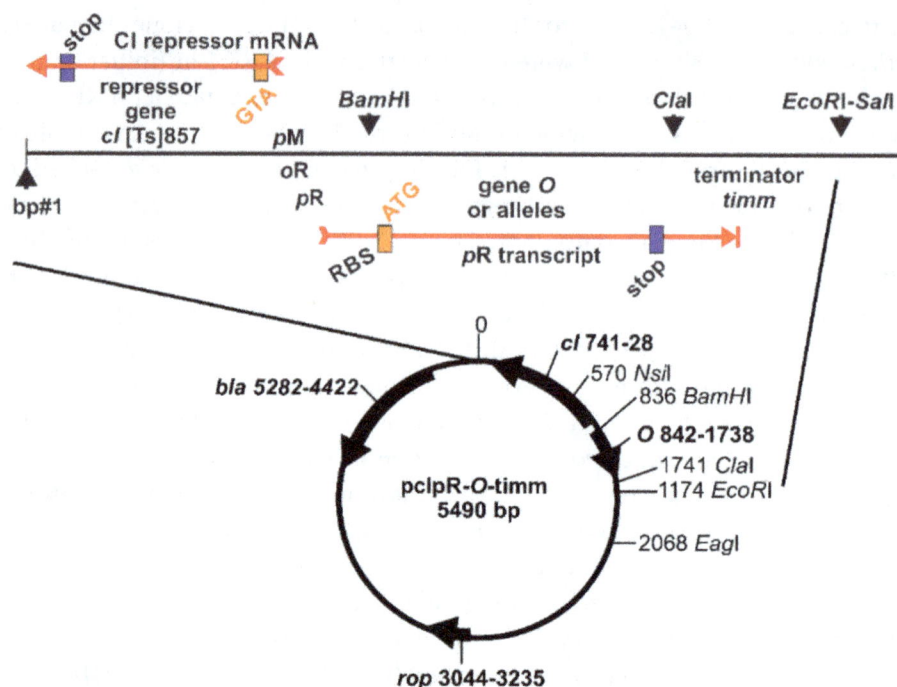

Figure 3. Expression vector pcIpR-(*O* alleles)-timm. Expression of gene *O* or an allele occurs upon inactivation of the CI repressor by raising cells grown at 30 °C to 42 °C. Immediately following the 299 codons of *O* is an ochre stop codon, where the last base in TAA represents the first base of the *Cla*I restriction site ATCGAT.

Each plasmid was transformed into 594 cells, creating strains as 594[pcIpR-*O*-timm] that were used as hosts for λ *O*am plating. The assays for *O* complementation were incubated at 30, 37, 39 and 42 °C. The results for plating assays at 42 °C, where the *O* allele is fully expressed, are shown in Table 2. Phages whose *O* allele produced 76 or 294 AA's of O were weakly complemented by O⁺, whereas the *O*am905 mutation expressing 37 AA of O was not complemented by O⁺. Complementation was improved 5- to 6-fold in two of the three λ *O*am suppression assays by the addition of a SPA tag to the COOH end of the wild type *O* sequence, i.e., the addition of a seven AA linker (GGSGAPM) joined to the 69 AA SPA tag [47] sequence. The *O-ori*:98 mutation removing ITN4 within *O* was incapable of complementing for O. Remarkably, *O* alleles with the *ori*:ti12 point mutation in ITN4 and those with *ori*:95 and *ori*:96 in-frame deletions, respectively, of 12 and 15 bp's within the High AT-rich region of *ori*λ, were each able to complement all three *O*am mutants. Any condition where P, or a portion of the N-terminal end of P was expressed, completely prevented O-complementation. Induced prophage strains with insertions within *P*, but with sequenced intact *O* genes that would be fully derepressed when shifted to 42 °C were incapable of providing for O complementation. The RK⁻ ilr mutants, previously designated phenotypically as *O*⁺ [11], proved to have insertions or deletions in *O* and should not complement, as was found for the cloned prophage *O* genes from mutants 208b, 223a and 541c (each of which could complement for *P* [36]).

Table 2. Complementation of λ *O*am mutants by alleleic forms of *O* expressed from plasmids.

Host Strains and [Plasmid] # [a]	EOP of λ Phage with *O*am Mutants [b]		
	λ *cI857* *O*am905 [c] (37 AA of *O*)	λ *cI857* *O*am29 [c] (76 AA of *O*)	λ *cI857* *O*am205 [c] (294 AA of *O*)
Pm⁺ *SupE* [d]	1.0	1.0	1.0
Pm⁻ *Sup*⁰	0	0	0
Complementation by *O* variations			
O⁺ combinations			
[O] [e], p465	0	0.2	0.1
[O-SPA] [f], p472	0	1.0	0.6
[oop-O] [g], p677	0.05	0.1	0.1
O null mutations [h]			
[O-ilr208b], p488	0	0	0
[O-ilr223a], p486	0	0	0
[O-ilr541c], p485	0	0	0
O-origin (*ori*λ) mutations [i]			
[O-ori:98], p489	0	0	0
[O-ori:95], p491	0.2	0.3	0.2
[O-ori:96], p492	0.3	1.0	0.3
[O-ori:ti12], p493	0.3	0.1	0.3
O-P combinations [j]			
[O-36P], p565	0	0.01	0
[O-63P], p566	0	0	0
[O-P], p569	0	0	0
[oop-O-P] [k] p567, p568	0	0	0
RK⁻ O⁺ P⁻ prophage derived from Y836 transduced into 594			
ilr 566a [l]	0	0	0.002
P::kan [m], Bib11t	0	0	0.001

[a] All of the complementation studies were undertaken in strains 594[pcIpR-Ovariant-timm] or with 594 cells transduced for the λ fragment mutants (ilr566a, BiB11t) from the original RK⁺ strain Y836. The host strain 594 is designated as being nonpermissive, Pm⁻ (sup⁰), without an amber suppressor). The precise sequences for each of the allelic forms of *O* were amplified by PCR, cloned into plasmid pcIpR-(..)-timm, between *Bam*HI and *Cla*I sites (designated by the internal brackets), and the inserted *O*-variant fragments were each verified by DNA sequence analysis. Each plasmid includes an allele of *O* positioned as is gene *cro* in WT λ, just downstream of promoter *pR* and the consensus ribosomal binding site (RBS) for *cro*. The initiation of transcription from *pR* is regulated by the Ts CI857 λ repressor encoded on the plasmid via binding to the operator site, *oR* that overlaps *pR*. For cells grown at 30 °C the CI Ts repressor remains active, binds to *oR* and blocks transcription initiation from *pR*. When the cells are shifted to 39–42 °C the CI Ts repressor transitions from partially to fully-inactive, allowing transcription initiation from *pR* and the expression of the downstream *O* allele. [b] The EOP value for "0" was set to <0.001. Thus, the difference between "0" and 0.1 is more than 100-fold. The efficiency of plating (EOP) was assessed at 30, 39 and 42 °C on cell lines containing plasmids. At 30 °C the results were all 0, i.e., the EOP was <0.001. In every situation, the plating results obtained at 42 °C showed an equivalent, or somewhat higher EOP than at 39 °C. All EOP data were calculated as: titer of *O*am phage on indicated host with plasmid containing *O* allele/titer of the same phage on the Pm⁺ SupE host at same temperature. The phage titer on the Pm⁺ SupE strain was set as EOP = 1.0. All values are rounded up and are relative so that standard error is not shown but represents ±10–20% of the values indicated. Each of the plating phage were sequenced throughout the *oop-O-P-ren* genes and shown to contain only the designated *O*am mutation. [c] Sequence designations for the *O* mutations are shown in Table 1 with mutations introducing amber stop codons: *O*am905 at 38797, *O*am29 at 38914, and *O*am205 at 39579. To have all phages include the *cI857* mutation the lysate #1023 was used for *O*am29 which includes a silent mutation at 38713 (Ser to Ser). The phage nonsense mutations in *O* truncate gene expression, producing polypeptides of the length shown in the heading of Table 2, each with the N-terminal end of the WT protein. [d] Permissive, Pm⁺, strain was TC600 *SupE*, where the efficiency for amber suppression (not complementation) was used as the baseline for full complementation. [e] Sequence for *O* (λ WT bases 38686–39582), representing 299 codons, plus an ochre stop codon was inserted to make plasmid pcIpR-*O*-timm. [f] Fusion construct represents WT *O*-(7 amino acid linker GGSGAPM)-69 amino acid SPA tag sequence-ochre stop codon. The SPA tag sequence at COOH end of *O* includes a calmodulin binding site, a TEV (tobacco etch virus) protease cleavage site and 3X FLAG sequence [47]. [g] Results approximate data for two plasmid constructs oop#1-*O*, representing λ WT bases 38559–39582, and oop#2-*O*, representing λ bases 38546–39582, each inserted between the BamHI and ClaI sites in pcIpR-(..)-timm. [h] Replicative-Killing defective (RK⁻) mutants in gene *O* (see Figure 2) isolated as survivors from induced cryptic λ prophage strain Y836 as described in [11,48]. [i] Removed *O* fragments from replicator mutants of M72(λ Nam7am53 *cI857* r95), M72(λ Nam7am53 *cI857* r96), and M72(λ Nam7am53 *cI857* r98) lysogens from Rambach [20] via WD. [j] Plasmids were described in [25]. Each plasmid includes the intact sequence of *O* (λ bases 38686–39582 plus the N-terminal portions of gene *P* followed by ochre stop codon: 38686–39687 = O-P36, 38686–39768 = O-P63, 38686–40280 = O-P. Note that *O* and *P* are in different reading frames. [k] Plasmids p567 oop#1-O-P and p568 oop#2-O-P include λ bases 38559–40280 and 38546–40280, respectively, cloned between the *Bam*HI and *Cla*I sites in the pcIpR-(..)-timm plasmid [25]. The oop-O-P line represents equivalent data for plasmids oop#1-O-P and oop#2-O-P. [l] The RK⁻ ilr mutant 566a derived from strain Y836 was transduced using P1 with the marker *nad57*::Tn*10* that was inserted contiguous to the chromosomal λ fragment. Then the Tet^R *imm*λ region was transduced into strain 594. [m] The *kan* marker was introduced into gene *P* in strain Y836 by recombineering (=strain Bib11t) and the defective λ fragment was transduced into 594 cells as indicated for moving mutation 566a (see [25] for additional details).

2.4. Influence of O-P Co-Expression on Cell Growth, P-Lethality, and Plasmid Loss

The expression of P, or N-terminal fragments of P, block O complementation (Table 2). If O and P expression can influence O complementation, does their co-expression negate P-lethality? Figure 4 shows that *O* expression alone, or the co-expression of WT genes *O* and *P* over a span of four doublings in culture absorbance (with 45 min per doubling) did not perturb cell growth for cultures shifted from growth at 30 °C to 42 °C. In contrast, expressing *P* alone, or constructs expressing *oop-O-P*, or constructs that were WT for *O* but could express a portion of the N-terminal region of *P* were each highly inhibitory to cell growth. Table 3 shows the effect of *O-P* constructs on cell viability and plasmid loss. We re-examined several of the observations reported in [25], where the expression of *P*, even in trace levels at 37 °C, kills about 99% of the transformed cells and all plasmids were lost in survivor CFU's. The lethality of P is completely suppressed by two missense mutations in *dnaB* that comprise the allele *dnaB*-GrpD55. Expressed by itself, O is not toxic and does not cause plasmid loss. Co-expression of *O-P* reduces the cellular toxicity of *P* expression alone by 12 to 15-fold at 37 and 39 °C. Co-expression of *oop-O-P* significantly prevents plasmid loss at 37 and 39 °C but exerts a minimal effect on cell viability. The inclusion of portions of the N-terminal end of *P* plus *O* significantly reduces cell viability and plasmid retention at 39 and 42 °C, compared to the expression of only *O*.

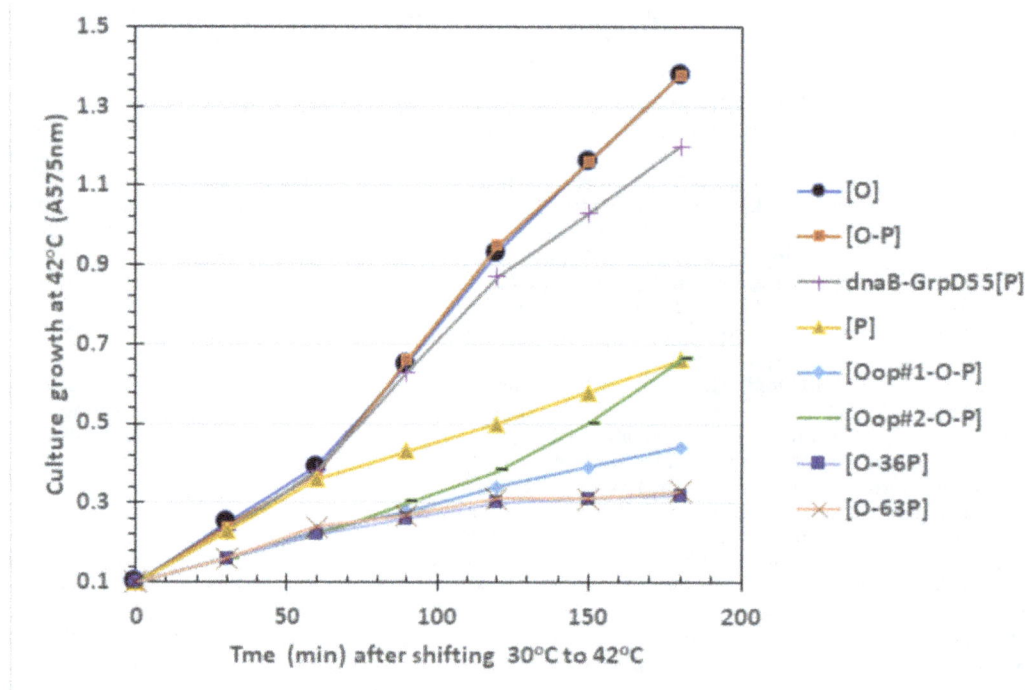

Figure 4. Influence of induced *O, P* gene expression on cell growth at 42 °C. All the strains were made by transforming hosts 594 or 594 *dnaB*-GrpD55 with pcIpR-(..)-timm plasmids that included the cloned *O*, *P* DNA fragment, and selecting the transformants on LBAmp50 agar (medium composition is described in footnote to Table 3). The plasmid inserts in each CFU employed were verified by DNA sequence analysis. Cells were inoculated from overnight cultures grown up overnight in LBAmp50 broth and then 0.4 mL of culture was added to triplicate 20 mL fresh LB cultures that were incubated at 30 °C for 30 min to reach an A575 = 0.1. Upon reaching an absorbance of 0.1 the cultures were transferred to a shaking 42 °C water bath. Aliquots were sampled every 30 min for 3 h. The average absorbance is shown, with a standard error for each culture time of less than 5% the averaged absorbance value.

Table 3. Does *O-P* co-expression temper P-lethality and plasmid loss?

Plasmid in 594 Host Cells	Cell Viability and (Plasmid Retention per CFU Assayed; %) at CFU Growth Temperature [a]			
	30 °C	37 °C	39 °C	42 °C
Only *P* expression				
[P]	1.0 (35/35; 100%)	0.01 (0/35; 0%)	0.008 (0/35; 0%)	0.07 (0/35; 0%)
dnaB-GrpD55 [P]	1.0 (35/35; 100%)	1.0 (35/35; 100%)	1.0 (35/35; 100%)	0.98 (35/35; 100%)
Only *O* expression				
[O]	1.0 (30/30; 100%)	1.0 (30/30; 100%)	1.0 (30/30; 100%)	0.61 (29/30; 97%)
O-P expression combinations				
[O-P]	1.0 (62/70; 89%)	0.12 (0/70; 0%)	0.12 (0/70; 0%)	0.022 (0/36; 0%)
[oop#1-O-P]	1.0 (120/120; 100%)	0.20 (98/101; 97%)	0.005 (115/120; 96%)	0.002 (0/36; 0%)
[oop#2-O-P]	1.0 (117/120; 98%)	0.055 (76/154; 49%)	0.048 (62/120; 52%)	0.008 (0/36; 0%)
[O-36P]	1.0 (30/30; 100%)	0.79 (30/30; 100%)	0.012 (1/30; 3%)	0.0005 (0/36; 0%)
[O-63P]	1.0 (30/30; 100%)	0.90 (30/30; 100%)	0.055 (14/40; 35%)	0.0023 (0/36; 0%)

[a] The 594 cultures with indicated plasmids were grown to stationary phase in LB (10 g Bacto-Tryptone, 10 g Bacto-Yeast Extract, 5 g NaCl per liter) plus 50 μg/mL ampicillin (=LBAmp50) for 48 h at 30 °C, diluted, spread on LB agar (includes the addition of 11 g/liter Bacto-Agar) plates (no ampicillin) that were incubated at 30, 37, 39, or 42 °C for 30 h and the average survivor titer for CFU per mL was determined for each plating temperature. Isolated survivor CFU were stabbed to LB and to LBAmp50 agar plates to estimate the proportion of CFU retaining the Amp^R plasmid. We tried to assay all the CFU per plate to avoid colony size discrimination, and minimally 30 CFU. The cell viability results shown in each column entry were determined by dividing the cell titer obtained for each incubation by the cell titer at 30 °C, and each value represents the average of duplicate plasmid isolates for each single experiment, with plating variations of about 10%. The results in parentheses represent the sum of results for all the CFU's assayed from isolates. These results represent independent determinations by KR to those reported in [25], where it was shown that 594[P] cells lost 100% of their plasmids when grown at 36 °C and higher, indicating that trace levels of *P* expression (where the CI[Ts] repressor still retains some ability to block *pR*-promoted transcription below about 38–39 °C) will cure cells of the plasmid.

The *oop* DNA sequence encodes a 77-base noncoding small RNA that is transcribed in an antisense orientation to *O*. Part of the *oop* sequence overlaps the sequence for gene *cII* preceding *O*, with the *pO* promoter for *oop* transcription overlapping the N-terminal end of the *O* sequence. The #1 and #2 *oop-O* or *oop-O-P* constructs are deleted for the N-terminal end of cII. Since *O* or *O-P* are directly transcribed from *pR* on the plasmid, we asked if the antisense *oop* transcript would influence O or P activity expressed from the plasmid. Except for its ability to support some low-level suppression of λOam905 plating, OOP RNA expression does not significantly influence O complementation (Table 2); however, it exhibits a profound effect on the ability of P expression to evoke plasmid loss (Table 3), over and above the quenching influence of *O-P* co-expression on cellular P-lethality. A hypothesis is that OOP RNA hybridization to the *pR-oop-O-P* mRNA expressed from the induced plasmid reduces downstream *P* translation/accumulation within the cell.

3. Discussion

3.1. O-Complementation

Our sequencing of Oam29 reveals that this *O* allele encodes 294 of 299 amino acids. Thus, the last five amino acids of O are essential for O activity, and yet 76 amino acids, i.e., a linker and the SPA tag sequence, can be added to its COOH-terminal end, with the effect of improving the ability of O to complement.

Until this report, no one appears to have determined if in-frame deletions within *O* can influence its ability to complement, or will simply nullify its activity. We show that the 24 bp deletion in ori98 (*r98*) removing ITN4 nullifies the ability of O to complement; however, the 12 and 15 bp deletions in ori95 and ori96 (*r95*, *r96*), each falling within the High-AT rich region of *ori*λ improved the ability of O to complement. In addition, the *ori*λ *ti*12 mutation, representing a mismatch changing threonine to lysine within the ITN4 interval seemed to improve, rather than reduce, O complementation.

We were unable to demonstrate O complementation or saw extremely poor complementation for two sequenced *O*^+ prophages in *N*^+ RK^− cells, each of which had acquired insertions within *P*, i.e., strains ilr566a and Bib11t. This result leads us to question whether it is possible to demonstrate complementation where the prophage for the RK⁻ cells carries a N^- mutation and would poorly express O, e.g., Rambach's conclusion that the $r96$ mutant isolated from an N^- prophage complemented for O. Indeed, full O^+ expression from the pcIpR-O-timm plasmid in cells plated at 42 °C did not complement (i.e., support plaque formation of) a phage with an Oam905 mutation.

3.2. O:P Interaction Effects

The functional cooperation of O and P in λ replication initiation was suggested by genetic studies [49]. The N-terminal region of O was suggested to contain a DNA binding domain and the COOH-terminal region to contain a P-binding domain [40,50,51], with the domains separated by a flexible linker region [52]. Tsurimoto and Matsubara [5] showed that O protein binds to each ITN as a dimer, thus $ori\lambda$ should bind four dimers, with higher order binding suggested [53] to form an O-some that produces torsional stress on the adjacent AT rich region causing the double-stranded DNA to become slightly destabilized and partially unwound [54]. The N-terminal portion of P was assumed to contain an O-binding domain [55], while its COOH-terminal domain was suggested to interact with the host DnaB replicative helicase [55,56]. It has been suggested that a complex between O and P is formed that can be independent of DnaB [51,57].

In essence, the idea was advanced that O bound to $ori\lambda$ is a display platform that is recognized by P:DnaB. However, we show that the co-expression of O-P results in several phenotypic effects which suggest that this idea is too simplistic. The co-expression of O-P nullifies the inhibitory effect of P expression on cell growth, for over four hours, and it reduces cell killing caused by prolonged expression of P (i.e., when expressed at 39 °C). In contrast, the co-expression of O-P nullifies the ability of O to complement. These opposed activities suggest that O and P physically interact without having O bound to $ori\lambda$. Combining O expression with the possibility for expression of the N-terminal portion of P eliminates O complementation, suggesting that O binding to the N-terminal portion of P prevents its useful binding to $ori\lambda$, which is presumably a requirement for O complementation activity. However, the co-expression O-P does not temper the ability of P to cause plasmid loss. Thus, while the expression of P, or N-terminal portions of P, can obviate O complementation, coordinate O expression does not fully nullify all the P-lethality phenotypes.

3.3. RK⁻ Mutant Selection Considerations

Dove and Blattner's laboratories collaborated in mapping [40] and sequencing [46] some of the nine r mutants selected by Rambach [20], who based his selection on the assumption that the "replicator" gene was different from initiator genes O or P. They concluded that regions of the initiator gene, i.e., O, overlap the replicator site, now termed $ori\lambda$. We show herein that regions of $ori\lambda$ are not essential for activity of the O initiator protein. We previously demonstrated [39] that λ Nam7am53 cI857 $r95$, or $r96$ prophages in su^+ hosts (hence the prophages were phenotypically N^+) were defective in $ori\lambda$ replication initiation, were 7- to 17-fold reduced in pR-Q transcription, and did not yield any increase in phage titer after prophage induction. Five of the nine r mutants have now been sequenced and each has a small, in-frame deletion within O. In contrast, among hundreds of RK⁻ ilr mutants isolated from a defective N^+ prophage (Figure 1), none were identified with in-frame deletions in O. Nor, have other instances involving use of the PDS, or similar selections resulted in small in-frame deletions within O being reported [12,16,17,58,59]. The major theme of those reports was that perturbing the expression of pR-O-P can influence replication initiation. The recent documentation on the lethal effect of P expression (see [25,36] and included references) may help to explain the selection differences, i.e., constitutive P expression is lethal to a cell, even if there is no replication initiation from $ori\lambda$. Rambach's study required several other unstated assumptions: (i) replication initiation will occur from an induced N mutant prophage with reduced transcription of O-P (we note above that this was not observed for the $r95$ and $r96$ mutants); (ii) in induced N-defective prophage, sufficient rightward transcription occurs across (or near to) the replicator ($ori\lambda$) site to provide the requirement for transcriptional activation (as noted above, even when the r-mutant prophages were made su^+ rightward transcription across pR-Q was significantly reduced); and (iii) the constitutive expression of the replication initiation proteins O and P or other de-repressed λ gene products will not be lethal to the host cell. Assumptions (i) and (ii) may still require additional study. A previous characterization of RK$^-$ ilr survivor mutations from N^+ prophage, revealed that all were defective in P or had insertions in O that could limit downstream P expression [48], suggesting that assumption (iii) is unlikely.

4. Materials and Methods

4.1. Complementation Assays and Initial Strategy for Characterizing RK$^-$ Mutants

Past studies have generated hundreds of RK$^-$ mutants capable of colony formation at 42 °C. Since almost all these mutants were selected prior to an ability to combine PCR with rapid DNA sequence analysis of the generated PCR fragment, the characterization of the genetic defect that permitted cell survival and growth at 42 °C required genetic analysis. This, in principle, involved complementation analysis for expression of genes N, cI, cro, cII, O, and P. Of those mutants that retained an active $imm\lambda$ region encoding a Ts CI repressor, the cells grown at 30 °C expressed an immune response to plating by $imm\lambda$ phage, but not to the heteroimmune phages as $\lambda imm434$. Shifting the cells to growth at 42 °C inactivated the Ts CI repressor and permitted the expression of N, cro, cII, O, and P. RK$^-$ clones were inoculated into 1.5 mL tryptone broth (TB: 10 g of Bacto Tryptone, 5 g of NaCl per liter) and grown to stationary phase at 30 °C. One-tenth mL of each culture was mixed with dilutions high titer lysates $imm\lambda$ or $imm434$ phages carrying an amber mutation in genes N, O, or P (none of which—at the time—were characterized by DNA sequence analysis) plus 2.5 mL of TB top agar (0.65%) agar. The mixture was poured on TB agar (1.1%) plates that were incubated at 42 °C. In the present study lysates of λ phage with Oam mutants were freshly prepared. A single colony of E. coli strain 594 or these cells transformed with different versions of O plasmids were grown in LBAmp50 broth (see footnote "a" Table 3) at 30 °C overnight. Then a mixture of cells and soft agar (3 mL of warm top agar, 0.25 mL of cells and 0.25 mL of 0.01 M MgCl$_2$) was poured on the top of LB plates. After agar solidification, diluted Oam λ phage lysates were spotted on the agar, allowed to dry, the plates were incubated inverted at 30, 37, 39 and 42 °C overnight and plaque forming units were counted. The appearance of plaques at elevated plating efficiency indicated complementation for the defective gene carried on the infecting phage by the thermally induced prophage in the RK$^-$ mutant cells or expressed from the plasmid. 100% plating efficiency was equated to the titer of the amber phage mutant on E. coli cells with a suppressor tRNA, e.g., on strain TC600 $supE$. Very low plating efficiency ($<10^{-4}$) suggested phage-prophage marker rescue. The ability of RK$^-$ cells to complement for the wild type functions expressed from N or P has always been very simple to assess. However, the interpretation of whether O expressed from the induced prophage was able to complement an Oam infecting phage proved problematic.

4.2. DNA Sequence Analysis of λ Phage, Prophage and Plasmid Constructs

The DNA sequencing results reported herein, for each plasmid construct and phage isolate were obtained by us using methods for colony PCR, plaque PCR, and PCR amplification of cloned regions from isolated plasmid constructs, as previously described [60]. The actual sequencing results were obtained from sequencing services at the NRC National Biotechnology Institute, Saskatoon, or were submitted to Eurofins Genomics. The oligonucleotide primers employed, Table 4, were obtained from Integrated DNA Technologies, Inc. Coralville, IA, USA. In every case, at minimum, four individual representative colony, plaque or plasmids were sequenced per construct or isolate.

4.3. Plasmid Constructs

The O gene alleles were amplified from E. coli strains with a prophage (e.g., each of the RK$^-$ mutants shown in Figure 2) or λ phage DNA, using PCR primers L-Bam-O and R-ClaI-O. The PCR fragments were cloned just downstream of promoter *pR* between the *Bam*HI and *Cla*I restriction sites in the pcIpR-(. . .)-timm plasmid isolated from a *dam* host strain, as drawn in Figure 3. The R-ClaI-O primer introduces an ochre stop codon at the COOH-terminal end of *O*. Primers L-Bam-P and R-ClaI-P were used for to clone gene *P*. Primers L-Bam-O and R-ClaI-P were used to clone genes *O-P*, which include the natural TGA stop codon for *O* and an ochre codon terminating *P*. The construction of plasmids pcIpR-*P*-timm, pcIpR-*O*-timm, pcIpR-*O-P*-timm, pcIpR-*O*-36*P*-timm, pcIpR-*O*-63-*P*-timm, pcIpR-*oop*#1-timm, and pcIpR-*oop*#2-timm was as reported in [25]. The plasmids oop-O and oop-O-P, Table 2, were constructed using primers L-Bam-oop#1 or L-Bam-oop#2 and R-ClaI-O to make oop-O and R-ClaI-P to make oop-O-P and the PCR fragments were cloned between the *Bam*HI and *Cla*I restriction sites in the unmethylated pcIpR-(. . .)-timm plasmid. Plasmid O-SPA was constructed by removing the *Bam*HI-*P*-*Asc*I fragment from pcIpR-*P*-SPA-timm [25] and inserting the fragment *Bam*HI-*O*-*Asc*I prepared using primers L-Bam-O and R-O-AscI. This construct is described in footnote "f" of Table 2. The DNA template used for amplifying wild type alleles of *oop-O-P* was from λ*cI*857 [25].

4.4. Bacterial and Phage Strains

The genotype, source and laboratory reference number for bacterial strains 594 (Pm$^-$), TC600 (Pm$^+$), 594 *dnaB*-grpD55 is described in Table 10 in reference [25] as are the reference phages (see also [41]). Y836, Y836 *P*:kan (Bib11t), Y836 RK$^-$ ilr566a are described in Table 8 in reference [36]. Examples showing the characterization of RK$^-$ mutants can be found in [11,48].

Table 4. Oligonucleotide primers employed for DNA sequence analysis and plasmid constructions.

Name	λ Map Position	Sequence (5′ to 3′) [a]
L-37904+18	37904–37922	GCTGCTCTTGTGTTAATGG
L-MH29	37905–37922	CGTCCTCAAGCTGCTCTTGTGTTAATGG
L20	39465–39484	ACTCCGCGATAAGTGGACCC
L-22	38517–38534	TGCTGCTTGCTGTTCTTG
L-PG30	38530–38547	TTGGAACTGAGAAGACAG
L-PG1	38784–38801	AAATATGCTGCTTGAGGC
L-38985p20	38985–39005	GCAGCAAGGCGGCATGTTTGG
L-MH32	39531–39550	CACAGATCTATAGCAAACCAAAACTCGACCTGA
L-18	39980–39996	TTGCCGGAAGCGAGGCC
L-21	40360–40377	CGCAACAGTAACCAGCAT
R-PG2	40747–40764	GGTTGCGTTCCTGAATGG
L-Bam-O	38686–38718	ATATGGATCCATGACAAATACAGCAAAAATACTCAACTTCGGC
L-Bam-P	39582–39606	ATATGGATCCATGAAAAACATCGCCGCACAGATGG
L-Bam-OOP#1	38559–38580	ATATGGATCCTGGCTCGATTGGCGCGACAAGT
L-Bam-OOP#2	38546–38577	ATATGGATCCGTTGACGACGACATGGCTCGAT
L-Bam-O	38686–38718	ATATGGATCCATGACAAATACAGCAAAAATACTCAACTTCGGC
L-Bam-P	39582–39606	ATATGGATCCATGAAAAACATCGCCGCACAGATGG
R-40769m22	40747–40769	GCTGCGGTTGCGTTCCTGAATGG
R-MH33	40315–40295	GCGACGTCCCCAGGTAATGAATAATTGC
R-17	40018–40002	TAAGACTCCGCATCCGG
R-MH25	39626–39609	CTGCTCACGGTCAAAGTT
R-39280m21	39259–39280	CTGCGGCGGTCAGGTCTTCTGC
R9+1	39191–39175	TGGTCAGAGGATTCGCC
R-PG6	38569–38552	CAATCGAGCCATGTCGTC
R-1536-19	pcIpR-()-timm	GAAGACAGTCATAAGTGCGG
R-ClaI-P	40280–40259	ATATATCGATTATACACTTGCTCCTTTCAGTCCG
R-ClaI-O	39582–39559	ATATATCGATTATAGATCCACCCCGTAAATCCAGTC
R-ClaI-36P	39687–39662	ATATATCGATTACCTGCTGTACCTGCGGCTTTTCGTCG
R-ClaI-63P	39768–39746	ATATATCGATTACTTCGTTCTGGTCACGGTTAGCC
R-AscI-O	39582–39559	ATATGGCGCGCCGCTGCCGCCTAGATCCACCCCGTAAATCCAGTC

[a] The portion of primer sequences shown in smaller font size contain restrictions sites used for cloning into plasmids and are not included within λ map sequence shown.

Acknowledgments: This work was supported by NSERC Canada Discovery grant 138296 to Sidney Hayes. The funder had no role in study design, data collection and analysis, decision to publish, or preparation of the manuscript.

Author Contributions: Performed the experiments and helped analyze the data: Connie Hayes and Karthic Rajamanickam. Conceived, designed the experiments, and wrote the paper: Sidney Hayes.

Abbreviations

Unique λ Terminology:Replicative Killing (RK⁺) competent phenotype: A property of *E. coli* cells that possess a "defective" λ prophage that is blocked by one of several means for chromosomal excision. The initiation of bi-directional replication from the prophage, which is normally prevented by an action of the prophage CI repressor—until repression is relieved, results in replication forks that move outward from the defective prophage into the *E. coli* chromosome. Massive cellular killing occurs, likely due to collisions between *E. coli*-initiated and λ-initiated opposing replication forks. **Replicative Killing (RK⁻) defective phenotype:** Mutants originating in RK⁺ cells that have lost the RK⁺ phenotype. There are numerous possibilities for **RK⁻ mutants**, but they all relate to being defective in a phage or host function required for the initiation of λ bi-directional replication. **RK⁻ Hd⁻ mutants** are defective in a host function required for λ replication initiation. **RK⁺ ilr mutants** are defective in a λ function required for the initiation of λ bi-directional replication, where ilr designates initiation of λ replication defective **RK⁻ FI⁻ mutants** represent RK⁻ mutants where the *immλ* region of the defective prophage cannot be rescued using a phage-prophage marker rescue recombination assay. The hundreds of mutants characterized have resulted from large chromosomal deletions where the deletion endpoints straddle or partially straddle the defective prophage; but they could also represent defects in *pR*, preventing *pR-cro-cII-O-P* transcription. *immλ* **region:** part of the λ genetic map between genes *N* and *cII* that includes the genetic elements *oL/pL-rexB-rexA-cI*[Ts857]-*oR/pR-cro*. *imm***434 region:** the region of a λ*imm*434 hybrid phage where the *immλ* region of λ is replaced by DNA from phage 434, but all the remaining portions of the phage genetic map are the same as for λ. **FI (functional immunity) assay:** a marker rescue assay where the *immλ* region of a prophage (in RK⁺ cells) is rescued by an infecting λ*imm*434 phage, where the recombinant λ*immλ* phage released can form plaques on cells lysogenized by a λ*imm*434 prophage. *oriλ* **region:** A region within λ gene *O* that contains four iteron (or ITN) sequences each containing an 18 bp inverted repeat of hyphenated symmetry (each bound by two O proteins) and an adjacent region of 39 bp termed the High-AT-RICH region that is sensitive to DNA unwinding. **PDS selection:** a selection for RK⁻ survivor mutants starting with lysogenic cells with an intact λ prophage that encodes a temperature sensitive *cI*[Ts857] repressor and is defective for *N*, such that prophage excision is prevented because genes *int-xis* are not expressed from the induced prophage, i.e., when the cells are shifted from growth at 30 °C (where the TS CI repressor is active, binds operator sites *oL* and *oR* and prevents transcription initiation from promoters *pL* and *pR*) to 42 °C where the TS CI repressor is thermally inactivated and transcription is de-repressed from promoters *pL* and *pR*. **RK⁻ selection:** same as the PDS selection except that the starting cells include an *N*⁺ cryptic λ prophage deleted for genes *int-xis-exo-bet-gam-kil* left of *immλ* (encoding a *cI* Ts857 repressor), and all λ late genes for cell lysis and phage morphogenesis. **riC mutation:** putative new promoters arising left or right of *oriλ* that enable transcription near to *oriλ*, thus suppressing "**replicative inhibition**" caused by the loss of a *cis*-requirement for transcription from *pR* (or in the vicinity of *oriλ*), which, in addition to the activities of λ replication initiator genes *O* and *P* is a requirement for bi-directional λ replication initiation.

References

1. Casjens, S.R.; Hendrix, R.W. Bacteriophage lambda: Early pioneer and still relevant. *Virology* **2015**, *479–480*, 310–330. [CrossRef] [PubMed]

2. Friedman, D.I.; Gottesman, M. Lytic mode of lambda development. In *Lambda II*; Hendrix, R.W., Roberts, J.W., Stahl, F.W., Weisberg, R.A., Eds.; Cold Spring Harbor Laboratory: Cold Spring Harbor, NY, USA, 1983; pp. 21–51.

3. Hendrix, R.W.; Casjens, S. Bacteriophage lambda and its genetic neighborhood. In *The Bacteriophages*, 2nd ed.; Calendar, R., Ed.; Oxford University Press: Oxford, UK, 2006; pp. 409–447.

4. Court, D.L.; Oppenheim, A.B.; Adhya, S.L. A new look at bacteriophage lambda genetic networks. *J. Bacteriol.* **2007**, *189*, 298–304. [CrossRef] [PubMed]

5. Tsurimoto, T.; Matsubara, K. Purified bacteriophage lambda O protein binds to four repeating sequences at the lambda replication origin. *Nucleic Acids Res.* **1981**, *9*, 1789–1799. [CrossRef] [PubMed]

6. Tsurimoto, T.; Matsubara, K. Purification of bacteriophage lambda O protein that specifically binds to the origin of replication. *Mol. Gen. Genet.* **1981**, *181*, 325–331. [CrossRef] [PubMed]

7. Biswas, S.B.; Biswas, E.E. Regulation of dnaB function in DNA replication in *Escherichia coli* by dnaC and lambda *P* gene products. *J. Biol. Chem.* **1987**, *262*, 7831–7838. [PubMed]

8. Alfano, C.; McMacken, R. Ordered assembly of nucleoprotein structures at the bacteriophage lambda replication origin during the initiation of DNA replication. *J. Biol. Chem.* **1989**, *264*, 10699–10708. [PubMed]

9. Zylicz, M.; Ang, D.; Liberek, K.; Georgopoulos, C. Initiation of lambda DNA replication with purified host- and bacteriophage-encoded proteins: The role of the dnaK, dnaJ and grpE heat shock proteins. *EMBO J.* **1989**, *8*, 1601–1608. [PubMed]

10. Thomas, R.; Bertani, L.E. On the Control of the Replication of Temperate Bacteriophages Superinfecting Immune Hosts. *Virology* **1964**, *24*, 241–253. [CrossRef]

11. Hayes, S.; Hayes, C. Spontaneous lambda OR mutations suppress inhibition of bacteriophage growth by nonimmune exclusion phenotype of defective lambda prophage. *J. Virol.* **1986**, *58*, 835–842. [PubMed]

12. Furth, M.E.; Dove, W.F.; Meyer, B.J. Specificity determinants for bacteriophage lambda DNA replication. III. Activation of replication in lambda *ric* mutants by transcription outside of *ori*. *J. Mol. Biol.* **1982**, *154*, 65–83. [CrossRef]

13. Moore, D.D.; Blattner, F.R. Sequence of lambda ric5b. *J. Mol. Biol.* **1982**, *154*, 81–83. [CrossRef]

14. Echols, H.; Guarneros, G. Control of Integration and Excision. In *Lambda II*; Hendrix, R.W., Roberts, J.W., Stahl, F.W., Weisberg, R.A., Eds.; Cold Spring Harbor Laboratory: Cold Spring Harbor, NY, USA, 1983; pp. 75–92.

15. Pereira da Silva, L.; Eisen, H.; Jacob, F. Sur la replication du bacteriophage. *C. R. Acad. Sci. Paris* **1968**, *266*, 926–928.

16. Brachet, P.; Eisen, H.; Rambach, A. Mutations of coliphage lambda affecting the expression of replicative functions O and P. *Mol. Gen. Genet.* **1970**, *108*, 266–276. [CrossRef] [PubMed]

17. Castellazzi, M.; Brachet, P.; Eisen, H. Isolation and characterization of deletions in bacteriophage lambda residing as prophage in *E. coli* K 12. *Mol. Gen. Genet.* **1972**, *117*, 211–218. [PubMed]

18. Dove, W.F.; Inokuchi, H.; Stevens, W.F. Replication control in phage lambda. In *The Bacteriophage Lambda*; Hershey, A.D., Ed.; Cold Spring Harbor Laboratory: Cold Spring Harbor, NY, USA, 1971; pp. 747–771.

19. Lieb, M. Studies of heat-inducible lambda-phage. 3. Mutations in cistron N affecting heat induction. *Genetics* **1966**, *54*, 835–844. [PubMed]

20. Rambach, A. Replicator mutants of bacteriophage lambda: Characterization of two subclasses. *Virology* **1973**, *54*, 270–277. [CrossRef]

21. Sly, W.S.; Eisen, H.A.; Siminovitch, L. Host survival following infection with or induction of bacteriophage lambda mutants. *Virology* **1968**, *34*, 112–127. [CrossRef]

22. Hayes, S. Mutations suppressing loss of replication control: Genetic analysis of bacteriophage lambda-dependent replicative killing, replication initiation, and mechanisms of mutagenesis. In *DNA Replication and Mutagenesis*; Moses, R.E., Summers, W.C., Eds.; American Society for Microbiology: Washington, DC, USA, 1988; pp. 367–377.

23. Greer, H. The *kil* gene of bacteriophage lambda. *Virology* **1975**, *66*, 589–604. [CrossRef]

24. Bull, H.J.; Hayes, S. The *grp*D55 locus of *Escherichia coli* appears to be an allele of *dnaB*. *Mol. Gen. Genet.* **1996**, *252*, 755–760. [PubMed]

25. Hayes, S.; Erker, C.; Horbay, M.A.; Marciniuk, K.; Wang, W.; Hayes, C. Phage Lambda P Protein: Trans-Activation, Inhibition Phenotypes and their Suppression. *Viruses* **2013**, *5*, 619–653. [CrossRef] [PubMed]

26. Hayes, S.; Duincan, D.; Hayes, C. Alcohol treatment of defective lambda lysogens is deletionogenic. *Mol. Gen. Genet.* **1990**, *222*, 17–24. [PubMed]

27. Hayes, S. Mapping ethanol-induced deletions. *Mol. Gen. Genet.* **1991**, *231*, 139–149. [CrossRef] [PubMed]

28. Hayes, S. Ethanol-induced genotoxicity. *Mutat. Res.* **1985**, *143*, 23–27. [CrossRef]

29. Hayes, S.; Hayes, C.; Taitt, E.; Talbert, M. A simple, forward selection scheme for independently determining the toxicity and mutagenic effect of environmental chemicals: Measuring replicative killing of *Escherichia coli* by an integrated fragment of bacteriophage lambda DNA. In *In Vitro Toxiciry Testing of Environmental Agents, Part A*; Kolber, A.R., Wong, T.K., Grant, L.D., DeWoskin, R.S., Hughes, T.J., Eds.; Plenum Publishing Corp.: New York, NY, USA, 1883.

30. Hayes, S.; Gordon, A.; Sadowski, I.; Hayes, C. RK bacterial test for independently measuring chemical toxicity and mutagenicity: Short-term forward selection assay. *Mutat. Res.* **1984**, *130*, 97–106. [CrossRef]

31. Hayes, S.; Gordon, A. Validating RK test: Correlation with Salmonella mutatest and SOS chromotest assay results for reference compounds and influence of pH and dose response on measured toxic and mutagenic effects. *Mutat. Res.* **1984**, *130*, 107–111. [CrossRef]

32. Kaiser, A.D. *Lambda DNA Replication*; Hershey, A.D., Ed.; Cold Spring Harbor Press: Cold Spring Harbor, NY, USA, 1971.

33. Rao, R.N.; Rogers, S.G. A thermoinducible lambda phage-ColE1 plasmid chimera for the overproduction of gene products from cloned DNA segments. *Gene* **1978**, *3*, 247–263. [PubMed]

34. Kleckner, N. Amber mutants in the *O* gene of bacteriophage lambda are not efficiently complemented in the absence of phage N function. *Virology* **1977**, *79*, 174–182. [CrossRef]

35. Campbell, A. Sensitive mutants of bacteriophage lambda. *Virology* **1961**, *14*, 22–32. [CrossRef]

36. Hayes, S.; Wang, W.; Rajamanickam, K.; Chu, A.; Banerjee, A.; Hayes, C. Lambda *gpP-DnaB* Helicase Sequestration and *gpP-RpoB* Associated Effects: On Screens for Auxotrophs, Selection for Rif(R), Toxicity, Mutagenicity, Plasmid Curing. *Viruses* **2016**, *8*, 172. [CrossRef] [PubMed]

37. Furth, M.E. *Specificity Determinants for Bacteriophage Lambda DNA Replication, and Structure of the Origin of Replication*; University of Wisconsin: Madison, WI, USA, 1978.

38. Thomas, R.; Leurs, C.; Dambly, C.; Parmentier, D.; Lambert, L.; Brachet, P.; Lefebvre, N.; Mousset, S.; Porcheret, J.; Szpirer, J.; et al. Isolation and characterization of new sus (amber) mutants of bacteriophage lambda. *Mutat. Res.* **1967**, *4*, 735–741. [CrossRef]

39. Hayes, S. Initiation of coliphage lambda replication, *lit, oop* RNA synthesis, and effect of gene dosage on transcription from promoters P_L, P_R, and P_R. *Virology* **1979**, *97*, 415–438. [CrossRef]

40. Furth, M.E.; Blattner, F.R.; McLeester, C.; Dove, W.F. Genetic structure of the replication origin of bacteriophage lambda. *Science* **1977**, *198*, 1046–1051. [CrossRef] [PubMed]

41. Hayes, S.; Asai, K.; Chu, A.M.; Hayes, C. NinR- and red-mediated phage-prophage marker rescue recombination in *Escherichia coli*: Recovery of a nonhomologous immlambda DNA segment by infecting lambdaimm434 phages. *Genetics* **2005**, *170*, 1485–1499. [CrossRef] [PubMed]

42. Daniels, D.L.; Schroeder, J.L.; Szybalski, W.; Sanger, F.; Blattner, F.R. Appendix I. A molecular map of coliphage lambda. In *Lambda II*; Hendrix, R.W., Roberts, J.W., Stahl, F.W., Weisberg, R.A., Eds.; Cold Spring Harbor Laboratory: Cold Spring Harbor, NY, USA, 1983; pp. 469–517.

43. Scherer, G. Nucleotide sequence of the *O* gene and of the origin of replication in bacteriophage lambda DNA. *Nucleic Acids Res.* **1978**, *5*, 3141–3156. [CrossRef] [PubMed]

44. Moore, D.D.; Denniston, K.; Kruger, K.E.; Furth, M.E.; Williams, B.G.; Daniels, D.L.; Blattner, F.R. Dissection and comparative anatomy of the origins of replication in lambdoid coliphages. In *Proceedings of the Cold Spring Harbor Symposium Quantitative Biology*; Cold Spring Harbor Laboratory: Cold Spring Harbor, NY, USA, 1979; pp. 155–163.

45. Zahn, K.; Blattner, F.R. Sequence-induced DNA curvature at the bacteriophage lambda origin of replication. *Nature* **1985**, *317*, 451–453. [CrossRef] [PubMed]

46. Denniston-Thompson, K.; Moore, D.D.; Kruger, K.E.; Furth, M.E.; Blattner, F.R. Physical structure of the replication origin of bacteriophage lambda. *Science* **1977**, *198*, 1051–1056. [CrossRef] [PubMed]

47. Zeghouf, M.; Li, J.; Butland, G.; Borkowska, A.; Canadien, V.; Richards, D.; Beattie, B.; Emili, A.; Greenblatt, J.F. Sequential Peptide Affinity (SPA) system for the identification of mammalian and bacterial protein complexes. *J. Proteome Res.* **2004**, *3*, 463–468. [CrossRef] [PubMed]

48. Hayes, S.; Hayes, C.; Bull, H.J.; Pelcher, L.A.; Slavcev, R.A. Acquired mutations in phage lambda genes *O* or *P* that enable constitutive expression of a cryptic lambdaN+cI[Ts]cro- prophage in *E. coli* cells shifted from 30 degreesC to 42 degreesC, accompanied by loss of immlambda and Rex+ phenotypes and emergence of a non-immune exclusion-state. *Gene* **1998**, *223*, 115–128. [PubMed]

49. Tomizawa, J. Functional cooperation of genes *O* and *P*. In *The Bacteriophage Lambda*; Hershey, A.D., Ed.; Cold Spring Harbor Laboratory: Cold Spring Harbor, NY, USA, 1971; pp. 549–552.

50. Furth, M.E.; Yates, J.L. Specificity determinants for bacteriophage lambda DNA replication. II. Structure of O proteins of lambda-phi80 and lambda-82 hybrid phages and of a lambda mutant defective in the origin of replication. *J. Mol. Biol.* **1978**, *126*, 227–240. [CrossRef]

51. Wickner, S.H.; Zahn, K. Characterization of the DNA binding domain of bacteriophage lambda O protein. *J. Biol. Chem.* **1986**, *261*, 7537–7543. [PubMed]

52. Gonciarz-Swiatek, M.; Wawrzynow, A.; Um, S.J.; Learn, B.A.; McMacken, R.; Kelley, W.L.; Georgopoulos, C.; Sliekers, O.; Zylicz, M. Recognition, targeting, and hydrolysis of the lambda *O* replication protein by the ClpP/ClpX protease. *J. Biol. Chem.* **1999**, *274*, 13999–14005. [CrossRef] [PubMed]

53. Dodson, M.; Echols, H.; Wickner, S.; Alfano, C.; Mensa-Wilmot, K.; Gomes, B.; LeBowitz, J.; Roberts, J.D.; McMacken, R. Specialized nucleoprotein structures at the origin of replication of bacteriophage lambda:

Localized unwinding of duplex DNA by a six-protein reaction. *Proc. Natl. Acad. Sci. USA* **1986**, *83*, 7638–7642. [CrossRef] [PubMed]

54. Alfano, C.; McMacken, R. The role of template superhelicity in the initiation of bacteriophage lambda DNA replication. *Nucleic Acids Res.* **1988**, *16*, 9611–9630. [CrossRef] [PubMed]

55. Reiser, W.; Leibrecht, I.; Klein, A. Structure and function of mutants in the *P* gene of bacteriophage lambda leading to the pi phenotype. *Mol. Gen. Genet.* **1983**, *192*, 430–435. [CrossRef] [PubMed]

56. Wickner, S.H. DNA replication proteins of *Escherichia coli* and phage lambda. *Cold Spring Harb. Symp. Quant. Biol.* **1979**, *43*, 303–310. [CrossRef] [PubMed]

57. Zylicz, M.; Gorska, I.; Taylor, K.; Georgopoulos, C. Bacteriophage lambda replication proteins: Formation of a mixed oligomer and binding to the origin of lambda DNA. *Mol. Gen. Genet.* **1984**, *196*, 401–406. [CrossRef] [PubMed]

58. Eisen, H.; Barrand, P.; Spiegelman, W.; Reichardt, L.F.; Heinemann, S.; Georgopoulos, C. Mutants in the y region of bacteriophage lambda constitutive for repressor synthesis: Their isolation and the characterization of the Hyp phenotype. *Gene* **1982**, *20*, 71–81. [CrossRef]

59. Fiandt, M.; Szybalski, W.; Malamy, M.H. Polar mutations in *lac, gal* and phage lambda consist of a few IS-DNA sequences inserted with either orientation. *Mol. Gen. Genet.* **1972**, *119*, 223–231. [CrossRef] [PubMed]

60. Hayes, S.; Horbay, M.A.; Hayes, C. A CI-Independent Form of Replicative Inhibition: Turn Off of Early Replication of Bacteriophage Lambda. *PLoS ONE* **2012**, *7*, e36498. [CrossRef] [PubMed]

6

The Membrane Steps of Bacterial Cell Wall Synthesis as Antibiotic Targets

Yao Liu and Eefjan Breukink *

Department of Membrane Biochemistry and Biophysics, Utrecht University, Utrecht 3584 CH, The Netherlands; y.liu3@uu.nl
* Correspondence: e.j.breukink@uu.nl

Academic Editor: Waldemar Vollmer

Abstract: Peptidoglycan is the major component of the cell envelope of virtually all bacteria. It has structural roles and acts as a selective sieve for molecules from the outer environment. Peptidoglycan synthesis is therefore one of the most important biogenesis pathways in bacteria and has been studied extensively over the last twenty years. The pathway starts in the cytoplasm, continues in the cytoplasmic membrane and finishes in the periplasmic space, where the precursor is polymerized into the peptidoglycan layer. A number of proteins involved in this pathway, such as the Mur enzymes and the penicillin binding proteins (PBPs), have been studied and regarded as good targets for antibiotics. The present review focuses on the membrane steps of peptidoglycan synthesis that involve two enzymes, MraY and MurG, the inhibitors of these enzymes and the inhibition mechanisms. We also discuss the challenges of targeting these two cytoplasmic membrane (associated) proteins in bacterial cells and the perspectives on how to overcome the issues.

Keywords: peptidoglycan; MraY; MurG; inhibition; antibiotics; mechanism; target

1. Introduction

Bacteria have evolved to survive a considerable variety of environments and can develop resistance to various antibacterial reagents rapidly. This ability of bacteria presents a big challenge in treating infections, especially in hospitals. The peptidoglycan layer that is in almost all bacteria lends structural strength and provides a protective barrier for the bacterium [1]. The peptidoglycan layer is composed of polysaccharides with alternating N-acetylglucosamine (GlcNAc) and N-acetylmuramic acid (MurNAc) saccharide groups. Between three and five amino acids, typically a pentapeptide with a sequence of L-Ala-γ-D-Glu-L-lysine (or -*meso*-diaminopimelic acid)-D-Ala-D-Ala [2], are attached to the MurNAc group. These peptide chains can be crosslinked with each other.

Peptidoglycan synthesis occurs in three distinctive compartments of bacteria, namely the cytoplasm, the cytoplasmic membrane and the periplasmic space [3]. It starts in the cytoplasm, where the nucleotide precursors are synthesized, i.e., UDP-GlcNAc is synthesized from fructose-6-phosphate by the Glm enzymes [4], and UDP-N-acetylmuramyl-pentapeptide (UDP-Mpp) is synthesized by the Mur enzymes (MurA, MurB, MurC, MurD, MurE and MurF) [5] from UDP-GlcNAc. The synthesis of the membrane-embedded undecaprenyl phosphate takes place on the cytoplasmic side. This is performed by undecaprenyl pyrophosphate synthase (UppS) catalyzing the consecutive condensation reactions of a farnesyl pyrophosphate (FPP) with eight isopentenyl pyrophosphates (IPP), in which new *cis*-double bonds are formed [6]. The resulting undecaprenyl pyrophosphate (C55-PP) is dephosphorylated by undecaprenyl pyrophosphate phosphatase (UppP) to produce undecaprenyl phosphate (C55-P) [7]. UDP-Mpp and C55-P are the two substrates of the integral membrane enzyme phospho-MurNAc-pentapeptide translocase (MraY). MraY catalyzes the first membrane step of peptidoglycan synthesis by transferring the phospho-MurNAc-pentapeptide moiety from UDP-Mpp to C55-P and yields uridine-monophosphate (UMP) and undecaprenyl-pyrophosphoryl-MurNAc-pentapeptide, typically referred to as Lipid I [8]. Although the use of C55-P as the lipid carrier is the common rule in bacteria, there is evidence that the shorter chain decaprenyl phosphate and nonaprenyl phosphate homologues assist glycan translocation in some species [9,10]. Moreover, C55-P is also shared by other cell wall pathways, such as the wall teichoic acid synthesis and capsular polysaccharide synthesis in *Staphylococcus aureus* [11–14]. Since C55-P exists in bacterial cells in very limited amounts, the synthesis of these different components is highly integrated and coordinated temporally.

After Lipid I synthesis, the glycosyltransferase MurG transfers a GlcNAc moiety from UDP-GlcNAc to Lipid I to produce undecaprenyl-pyrophosphoryl-MurNAc-(pentapeptide)- GlcNAc. This is usually referred to as Lipid II, which is subsequently transported by a flippase from the inner side of the membrane to the outer side [15–18] where polymerization to give a peptidoglycan layer takes place. The proteins that catalyze the last steps of the formation of the peptidoglycan layer have been researched in detail and include the bifunctional penicillin binding proteins (PBPs), e.g., PBP1A and PBP1B of Gram-negative *Escherichia coli* [19] and PBP4 of Gram-positive *Listeria monocytogenes* [20]. The transglycosylase domain of the PBPs polymerizes the sugar moieties of Lipid II to produce glycan strands, where the transpeptidase domain links the peptides to form a 3D network. These actions ultimately result in the peptidoglycan layer that is responsible for the shape and rigidity of the bacterial cell [21].

Destruction of the peptidoglycan layer brings about loss of integrity and can lead to cell death by bursting. Some most successful and widely-used antibiotics, such as the β-lactams and glycopeptide antibiotics [22–26], have targets in the peptidoglycan synthesis pathway. Although studied in some detail, this pathway can still be exploited for novel antibacterial compounds. Research into the peptidoglycan biogenesis can therefore form part of our response to the ever-present problem of resistance to antibiotics, as well as improve our understanding of bacterial physiology.

Several reviews have been published dealing with different stages of peptidoglycan biogenesis; the present review focuses on the membrane steps of this pathway, summarizing the recent advances in the research of structure, function, inhibition mechanisms and the attempts to develop inhibitors of the essential enzymes, MraY and MurG. There are several enzymes, including WecA, TagO and WbcO, of the PNPT family that fulfill similar roles as MraY or MurG, in some bacterial species. These will not be discussed in the present review to focus on the more commonplace types of bacterium and to keep our messages concise. Extensive reviews dealing with similar topics, such as MraY inhibitors and peptidoglycan lipid intermediates, have been published by different groups in 2006 [27] and 2007 [2]; the present review therefore focuses on the advances that were made thereafter with a brief introduction and overview of the earlier knowledge.

2. MraY

The first evidence of phospho-MurNAc-pentapeptide translocase (MraY) and its function was collected in 1965 when an active membrane fraction was prepared in vitro that could successfully produce Lipid I (Figure 1) [28]. The enzyme that was responsible for the production of Lipid I was often referred to as translocase I until 1991, when the *MraY* (mra: murein synthesis gene cluster a) gene for the enzyme responsible was identified in *E. coli* [29].

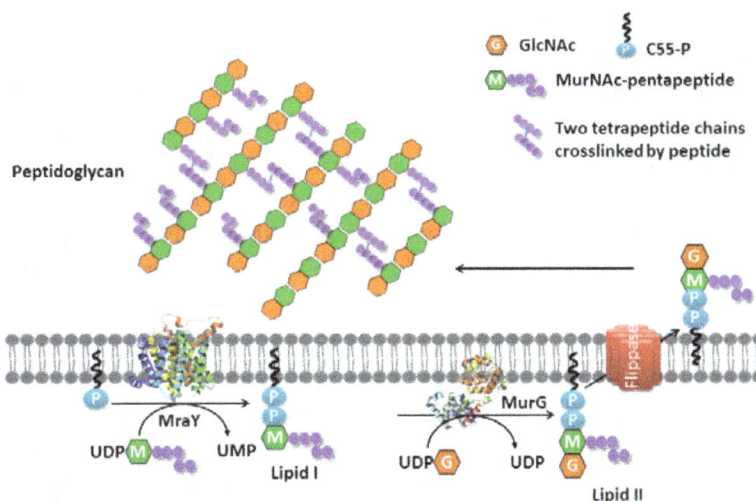

Figure 1. Membrane steps of the bacterial peptidoglycan synthesis pathway.

2.1. Biochemical Characterization of MraY

In-depth biochemical analysis of protein function relies on the overexpression and purification of the desired protein and in a manner that retains its enzymatic activity. Early studies on MraY relied on crude membrane preparations of MraY, because production, as well as detailed investigations of the biochemical properties of MraY had been long held back by the hydrophobic nature of this enzyme. For example, a method of overexpressing *E. coli* MraY and solubilizing the membranes using Triton X-100 was reported [30,31]. It was demonstrated that the protein was produced at a concentration of 4 mg/mL, but it did not undergo a purification step. Using these protein-enriched membrane preparations, the binding modes of several MraY inhibitors, such as mureidomycin A, tunicamycin and liposidomycin B (see Section 2.3), were studied [30]. It was found that the nucleoside antibiotics displayed different modes of action, being competitive either with the nucleotide substrate UDP-Mpp or the lipid substrate C55-P. The information was yet limited on the binding mode since no structural model of the protein was available.

The purification of the Gram-positive *Bacillus subtilis* MraY (BsMraY) to homogeneity in the milligram range (from a 5-L cell culture) was first achieved by using an *n*-dodecyl-β-D-maltoside (DDM) detergent system [32]. Bouhss et al. [32] tested different detergent systems for their influence on the MraY activity; the ionic detergent with a low aggregation number, i.e., *N*-lauroyl sarcosine, was identified as the best detergent for a Lipid I synthesis assay using radiolabeled UDP-MurNAc-[^{14}C]pentapeptide. The development of the purification method for BsMraY allowed the study of its kinetics. The K_M value of BsMraY was obtained by varying the concentration of either substrate while keeping the other at a fixed value. It was reported that the K_M values of pure BsMraY for its substrates UDP-Mpp and C55-P were 1.0 ± 0.3 mM and 0.16 ± 0.08 mM, respectively [32]. The catalytic constant K_{cat} was 320 ± 34 min^{-1}. This result was later challenged by a report of a K_M value of pure BsMraY for UDP-Mpp being 36.2 ± 3.6 µM [33]. However, the two studies used different concentrations of the lipid carrier C55-P in the synthesis reaction, namely 1.1 mM in [32] and 50 µM in [33], suggesting that the true K_M value of BsMraY for UDP-Mpp is different from these apparent K_M values. Indeed, more recent kinetics studies on BsMraY showed that the apparent affinity of either substrate to the enzyme is dependent on the concentration of the other [34,35]. This characteristic has been overlooked by the other published studies.

Further investigations on the enzymatic mechanism of BsMraY were carried out using single mutants of invariant or highly-conserved polar residues (all in the cytoplasmic loops) using site-directed mutagenesis followed by detailed analysis of the mutant proteins [36]. The importance of highly-conserved aspartate residues, namely D98 and D99 in BsMraY (corresponding to D115 and D116 in *E. coli* MraY (EcMraY)), were addressed in this study [36]. It was the first time that MraY catalysis was studied with purified enzyme, both the wild-type and its mutants, without the interference of other contaminant enzymes or traces of C55-P in a membrane preparation. Fourteen single mutations that led to significant loss of activity revealed the involvement of these residues in the catalytic role of MraY. However, it was also observed that these mutants did not impair the binding of MraY to its nucleotide substrate, UDP-Mpp. Al-Dabbagh et al. [36] also proposed the involvement of D98 in deprotonation of the lipid substrate, C55-P, due to the clear influence of pH on the D98N mutant, as this mutant showed maximum activity at pH 9.0–9.4, where the wild-type worked optimally at pH 7.6. This suggests that the translocase reaction proceeds through a nucleophilic attack of phosphate oxyanion from the deprotonated C55-P onto the β-phosphate via the acidic residue (D98). Based on these findings, the authors support the proposed one-step catalytic mechanism for MraY. It is worth noting that in this study, the kinetic values of BsMraY and its mutants were obtained by varying UDP-Mpp concentration between 3 and 6 mM while keeping C55-P at 1.1 mM. These concentrations are very high, and the K_M values obtained were much higher than those of our own kinetic study [34]. The K_{cat} value of the H289R mutant reported in this study decreased by three orders of magnitude. However, in our own studies, the H289R mutant is virtually inactive, and it was impossible to determine the kinetic values.

The success of isolating and purifying BsMraY from Gram-positive species was not matched in studies of Gram-negative ones. A cell-free overexpression system coupled with detergent solubilization increased the yield of EcMraY considerably, giving yields in the milligram range from just a few milliliters of the cell-free reaction volumes [33,37,38]. However, EcMraY was found to form aggregates in the presence of a range of detergents, and any purified material was inactive [38]. The cell-free expression system was useful for investigating the role of lipid composition on EcMraY function. It was discovered that the activity of EcMraY is highly dependent on the presence of particular phospholipids [33]. Anionic and glycerol-containing lipid head groups, such as phosphatidylglycerol and cardiolipin, were shown to be essential for the functionality of EcMraY [39]. This was consistent with the research from the 1970s that showed MraY from *Micrococcus luteus* that was solubilized with Triton X-100 required neutral and polar lipids in order to remain active [40]. Notably, although a polar lipid was required for the synthesis of Lipid I, neither was required for the exchange reaction between UMP and UDP-Mpp [40]. The lack of structural information at the time limited the understanding of the mechanism of MraY, which made the reasons for the dependence on polar lipids unclear. Recent observations [34,35] indicate that an exchange reaction between UMP and UDP-Mpp does not occur unless C55-P is present, and the previously-suggested covalent enzyme-substrate intermediate, MraY-phospho-MurNAc-pp, is questionable [41]. Lloyd et al. [41] claimed that an intermediate was trapped in the reaction mixture without the addition of C55-P, an *E. coli* membrane preparation was used instead of pure MraY enzyme; therefore, the presence of a small amount of C55-P cannot be excluded.

2.2. Structural Characterization of MraY

There was almost a 20-year gap between the discovery of the MraY enzyme (from *Staphylococcus aureus*) [42] in 1973 and the elucidation of the exact sequence of this protein (from *E. coli*) [29] in 1991. Alternating hydrophobic and hydrophilic fragments of amino acid sequences in MraY indicate that the enzyme spans the cytoplasmic membrane several times [29]. The topology maps of MraY from two different species, namely the Gram-positive *Staphylococcus aureus* and the Gram-negative *E. coli*, were later reported [43]. β-Lactamase fusions to different domains of MraY were constructed and expressed in *E. coli* DH5α cells. The resistance or sensitivity of the cells expressing different hybrids to ampicillin revealed the orientation of the different domains of MraY. It became clear that MraY has 10 transmembrane domains, and both its N- and C-termini are located in the periplasm across species (Figure 2). Since the precursors for Lipid I are synthesized in the cytoplasm, it follows that the active site of MraY is exposed to the cytoplasm, as well. It was proposed that cytosolic loops II, III and IV are responsible for the binding to UDP-Mpp, as they contained highly-conserved residues that are common for the polyprenyl-phosphate N-acetyl hexosamine 1-phosphate transferase (PNPT) super family, while loops I and V were likely involved in the interaction with other proteins of the peptidoglycan synthesis pathway given that the sequences were strictly specific to MraY orthologues.

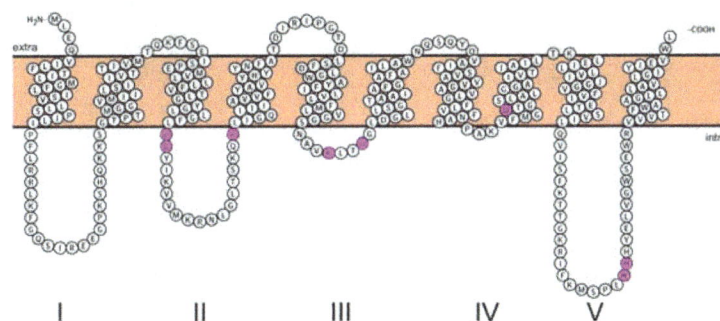

Figure 2. Topology maps of MraY from *B. subtilis*. Highly-conserved residues (D98, D99, K116, N171, D174, D231, H289 and H290) are highlighted in pink. The figure is rendered with the Protter web service [44]. Topology of other MraY species can be found in the Supplementary Information.

As briefly mentioned in the previous section, a number of conserved residues distributed all over the cytoplasmic loops of MraY were proven to be catalytically important taking BsMraY as a model (D98, D99, K116, N171, D174, D231, H289 and H290) (Figure 2) [36]. This suggests that all of the cytoplasmic loops are involved in maintaining the UDP-Mpp in an efficient configuration for catalysis. Two biochemistry-based catalytic models were proposed. One is a two-step model in which the MraY-p-MurNAc-pentapeptide intermediate is formed very rapidly to account for an exchange reaction [45,46]; the second is a one-step model that involves a direct attack of the phosphate oxyanion onto UDP-Mpp [36]. Unfortunately, as no 3D structure of any MraY isoform or even any member of the PNPT super family was available, it was not possible to be conclusive about by which mechanism this reaction proceeds. Many unanswered questions remained regarding how the other important residues affect the substrate binding and the catalytic process of MraY. Recently, Chung and his co-workers [8] reported the crystal structure of MraY from *Aquifex aeolicus* (AaMraY) at 3.3 Å resolution. The observation that the N and C termini are on the periplasmic side is consistent with previous studies of the topology of EcMraY, SaMraY and BsMraY. They also showed that AaMraY was crystallized as a dimer, and a large tunnel formed by the helices of the dimer interface could facilitate positioning of the lipid carrier C55-P. Moreover, the evidence for a cleft formed by the cytoplasmic and inner leaflet regions of transmembrane helices 3, 4, 5, 8 and 9b led to the suggestion that this was the active site of AaMraY. The cleft is deepened by the amphipathic helix TM9b protruding towards the cytoplasmic membrane, which is connected with a highly-conserved HHH motif (amino acid sequence: PXHHHXEXXG) in the fifth cytoplasmic loop, pointing towards the region where Mg^{2+} is bound (Figure 3). The activity of MraY is highly dependent on the presence of its co-factor Mg^{2+} [27,47]. Mg^{2+} binds close to D265 (Figure 3), which is a catalytic residue corresponding to D265 of BsMraY, D267 of EcMraY and D229 of SaMraY (Figure 4). It was suggested that the cleft is the essential binding site for the nucleotide substrate, UDP-Mpp. Mutagenesis of the residue showed the importance of D117 (corresponding to D98 in BsMraY and D115 in EcMraY) in binding to the lipid substrate, C55-P. Based on these findings, the study of Chung et al. supported the proposal that D117 deprotonates the phosphate moiety of C55-P allowing a direct nucleophile attack on UDP-Mpp. This evidence suggests that a one-step MraY catalysis mechanism is more likely than a two-step mechanism. Chung et al. [8] predicted that C55-P with a lipid chain longer than the thickness of the membrane needs to bend sharply to allow the phosphate moiety to reach D117, though there is no direct evidence as to how this is actually achieved. Furthermore, no clear catalytic role was attributed to the highly-conserved H324 (corresponding to H289 in BsMraY). It was proposed that 13 amino acids, including the HHH motif in the cytoplasmic loop, are unique to the MraY family and contribute to the substrate specificity towards UDP-Mpp instead of other nucleotide substrates utilized by the other UDP-d-N-acetylhexosamine: polyprenol phosphate d-N-acetylhexosamine 1-phosphate transferases [48].

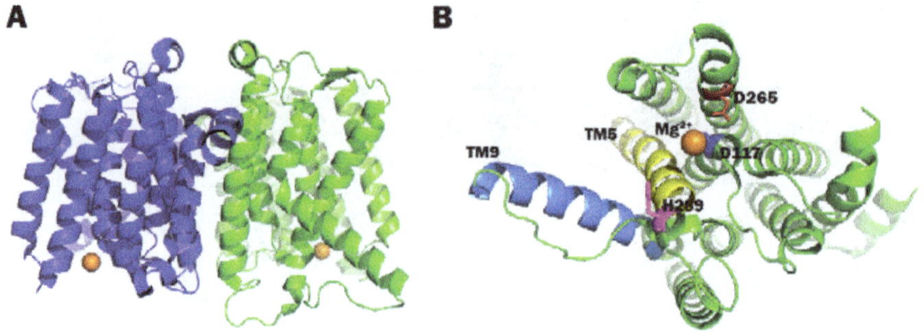

Figure 3. (**A**) 3D structure of AaMraY; (**B**) Close-up view of TM5 (helix shown in blue), TM9b (helix shown in cyan), the HHH motif (shown as rainbow sticks) in loop E, the Mg^{2+} (shown as an orange sphere) and the essential D265 of AaMraY. Images obtained and rendered with Pymol using 4J72.pdb.

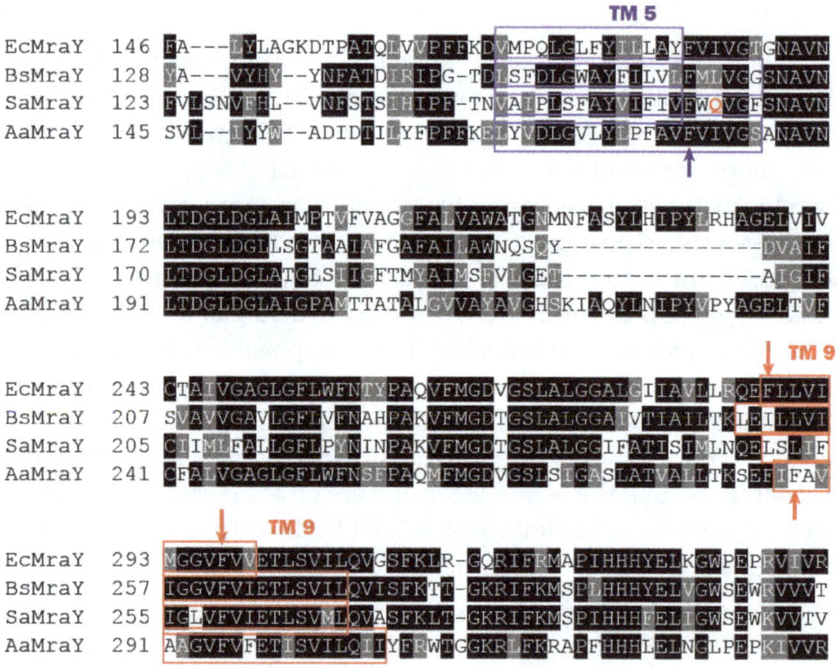

Figure 4. Partial sequence alignment of MraY from four different species (Ec = *E. coli*; Sa = *S. aureus*; Bs = *B. subtilis*; Aa = *A. aeolicus*). Some essential phenylalanine residues are indicated with an arrow. The polar Gln residue in *S. aureus* MraY is marked in red.

Chung et al. used a chemical cross-linking experiment on detergent-solubilized AaMraY and structure-guided disulfide cross-bridge experiments (based on cysteines) on membrane-embedded AaMraY in order to show that AaMraY forms a dimer both in detergent micelles and in the membranes. It was suggested that this finding is in agreement with a previous study where bacterial two-hybrid studies were performed in the Gram-negative *Caulobacter crescentus* cells [49]. However, no clear indication in the original paper was found [49]. The fact that MraY was crystallized as a dimer and that dimerization of AaMraY was found in micelles and membranes was not given further explanation or analysis. Notably, the Gram-positive BsMraY comprises no cysteine residues. Remaining questions in this area include whether or not MraY always functions as a dimer, and how the oligomeric status influences the enzyme activity in different species would be an interesting topic for further studies on this system.

2.3. MraY Inhibitors and Inhibition Mechanism

MraY is regarded as an ideal target for novel antibiotics both because it is an essential molecular tool for generating the cellular envelope and because it has no counterparts in mammalian cells. A few different classes of MraY inhibitors have been studied to date. However, none of these has entered clinical development, to a large extent ascribed to the difficulties to deliver the compounds across the membranes. MraY inhibitors discovered thus far have come from either screening assays [50,51] or synthesis of compounds mimicking existing (natural) MraY inhibitors, such as mureidomycin A [52]. In this section, the methods for screening MraY inhibitors and the currently documented inhibitory compounds are discussed.

2.3.1. Method Development for MraY Inhibitor Screening

Competitive binding to MraY was believed to be the key to the discovery of novel MraY inhibitors. The main assays designed to explore such compounds involved the use of a radiolabeled UDP-Mpp or a fluorescent variant of this substrate [27,51,53–56].

Formative experiments required the extraction of products or repeated filtration or washing steps that are not suitable for high throughput testing [57]. In other cases, the assays were coupled with other enzyme activities, such as MurG, transglycosylase or transpeptidase [54,55,58,59]. The first assay targeted only at MraY [57] is a microplate-based scintillation proximity assay (SPA) using a radiolabeled UDP-MurNAc-[^{3}H]-propionate-pentapeptide. Unique features of this assay include: it used E. coli membranes instead of purified MraY, but still, the assay was selective towards MraY inhibition, as the radioactive product of the assay was identified as Lipid I, and the substrate can be synthesized easily in large quantity. A major disadvantage, however, is that 3 h of incubation of the wheat germ agglutinin (WGA)-coated SPA beads was necessary to capture the radioactive product, although the product was claimed to remain stable for up to 12 h.

The early assays used membrane preparations containing the lipid substrate C55-P implying that the activity of other enzymes, such as WecA, could not be excluded. Furthermore, radioactive waste disposal and equipment contamination are the general concerns when using a radioisotope-dependent assay. Later, a relatively inexpensive fluorescence-detection-based assay was developed that could avoid the involvement of any radioactive compounds [50]. In this assay, using the fluorescent substrate UDP-MurNAc-N^ε-dansylpentapeptide (DNS-UDP-Mpp), the dansyl group is transferred to a hydrophobic environment upon synthesis of Lipid I, resulting in a blue shift and concomitant enhanced intensity of the fluorescent signal. This assay was validated by HPLC analysis where the product (DNS-Lipid I) could be clearly separated from the substrate (DNS-UDP-Mpp) [50]. Furthermore, a crude enzyme preparation of EcMraY-Enterobacter cloacae P99 β-lactamase protein fusion was used in this assay. The authors claimed that this protein fusion showed favorable activity over the wild-type EcMraY. This may raise the concern of whether the values determined in this assay represent the behavior of the MraY inhibitors correctly. IC_{50} values of known inhibitors such as mureidomycin B (IC_{50} = 0.038 μM) and synthetic riburamycin RU88110 (IC_{50} = 0.033 μM) determined by this assay were lower than those determined in an earlier cell-based assay that used toluene-permeabilized E. coli bacteria (0.065 μM and 0.33 μM, respectively) [60]. However, the IC_{50} value of tunicamycin determined in [50] (1.9 μM) was higher than by the cell-based assay (0.5 μM) [60]. The authors ascribed this to the difference in the mode of action of tunicamycin (reversible) with the other two compounds (slow binding) reported elsewhere [30] and/or its higher affinity to MraY in a membrane environment. In an early study, the MIC value of mureidomycin B was determined to be over 200 μg/mL (= 0.237 mM) against the E. coli NIHJ JC-2 strain, and its highest antibacterial activity was against the Pseudomonas aeruginosa SANK 70579 strain with an MIC value of about 0.24 μM [61]. These MIC values are not comparable with the IC_{50} values determined by either the fluorescence-based assay or the whole cell assay described above. This indicates the importance of cell/membrane penetration for inhibitors to reach their targets in order to be at their most effective [50,51,53,62].

Shapiro et al. [56] developed a fluorescence resonance energy transfer (FRET)-based assay to screen MraY inhibitors. In this assay, the FRET donor fluorophore BODIPY-FL was attached to labeled UDP-Mpp, and the FRET acceptor lipid lissamine rhodamine B dipalmitoyl phosphatidylethanolamine (LRPE) was embedded in the lipid micelle mix containing MraY and C55-P (Figure 5). When the UDP-Mpp labeled with the FRET donor is mixed with the detergent micelles containing active EcMraY and C55-P, the FRET donor is transferred to C55-P, yielding Lipid I labeled with the donor. Hence, the FRET donor and the acceptor are brought into close proximity yielding a FRET signal where the acceptor fluorescence increases when the donor fluorescence is excited. This assay used C55-P dissolved in detergent micelles and a membrane preparation of EcMraY. It was found that increase of C55-P concentration increased the sensitivity of the assay to inhibition by tunicamycin. This finding corresponds to the Km discrepancies of MraY between different studies when different C55-P concentrations were used, which is addressed as the major message in our own study [34]. This FRET assay allowed the measurement of the fluorescence intensity ratio of the donor and acceptor, hence fluctuations in measurements that influence both the donor and acceptor fluorescence could be ruled out. This way, the assay provided a more precise determination of percentage inhibition compared with the single fluorescence detection assay described above. This assay is sensitive to competitive inhibitors of UDP-Mpp. The IC_{50} values of tunicamycin determined by this assay were in the nanomolar range, apparently at odds with that determined by the other fluorescence assay described above. It should be noted that what proceeds in vitro, where both the substrate and the enzyme are dissolved in mixed micelles, is not comparable with what proceeds in vivo, where both C55-P and MraY are embedded in the membrane and can find each other through 2D diffusion. This means that discrepancies between IC_{50} and MIC values may be expected. The fact that MraY has a substrate embedded in the membrane, as well as a soluble nucleotide substrate presents a considerable challenge in designing a representative laboratory-based in vitro assay.

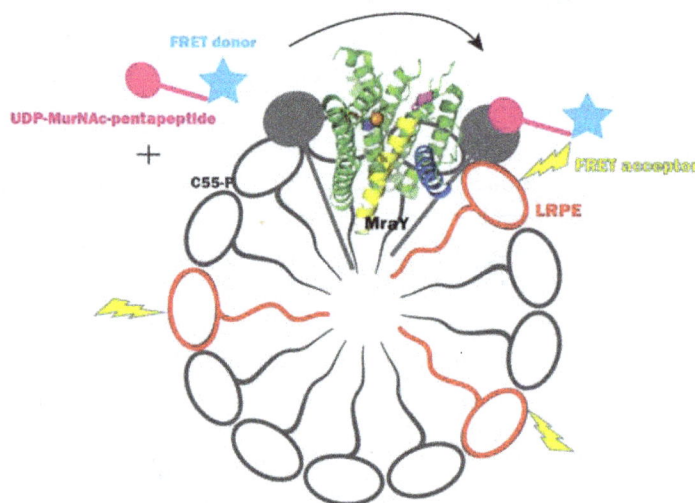

Figure 5. Fluorescence resonance energy transfer assay for MraY. The figure is adapted from [56].

2.3.2. Small Molecules that Inhibit MraY Activity

The best-known small molecule MraY inhibitors are the uridyl peptide antibiotics (UPAs), such as muraymycin, tunicamycin, mureidomycin, capuramycin and liposidomycin [27,30,31,41,63,64]. These small molecules share a common aminoribosyl-*O*-uridine skeleton, which was believed to be essential for their inhibitory activity, as it suggests that these compounds recognize and competitively bind to the UDP-Mpp binding sites on MraY [27,60,63–65]. A more detailed review has been published [27]. Here, we focus on the new discoveries, as well as a brief summary of the implications and challenges in developing such inhibitors.

Through detailed kinetics studies, UPA inhibitors were found to act against MraY in several ways. It was previously reported that mureidomycin A is competitive with both UDP-Mpp and C55-P, as the Km values of MraY for both substrates altered upon changing the inhibitor concentration [31]. This conclusion should be re-visited since the K_M value of either substrate is directly influenced by changing the concentration of the other [34]. This suggests that the inhibition of one substrate could indirectly influence the Km value for the other substrate without competitively inhibiting it. Tunicamycin was found to be only competitive with UDP-Mpp; liposidomycin B is non-competitive with UDP-Mpp [30]. It was also found that prolonged exposure of EcMraY to mureidomycin A [31] and liposidomycin B [30] did not alter the potency of these two inhibitors, indicating that the inhibition by these two molecules is reversible and that they are not consumed during the time of incubation, namely a slow-binding inhibitory mechanism.

Muraymycins (MRYs) are UPAs that have been studied extensively [65–68], and some exhibit antibacterial activity against Gram-positive pathogens, such as *S. aureus* and *Enterococcus* strains. MRY D2 and its epimer exhibit excellent anti-BsMraY activity with IC_{50} values of 0.01 µM and 0.09 µM, respectively, but both compounds showed very weak antibacterial activity against *S. aureus*, *E. faecalis* and *E. faecium* with MIC values over 64 µg/mL [65]. In contrast, two lipophilic analogues of MRY D2 with long lipid side chains showed excellent antibacterial activity against the same Gram-positive strains with MIC values between 0.5 and 4 µg/mL, although their IC_{50} values are about 10-fold higher than that of MRY D2 [65]. Apparently, adding lipophilic substituents [60,69–71] increased the accessibility of the active site of MraY for the MRY analogues, thereby improving their antibacterial activity. Further evidence remains to be established to explain this. A more recent study tested analogues of MRY D2 in the Gram-negative bacterium *P. aeruginosa*. Among all of the compounds tested, two analogues with a long lipid side chain and a positively-charged guanidinium group significantly increased the anti-*P. aeruginosa* activity [66]. Very recently, it was demonstrated through crystallography that AaMraY undergoes a large conformational change upon binding to MRY D2. This is the only structure of an MraY-inhibitor complex available at present. The structure shows that MraY is highly plastic and binds to its inhibitor MRY D2 in an overlapping, yet distinctive manner with respect to its natural nucleotide substrate. Such flexibility of MraY was also reported for MraY from *B. subtilis* [34], where it was demonstrated that BsMraY changes its conformation upon binding of C55-P to facilitate the nucleophilic attack on UDP-Mpp, involving an essential histidine residue.

How natural UPAs flip to the inner leaflet of cytoplasmic membrane and act against MraY as competitive inhibitors is not yet known. One hypothesis is that MraY is plastic and undergoes a conformational change upon periplasmic binding to UPAs. If correct, one could expect this to create a hydrophobic channel next to TM9, which may facilitate the uptake of these high molecular weight molecules to the cytoplasmic side and eventually allow them to bind to the active sites of MraY [63]. This hypothesis is based on some findings regarding the inhibition of EcMraY by protein E from bacteriophage ΦX174, which will be discussed in more detail in the next section. However, this implies that UPAs can bind to the periplasmic loops of MraY specifically, which seems not a likely mechanism.

Structural modification of known inhibitors provides a useful approach in developing novel inhibitors. An interesting example of this is the synthesis of 5'-triazole-substituted-aminoribosyl uridines (liposidomycin, caprazamycin or muraymycin) through Cu-catalyzed azide-alkyne cycloaddition (click chemistry) [72]. The 14 molecules investigated in this study exhibited IC_{50} values typically between 50 and 100 µM. Follow-up investigation using docking models showed that the activity of the most potent inhibitors correlates with their interaction with Leu191 in TM3 of AaMraY [73]. It was suggested that the introduction of a long lipid chain on the triazole substituent drastically improved the inhibitory activity. This lipid "anchor" may have helped in binding to TM3, given its possible involvement, hence locating the uridine close to the active sites of MraY. However, tests in vivo revealed that these molecules only showed bioactivity against Gram-positive bacteria with MICs between 8 and 32 μg/mL, including MRSA. Compared with the other studies on UPA-based MraY inhibitors, these two papers provide evidence for the involvement of an inhibition site (Leu191 of TM3) that was previously unknown.

Inhibitors developed through synthetic routes have only given high IC_{50} values thus far, e.g., 580 μM of an aminoribosyl-O-uridine based compound, limiting their application in vivo at present [72]. Nevertheless, a recently-discovered new MraY inhibitor through compound library screening, michellamine B, was found with a very high IC_{50} value (~0.5 mM against both EcMraY and BsMraY) and a reasonable MIC value (16 μg/mL against *B. subtilis*) [51]. Docking studies of the compound to the structure of AaMraY suggested that michellamine B inhibits MraY by binding to a hydrophobic groove formed between TM5 and TM9 of EcMraY (sequence alignment with MraY from other species shown in Figure 4). The authors addressed the importance of some phenylalanine residues in TM5 and TM9, which are known to make the TM interactions stronger [74]. It was also suggested that the presence of the polar glutamine residue that is close to a crucial phenylalanine (TM5) in *Staphylococcus aureus* MraY (SaMraY) was responsible for it becoming insensitive to michellamine B. However, this conclusion may require further evidence, as no mutant of these suggested residues was made to test this. Moreover, the docking study was carried out using the structure of AaMraY, while the antibacterial tests were performed on *B. subtilis*, which further complicates this issue. The possibility that MraY from different species may have different oligomeric states and that BsMraY is not necessarily present as a dimer have not yet been investigated. It is possible that the hydrophobic groove at the dimer interface of AaMraY proposed as the binding site of michellamine B may not even exist in BsMraY.

In summary, although some molecules show promising activity against MraY in tests carried out in vitro, applying these compounds in vivo, especially against Gram-negative pathogens, remains a challenge because keeping the compounds at low molecular weight while maintaining their antibacterial activity is not straightforward. Furthermore, some molecules, e.g., tunicamycin, possess other disadvantages, such as inhibiting other targets, e.g., GlcNAc-1-phosphate transferases, that are present in mammalian cells, which have hampered their clinical development [30,75,76].

2.3.3. MraY Inhibition by ΦX174 Protein E

Bacteriophages provide another therapeutic source of antibiotic lead compounds to treat bacterial infections. Early studies have found that protein E of a small single-stranded DNA phage ΦX174 causes *E. coli* cell lysis [77]. The exact mechanism was later revealed that protein E interferes with MraY function in *E. coli* and disrupts peptidoglycan synthesis [78]. Interestingly, this E-mediated lysis does not occur in Gram-positive bacteria [79].

Protein E is a 91-amino acid membrane protein with one transmembrane helix with 35 amino acids followed by a cytoplasmic domain. Both genetic and biochemical studies have found that the 29 amino acids from its N-terminus, which form the transmembrane domain of protein E, are responsible for the inhibition of MraY [77,80–83]. E is non-competitive with either substrate of MraY. Site-directed mutagenesis revealed that a proline at the 21 position of the TM domain of E is critical for its lytic activity; moving this proline along the membrane helix resulted in it being unable to inhibit MraY, suggesting that the kink at position 21 in the protein E helix caused by the proline is absolutely crucial [82]. It is unclear which binding pocket or helix of MraY binds to protein E because a structural model of MraY bound to protein E has not yet been produced. Genetic screening showed that Phe288 in TM9 of EcMraY (Phe286 on TM9 in AaMraY, Figure 5) is essential for its sensitivity towards protein E, as a single site mutation of F288L caused resistance against protein E. However, this phenylalanine residue is however missing in the E-insensitive Gram-positive BsMraY and SaMraY (Figure 4). TM9 is a titled helix in the AaMraY structure that breaks into two helices (TM9a and TM9b), while E has a kink caused by a proline [8,82]. In this respect, it is interesting to note that docking studies of protein E with a structural model of EcMraY suggested that TM9 (near the dimer interface) of MraY is involved in the binding to protein E indicating that this kinking of the helices may be important for their mutual interaction (Figure 6 [84]). In terms of a hypothesis, MraY presents a unique configuration when bound to protein E. In addition, we observed that there was no favored binding of E to the dimer interface when we tried to dock protein E to a structural model of BsMraY. This is an interesting observation given that BsMraY is not inhibited by protein E. Again, it is not clear whether BsMraY functions as a dimer at all in vivo. The reason why protein E does not interact strongly with the Gram-positive MraY homologues remains unresolved. Rodolis et al. [64] synthesized small peptides sharing a partial sequence of protein E and explored their inhibition of MraY homologues from both Gram-positive and -negative species. It was reported that an RWXXW motif found in E and other cationic antimicrobial peptides is essential for MraY inhibition. However, the small synthetic peptides reported in this paper all have a much lower inhibition, with an MIC value about 10–20-fold higher than protein E or the synthetic Epep (with the first 37 amino acid residues of protein E) against *E. coli*. Another study from the same group [63] presented the hypothesis that some UPAs, which show structural resemblance to the RWXXW motif, may bind to the protein E binding site on MraY near the periplasmic side initially before crossing the membranes and eventually bind to the active sites of MraY. Yet, evidence for this is lacking. Besides, protein E is synthesized in the cytoplasm of bacterial cells, while the other small molecule inhibitors of MraY must penetrate the cell envelope. This may result in a completely different mode of action in terms of how and where the molecules start binding to MraY. Therefore, it may be simplistic to attribute the inhibitory activity of protein E to a short peptide sequence.

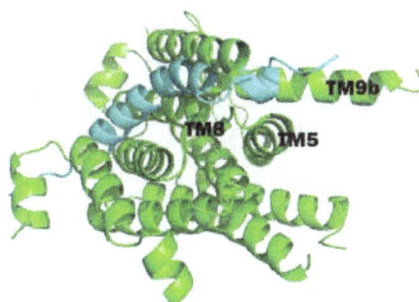

Figure 6. Cytoplasmic view of the docking model of protein E (the light blue helix) to an *E. coli* MraY structure model (modeled based on 4J72.pdb). The protein E helix binds closely to the hydrophobic groove formed by TM5, TM8 and TM9 and is bent towards the TM9b. The figure is rendered with Pymol.

MraY remains an interesting target for antibiotic discovery and development, although it still faces many challenges, particularly the penetration of the cell envelope. This holds true for all of the antibiotic targets that reside in the bacterial cytosol. The Lipid I synthesis catalyzed by MraY in vivo is drawn by the subsequent reaction of Lipid II synthesis, for which MurG is the responsible enzyme. Interestingly, these two enzymes interact as was shown by co-immunoprecipitation experiments [85]. In the following section, we will review its discovery, characterization and the advances made in inhibiting this important bacterial enzyme.

3. MurG

The earliest work on the *murG* gene indicated that it was involved in the cell envelope biogenesis and, in particular, peptidoglycan metabolism [86]. Later, it was identified that *murG* codes for an *N*-acetylglucosamine (GlcNAc) transferase, from then on referred to as MurG [87]. This enzyme belongs to the glycosyltransferase family and catalyzes an irreversible essential step on the membrane after MraY. MurG attaches the GlcNAc from UDP-GlcNAc to Lipid I and produces Lipid II [88]. MurG is an essential enzyme and is conserved across almost all bacterial species, which makes MurG a great target for novel antibiotics. However, MurG is a paradigm for glycosyltransferases that are present in the vast majority of both prokaryotic and eukaryotic cells. This implies that only inhibitors that compete with Lipid I bear the potential of further clinical development. The structural information regarding the substrate selectivity and the inhibition mechanism of MurG will be discussed in the following sections.

3.1. Biochemical Characterization of MurG

An early study demonstrated that *E. coli* MurG (EcMurG) is a membrane-associated protein [87]. Later, it was reported that EcMurG is exposed to the cytoplasm of *E. coli* by showing that the enzyme in spheroplasts was not sensitive to trypsin treatment [89]. With this knowledge combined, it could be concluded that MurG is peripherally associated with the inner leaflet of the plasma membrane.

Crouvoisier et al. described a purification of EcMurG to greater than an 80% yield using immobilized affinity beads [90], suggesting that the production and purification of MurG was much easier compared with the membrane-embedded MraY. N-terminally His-tagged MurG showed higher yield and purity with respect to wild-type or C-terminally His-tagged MurG. The authors concluded that MurG is a peripheral membrane protein according to a few criteria: partial solubilization by salt treatments, purification without detergent, localization on the inner side of the cytoplasmic membrane, a cationic theoretical pI value of 9.7 and a lack of significant hydrophobic regions in its amino acid sequence. It was yet unknown how exactly MurG associates with the bacterial membrane.

The kinetics of MurG had been difficult to measure because the lipid substrate Lipid I typically has a low abundance in vivo [54]. A series of water-soluble Lipid I analogues were used to determine EcMurG activity and kinetics in a biotin-capture assay (Figure 7) [91]. In this assay, a radiolabeled UDP-(^{14}C)-GlcNAc and a functional biotinylated GlcNAc acceptor analogue of Lipid I were incubated together with cell lysate enriched in MurG enzyme for a period of time. The reaction was quenched by adding SDS to a final concentration of 0.33%. Radioactivity was captured by an avidin-derivatized resin and counted after the unbound radioactivity was washed away.

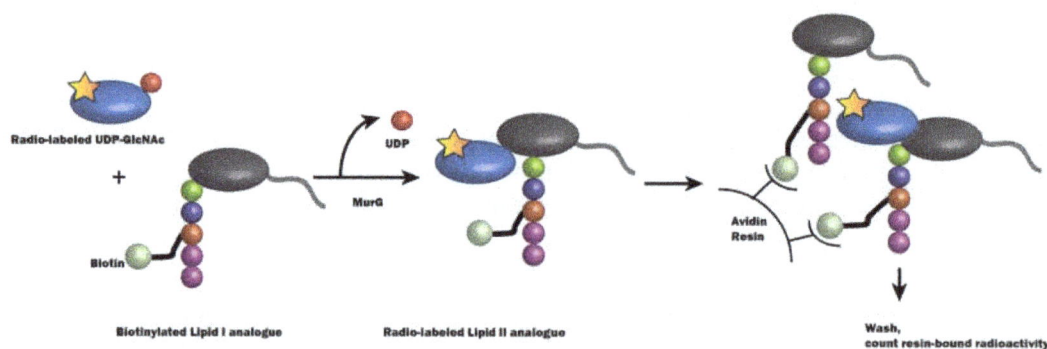

Figure 7. Schematic illustration of the biotin-capture assay for MurG activity [91]. In this assay, MurG catalyzes a reaction between radiolabeled (depicted by a yellow star) UDP-GlcNAc and biotinylated Lipid I analogue, and Lipid II with the radiolabel is synthesized. The avidin resin, which binds to biotin, therefore catches the radioactivity, which can be counted to indicate the MurG activity.

Production of pure MurG without the need of using detergent [90] led to speculation that MurG activity did not require membranes and could be assayed with soluble substrates instead of the natural long chain Lipid I [88]. A fluorescence assay for MurG coupled with pyruvate kinase activity was developed [88], which measures the decrease of the fluorescence signal from NADH (Figure 8). This study revealed that MurG accepted soluble substrates with short chains (two prenyl units) and preferred substrates that have a *cis*-allylic double bond. These findings built the foundation of using synthetic soluble substrates (Lipid I mimics) to assay MurG activity. It should be noted that in such a reaction system, MurG is not associated with any membranes, unlike its natural status. This will require that the Lipid I substrate finds the enzyme via three-dimensional diffusion. In vivo, Lipid I, and MurG likely as well, is membrane bound. Hence, they are able to find each other via two-dimensional diffusion, which is much more effective than diffusion in three dimensions, which normally occurs in solutions [92].

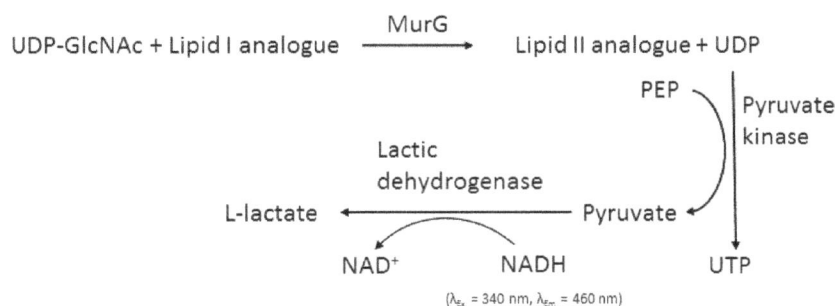

Figure 8. Fluorescence coupled assay for MurG. The figure is adapted from [88].

Later, it was reported that lipid vesicles enriched in the negatively-charged cardiolipin co-purified with EcMurG and the presence of cardiolipin also enhanced MurG activity [93]. This study provided the first direct evidence that MurG was linked to the cytoplasmic membrane by direct interaction with lipids and preferably with cardiolipin.

Besides the (naturally-occurring) polyisoprenyl-bound Lipid I mentioned above, it was also reported that the saturated C14 alkyl-Lipid I was a substrate of MurG, which was even the best performing analogue in this study [94]. Nevertheless, both studies showed that MurG prefers shorter Lipid I analogues than its natural Lipid I substrate in an in vitro set-up, possibly due to solubility problems because of the long lipid chains and the 3D diffusion mode in vitro instead of the 2D diffusion mode in vivo, as mentioned above. This is the first assay for MurG that did not rely on end point measurement or any radioisotope.

3.2. Structural Characterization of MurG

Soon after the first report on its purification, the crystal structure of EcMurG at 1.9 Å (PDB ID: 1F0K) emerged [95]. The crystal structure revealed two major domains of MurG and a hydrophobic cleft formed in between the domains. Although the homology is relatively low, the two domains of MurG are structurally similar. Both domains have Rossman-like folds, which is typical for nucleotide binding domains [96,97]. In particular, the C-domain of EcMurG shares significant structural homology with the C-domain of phage T4 β-glucosyltransferase (BGT) containing a UDP binding pocket. It is therefore suggested that the C-domain of MurG is the binding site of UDP-GlcNAc and transfers the GlcNAc moiety to Lipid I. Moreover, it was proposed that MurG is associated with the negatively-charged bacterial membrane via a hydrophobic patch surrounded by basic residues through hydrophobic and electrostatic interactions, which inspired the later finding that MurG associates with the membrane preferably via cardiolipin, described in Section 3.1 [93].

A co-crystal structure of EcMurG with UDP-GlcNAc (PDB ID: 1NLM) [98] confirmed that UDP-GlcNAc binds tightly to the C-domain. Moreover, substrate specificity studies revealed that EcMurG is highly selective for the nucleotide attached to its donor sugar substrate unlike most other GTases that do not discriminate between UDP and TDP [99]. EcMurG showed no activity when TDP-GlcNAc was used as the substrate [98]. The affinity of MurG to other nucleotide diphosphates, such as CDP, ADP and GDP, is at least 10-times lower than to UDP [91]. This substrate specificity may be sufficient for developing inhibitors for the UDP-binding site on MurG.

Many conserved residues of MurG are located in between the two major domains situated in the cleft. Crouvoisier et al. [100] aligned over 70 MurG orthologues from different bacterial species and performed site-directed mutagenesis to explore the functional significance of those conserved residues. Their studies have identified 13 residues located near the cleft that are somehow important for MurG's activity. The mutation of these amino acids into alanine has either caused significant loss of MurG activity or resulted in a highly unstable protein.

The different MurG homologues have moderate sequential homology, while their structural homology is thought to be high among different species that make peptidoglycan. This was demonstrated when the structure of *P. aeruginosa* MurG (PaMurG) bound to UDP-GlcNAc was also solved by a different group [101]. Although the sequence homology between these two MurG homologues was only 45%, the structures and the mode of binding to the donor substrate are very similar. The authors noted that one major difference between the structures was that the N-domain of *E. coli* MurG swung further away from the C-domain, causing the cleft between the two domains to be larger than that of PaMurG. For EcMurG, UDP-GlcNAc is situated closely to the cleft, which is not large enough to accommodate TDP-GlcNAc. An even narrower cleft in PaMurG confirms the substrate specificity regarding the nucleotide, but this knowledge does not seem to add any other significance, since EcMurG already has a sufficiently narrow cleft that facilitates only specific binding to UDP other than other nucleotide or nucleoside substrates. In the structure of PaMurG, H15 (equivalent of H19 in EcMurG) is present, as well. This residue is not only positioned very close to the bound UDP-GlcNAc, but also points towards the proposed Lipid I binding site (Figure 9B). This indicates the importance of this histidine residue in coupling the donor sugar to the acceptor Lipid I. To date, there is no crystal structure of MurG (from any bacterial species) bound to Lipid I available. Research in understanding the precise nature of the Lipid I-substrate interaction is essential for furthering our understanding of the mode of action of this enzyme.

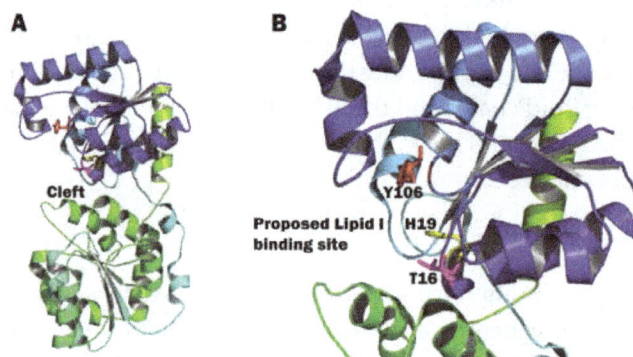

Figure 9. *E. coli* MurG structure. (**A**) The complete view of *E. coli* MurG, N-domain in blue, C-domain in green. The cleft in between the two domains is indicated by an arrow; (**B**) A close-up view of the cleft between the N- and C-domains of MurG. Residues T16 (pink), H19 (yellow) and Y106 (red) are shown as sticks. The proposed Lipid I binding site is indicated by an arrow. The image was obtained and rendered using Pymol.

3.3. MurG Inhibitors

To date, the discovery of selective MurG inhibitors typically relies on two approaches. One approach is to synthesize UDP-GlcNAc-mimicking compounds either by elaborating the nucleotide group or to use existing inhibitors to design similar molecules. The alternative approach relies on screening of a compound library to generate leads that can competitively bind to MurG using an assay that exploits the purified enzyme [98,102,103]. The compounds discovered through this channel require further modification to avoid two scenarios: (1) binding to other glycosyltransferases that are also present in eukaryotic cells; (2) poor penetration of the cell wall.

Since the elucidation of the structure of MurG-UDP-GlcNAc, efforts to identify competitive inhibitors by screening analogues of UDP-GlcNAc-mimicking compounds have been under way [103]. The ligand-bound MurG structure revealed that the methyl of the *N*-acyl group of UDP-GlcNAc was exposed, which suggests that modification of this group will not affect the binding of UDP-GlcNAc to MurG. A fluorescently-labeled UDP-GlcNAc was made based on this hypothesis. It was found that the fluorescent modification slowed rather than abolished substrate binding. The fluorescence decreased when the binding was inhibited by the addition of MurG inhibitors, as the substrate was displaced from MurG. A high throughput screening based on the substrate displacement was established. Using this method, the authors screened 64,000 molecules that came from a variety of compound libraries, and less than 0.6% of the molecules were found as hits. To validate the selectivity, kinetics assays as described in Section 3.1 (Figure 7) were used, and eventually, seven compounds were identified as selective MurG inhibitors with IC_{50} values ranging between 1 and 7 μM. However, all seven compounds showed an inhibitory effect against another glycosyltransferase GtfB (structurally related to MurG), with IC_{50} values of between two- and 10-fold higher. This indicates that the UDP-binding site is a relatively poor target for inhibitors despite MurG's specificity for UDP-GlcNAc over TDP-GlcNAc (vide supra). This suggests that the substrate displacement assay can only be used for identifying hit compounds. Inhibitor selectivity must be verified using another assay that is specific for MurG. However, such specificity will have to rely on blocking the binding of Lipid I to MurG.

Another interesting assay is based on a dansylated Lipid I analogue (MurNAc($N\varepsilon$-dansylpentapeptide)-pyrophosphoryl (R, S)-α-dihydroheptaprenol, C35-Lipid I) and a radiolabeled UDP-(^{14}C)-GlcNAc [104]. The radioactive substrate and product were separated using reverse-phase HPLC. Although this assay was shown to be rapid and specific for MurG, the authors could not separate the product (Lipid II) from the substrate (Lipid I) based on the dansyl fluorescent label. This assay could therefore not be optimized to a high throughput format easily. Nevertheless, this study showed for the first time that, via observations of the transfer of the radiolabel, a reverse reaction from Lipid II and UDP to UDP-GlcNAc can happen at a very low rate.

Several MraY-MurG coupled assays were also made available to discover lead compounds that can inhibit either or both enzymes in vitro [54,55,58,59]. Besides a higher efficiency in finding useful leads, the other advantage of such an assay is that there is no need to synthesize Lipid I analogues prior to the assay and thereby lower the cost.

It was reported that a vancomycin derivative with N-chlorobiphenyl-N-methyl leucine was a potent inhibitor of MurG in vitro [94]. Moenomycin, a known antibiotic that interferes with the function of the transglycosylase domain of PBP1B [105], was also found to inhibit MurG. However, neither vancomycin nor moenomycin inhibits MurG in vivo, as neither can penetrate the bacterial membranes and, therefore, do not encounter MurG [94].

The most recently-found inhibitor of MurG is a narrow-spectrum compound called murgocil [106]. While screening for antibacterial compounds that inactivate MRSA, the steroid-like molecule murgocil was identified to bind to MurG specifically. An assay in vitro showed that Lipid II synthesis was inhibited by murgocil in a dose-dependent manner. Interestingly, the bioactivity of murgocil against *Staphylococci* (MIC = 2–4 μg/mL) was considerably higher than its activity in vitro against purified *S. aureus* MurG (IC50 = 115 μM $\approx$ 51 μg/mL). Taken together with docking studies of the homology model of SaMurG based on the EcMurG structure, murgocil appears to inhibit peptidoglycan synthesis more efficiently in whole cells and has a synergistic activity with a β-lactam partially by delocalizing PBP2 from the division septum during peptidoglycan synthesis. The binding site of murgocil to MurG was revealed by several murgocil-resistant staphylococci of which the resistance could be mapped in the previously-mentioned cleft region between the N- and C-domains of MurG. Docking studies confirmed that murgocil can bind to this cleft of MurG and may lock the enzyme in an inflexible conformation. The significantly higher IC_{50} value of murgocil may be ascribed to the difference between the measurements taken from in vitro and in vivo systems. Lipid I is always embedded in the phospholipid bilayer membranes in vivo, where MurG can reach it via lateral diffusion. This is not the case for activity tests in vitro, where the substrate Lipid I is often presented in micelles, and in some cases, water-soluble Lipid I analogues are used [107]. Again, murgocil activity in vivo is strictly restricted to *Staphylococci*, the possibility of expanding its use to other Gram-positive or -negative bacteria seems rather limited, since it was found that murgocil activity depends on some amino acid residues that are unique in SaMurG, including M45 and D168. However, further work is required to confirm this.

The development on MurG inhibitors has reached a plateau by comparison to MraY. The potential toxicity of MurG inhibitors in vivo that compete with UDP-GlcNAc remains the biggest concern in terms of further clinical development.

4. Conclusions

Recent work has led to a substantial growth in our understanding of the structural and biochemical characteristics of MraY and MurG, which led to the gradual unraveling of the mode of action of these enzymes. It is evident that previous studies have put much effort in investigating the nucleotide substrate of both MraY and MurG, while many questions regarding the lipid substrate for both enzymes have yet to be answered. Once we understand the molecular details of their mutual interaction, novel inhibitors can be designed to block the enzymatic activity. The search for combination therapies that involve a synergistic effect of a cell wall inhibitor with another class of antibiotics, e.g., a β-lactam, might form part of the therapy yet to come.

Acknowledgments: Yao Liu is supported by a ZonMW grant (No. 205.100.008) from The Netherlands Organization for Scientific Research (NWO). The authors are grateful for the language editing and constructive feedback from Samuel Furse, University of Bergen, Norway. The authors also would like to acknowledge Joao Rodrigues (Stanford University) and Alexandre Bonvin (Utrecht University) for their effort in the unpublished docking studies.

Author Contributions: Yao Liu and Eefjan Breukink read, analyzed the literature and wrote the manuscript.

References

1.   Sobhanifar, S.; King, D.T.; Strynadka, N.C. Fortifying the wall: Synthesis, regulation and degradation of bacterial peptidoglycan. *Curr. Opin. Struct. Biol.* **2013**, *23*, 695–703. [CrossRef] [PubMed]

2.   Al-Dabbagh, B.; Mengin-Lecreulx, D.; Bouhss, A. Purification and characterization of the bacterial UDP-GlcNAc: Undecaprenyl-phosphate GlcNAc-1-phosphate transferase WecA. *J. Bacteriol.* **2008**, *190*, 7141–7146. [CrossRef] [PubMed]

3.   Typas, A.; Banzhaf, M.; Gross, C.A.; Vollmer, W. From the regulation of peptidoglycan synthesis to bacterial growth and morphology. *Nat. Rev. Microbiol.* **2012**, *10*, 123–136. [CrossRef] [PubMed]

4.   Rani, C.; Khan, I.A. UDP-GlcNAc pathway: Potential target for inhibitor discovery against *M. tuberculosis*. *Eur. J. Pharm. Sci.* **2015**, *83*, 62–70. [CrossRef] [PubMed]

5.   Lovering, A.L.; Safadi, S.S.; Strynadka, N.C. Structural perspective of peptidoglycan biosynthesis and assembly. *Annu. Rev. Biochem.* **2012**, *81*, 451–478. [CrossRef] [PubMed]

6.   Guo, R.T.; Ko, T.P.; Chen, A.P.; Kuo, C.J.; Wang, A.H.; Liang, P.H. Crystal structures of undecaprenyl pyrophosphate synthase in complex with magnesium, isopentenyl pyrophosphate, and farnesyl thiopyrophosphate: Roles of the metal ion and conserved residues in catalysis. *J. Biol. Chem.* **2005**, *280*, 20762–20774. [CrossRef] [PubMed]

7.   Chang, H.Y.; Chou, C.C.; Hsu, M.F.; Wang, A.H. Proposed carrier lipid-binding site of undecaprenyl pyrophosphate phosphatase from *Escherichia coli*. *J. Biol. Chem.* **2014**, *289*, 18719–18735. [CrossRef] [PubMed]

8.   Chung, B.C.; Zhao, J.; Gillespie, R.A.; Kwon, D.Y.; Guan, Z.; Hong, J.; Zhou, P.; Lee, S.Y. Crystal structure of MraY, an essential membrane enzyme for bacterial cell wall synthesis. *Science* **2013**, *341*, 1012–1016. [CrossRef] [PubMed]

9.   Ishii, K.; Sagami, H.; Ogura, K. A novel prenyltransferase from paracoccus denitrificans. *Biochem. J.* **1986**, *233*, 773–777. [CrossRef] [PubMed]

10.   Kaur, D.; Brennan, P.J.; Crick, D.C. Decaprenyl diphosphate synthesis in *Mycobacterium tuberculosis*. *J. Bacteriol.* **2004**, *186*, 7564–7570. [CrossRef] [PubMed]

11.   Guo, H.; Yi, W.; Song, J.K.; Wang, P.G. Current understanding on biosynthesis of microbial polysaccharides. *Curr. Top. Med. Chem.* **2008**, *8*, 141–151. [PubMed]

12. Xia, G.; Maier, L.; Sanchez-Carballo, P.; Li, M.; Otto, M.; Holst, O.; Peschel, A. Glycosylation of wall teichoic acid in *Staphylococcus aureus* by tarm. *J. Biol. Chem.* **2010**, *285*, 13405–13415. [CrossRef] [PubMed]

13. Bouhss, A.; Trunkfield, A.E.; Bugg, T.D.; Mengin-Lecreulx, D. The biosynthesis of peptidoglycan lipid-linked intermediates. *FEMS Microbiol. Rev.* **2008**, *32*, 208–233. [CrossRef] [PubMed]

14. Weidenmaier, C.; Lee, J.C. Structure and function of surface polysaccharides of *Staphylococcus aureus*. *Curr. Top. Microbiol. Immunol.* **2016**. [CrossRef]

15. Mohammadi, T.; van Dam, V.; Sijbrandi, R.; Vernet, T.; Zapun, A.; Bouhss, A.; Diepeveen-de Bruin, M.; Nguyen-Disteche, M.; de Kruijff, B.; Breukink, E. Identification of FtsW as a transporter of lipid-linked cell wall precursors across the membrane. *EMBO J.* **2011**, *30*, 1425–1432. [CrossRef] [PubMed]

16. Mohammadi, T.; Sijbrandi, R.; Lutters, M.; Verheul, J.; Martin, N.I.; den Blaauwen, T.; de Kruijff, B.; Breukink, E. Specificity of the transport of lipid II by FtsW in *Escherichia coli*. *J. Biol. Chem.* **2014**, *289*, 14707–14718. [CrossRef] [PubMed]

17. Sham, L.T.; Butler, E.K.; Lebar, M.D.; Kahne, D.; Bernhardt, T.G.; Ruiz, N. Bacterial cell wall. MurJ is the flippase of lipid-linked precursors for peptidoglycan biogenesis. *Science* **2014**, *345*, 220–222. [CrossRef] [PubMed]

18. Kahrstrom, C.T. Bacterial physiology: Flipping out over MurJ. *Nat. Rev. Microbiol.* **2014**. [CrossRef] [PubMed]

19. Egan, A.J.; Biboy, J.; van't Veer, I.; Breukink, E.; Vollmer, W. Activities and regulation of peptidoglycan synthases. *Philos. Trans. R. Soc. Lond. B Biol. Sci.* **2015**. [CrossRef] [PubMed]

20. Jeong, J.H.; Kim, Y.S.; Rojviriya, C.; Ha, S.C.; Kang, B.S.; Kim, Y.G. Crystal structures of bifunctional penicillin-binding protein 4 from listeria monocytogenes. *Antimicrob. Agents Chemother.* **2013**, *57*, 3507–3512. [CrossRef] [PubMed]

21. Sung, M.T.; Lai, Y.T.; Huang, C.Y.; Chou, L.Y.; Shih, H.W.; Cheng, W.C.; Wong, C.H.; Ma, C. Crystal structure of the membrane-bound bifunctional transglycosylase PBP1b from *Escherichia coli*. *Proc. Natl. Acad. Sci. USA* **2009**, *106*, 8824–8829. [CrossRef] [PubMed]

22. Slusarz, R.; Szulc, M.; Madaj, J. Molecular modeling of gram-positive bacteria peptidoglycan layer, selected glycopeptide antibiotics and vancomycin derivatives modified with sugar moieties. *Carbohydr. Res.* **2014**, *389*, 154–164. [CrossRef] [PubMed]

23. Yarlagadda, V.; Akkapeddi, P.; Manjunath, G.B.; Haldar, J. Membrane active vancomycin analogues: A strategy to combat bacterial resistance. *J. Med. Chem.* **2014**, *57*, 4558–4568. [CrossRef] [PubMed]

24. Chawla-Sarkar, M.; Bae, S.I.; Reu, F.J.; Jacobs, B.S.; Lindner, D.J.; Borden, E.C. Downregulation of Bcl-2, FLIP or IAPs (XIAP and survivin) by siRNAs sensitizes resistant melanoma cells to Apo2L/TRAIL-induced apoptosis. *Cell Death Differ.* **2004**, *11*, 915–923. [CrossRef] [PubMed]

25. Worthington, R.J.; Melander, C. Overcoming resistance to beta-lactam antibiotics. *J. Org. Chem.* **2013**, *78*, 4207–4213. [CrossRef] [PubMed]

26. Hamed, R.B.; Gomez-Castellanos, J.R.; Henry, L.; Ducho, C.; McDonough, M.A.; Schofield, C.J. The enzymes of beta-lactam biosynthesis. *Nat. Prod. Rep.* **2013**, *30*, 21–107. [CrossRef] [PubMed]

27. Bugg, T.D.; Lloyd, A.J.; Roper, D.I. Phospho-murnac-pentapeptide translocase (MraY) as a target for antibacterial agents and antibacterial proteins. *Infect. Disord. Drug Targets* **2006**, *6*, 85–106. [CrossRef] [PubMed]

28. Anderson, J.S.; Matsuhashi, M.; Haskin, M.A.; Strominger, J.L. Lipid-phosphoacetylmuramyl-pentapeptide and lipid-phosphodisaccharide-pentapeptide: Presumed membrane transport intermediates in cell wall synthesis. *Proc. Natl. Acad. Sci. USA* **1965**, *53*, 881–889. [CrossRef] [PubMed]

29. Ikeda, M.; Wachi, M.; Jung, H.K.; Ishino, F.; Matsuhashi, M. The *Escherichia coli* mraY gene encoding UDP-N-acetylmuramoyl-pentapeptide: Undecaprenyl-phosphate phospho-N-acetylmuramoyl-pentapeptide transferase. *J. Bacteriol.* **1991**, *173*, 1021–1026. [PubMed]

30. Brandish, P.E.; Kimura, K.I.; Inukai, M.; Southgate, R.; Lonsdale, J.T.; Bugg, T.D. Modes of action of tunicamycin, liposidomycin B, and mureidomycin A: Inhibition of phospho-N-acetylmuramyl-pentapeptide translocase from *Escherichia coli*. *Antimicrob. Agents Chemother.* **1996**, *40*, 1640–1644. [PubMed]

31. Brandish, P.E.; Burnham, M.K.; Lonsdale, J.T.; Southgate, R.; Inukai, M.; Bugg, T.D. Slow binding inhibition of phospho-N-acetylmuramyl-pentapeptide-translocase (*Escherichia coli*) by mureidomycin A. *J. Biol. Chem.* **1996**, *271*, 7609–7614. [PubMed]

32. Bouhss, A.; Crouvoisier, M.; Blanot, D.; Mengin-Lecreulx, D. Purification and characterization of the bacterial MraY translocase catalyzing the first membrane step of peptidoglycan biosynthesis. *J. Biol. Chem.* **2004**, *279*, 29974–29980. [CrossRef] [PubMed]

33. Ma, Y.; Munch, D.; Schneider, T.; Sahl, H.G.; Bouhss, A.; Ghoshdastider, U.; Wang, J.; Dotsch, V.; Wang, X.; Bernhard, F. Preparative scale cell-free production and quality optimization of MraY homologues in different expression modes. *J. Biol. Chem.* **2011**, *286*, 38844–38853. [CrossRef]

34. Liu, Y.; Rodrigues, J.P.; Bonvin, A.M.; Zaal, E.A.; Berkers, C.R.; Heger, M.; Gawarecka, K.; Swiezewska, E.; Breukink, E.; Egmond, M.R. New insight in the catalytic mechanism of bacterial MraY from enzyme kinetics and docking studies. *J. Biol. Chem.* **2016**. [CrossRef] [PubMed]

35. Al-Dabbagh, B.; Olatunji, S.; Crouvoisier, M.; El Ghachi, M.; Blanot, D.; Mengin-Lecreulx, D.; Bouhss, A. Catalytic mechanism of MraY and WecA, two paralogues of the polyprenyl-phosphate *N*-acetylhexosamine 1-phosphate transferase superfamily. *Biochimie* **2016**, *127*, 249–257. [CrossRef] [PubMed]

36. Al-Dabbagh, B.; Henry, X.; Ghachi, M.E.; Auger, G.V.; Blanot, D.; Parquet, C.; Mengin-Lecreulx, D.; Bouhss, A. Active site mapping of MraY, a member of the polyprenyl-phosphate *N*-acetylhexosamine 1-phosphate transferase superfamily, catalyzing the first membrane step of peptidoglycan biosynthesis. *Biochemistry* **2008**, *47*, 8919–8928. [CrossRef] [PubMed]

37. Roos, C.; Zocher, M.; Müller, D.; Münch, D.; Schneider, T.; Sahl, H.-G.; Scholz, F.; Wachtveitl, J.; Ma, Y.; Proverbio, D.; et al. Characterization of co-translationally formed nanodisc complexes with small multidrug transporters, proteorhodopsin and with the *E. coli* MraY translocase. *BBA—Biomembranes* **2012**, *1818*, 3098–3106. [CrossRef] [PubMed]

38. Henrich, E.; Dotsch, V.; Bernhard, F. Screening for lipid requirements of membrane proteins by combining cell-free expression with nanodiscs. *Methods Enzymol.* **2015**, *556*, 351–369. [PubMed]

39. Henrich, E.; Ma, Y.; Engels, I.; Munch, D.; Otten, C.; Schneider, T.; Henrichfreise, B.; Sahl, H.G.; Dotsch, V.; Bernhard, F. Lipid requirements for the enzymatic activity of MraY translocases and in vitro reconstitution of the lipid II synthesis pathway. *J. Biol. Chem.* **2016**, *291*, 2535–2546. [CrossRef] [PubMed]

40. Umbreit, J.N.; Strominger, J.L. Complex lipid requirements for detergent-solubilized phosphoacetylmuramyl-pentapeptide translocase from micrococcus luteus. *Proc. Natl. Acad. Sci. USA* **1972**, *69*, 1972–1974. [CrossRef] [PubMed]

41. Lloyd, A.J.; Brandish, P.E.; Gilbey, A.M.; Bugg, T.D.H. Phospho-*N*-acetyl-muramyl-pentapeptide translocase from *Escherichia coli*: Catalytic role of conserved aspartic acid residues. *J. Bacteriol.* **2004**, *186*, 1747–1757. [CrossRef] [PubMed]

42. Pless, D.D.; Neuhaus, F.C. Initial membrane reaction in peptidoglycan synthesis. Lipid dependence of phospho-*N*-acetylmuramyl-pentapeptide translocase (exchange reaction). *J. Biol. Chem.* **1973**, *248*, 1568–1576. [PubMed]

43. Bouhss, A.; Mengin-Lecreulx, D.; le Beller, D.; van Heijenoort, J. Topological analysis of the MraY protein catalysing the first membrane step of peptidoglycan synthesis. *Mol. Microbiol.* **1999**, *34*, 576–585. [CrossRef] [PubMed]

44. Omasits, U.; Ahrens, C.H.; Muller, S.; Wollscheid, B. Protter: Interactive protein feature visualization and integration with experimental proteomic data. *Bioinformatics* **2014**, *30*, 884–886. [CrossRef] [PubMed]

45. Heydanek, M.G., Jr.; Struve, W.G.; Neuhaus, F.C. On the initial stage in peptidoglycan synthesis. 3. Kinetics and uncoupling of phospho-*N*-acetylmuramyl-pentapeptide translocase (uridine 5′-phosphate). *Biochemistry* **1969**, *8*, 1214–1221. [CrossRef] [PubMed]

46. Umbreit, J.N.; Strominger, J.L. Isolation of the lipid intermediate in peptidoglycan biosynthesis from *Escherichia coli*. *J. Bacteriol.* **1972**, *112*, 1306–1309. [PubMed]

47. Maillard, A.P.; Biarrotte-Sorin, S.; Villet, R.; Mesnage, S.; Bouhss, A.; Sougakoff, W.; Mayer, C.; Arthur, M. Structure-based site-directed mutagenesis of the UDP-MurNAc-pentapeptide-binding cavity of the FemX alanyl transferase from *Weissella viridescens*. *J. Bacteriol.* **2005**, *187*, 3833–3838. [CrossRef] [PubMed]

48. Price, N.P.; Momany, F.A. Modeling bacterial UDP-HexNAc: Polyprenol-P HexNAc-1-P transferases. *Glycobiology* **2005**, *15*, 29R–42R. [CrossRef] [PubMed]

49. White, C.L.; Kitich, A.; Gober, J.W. Positioning cell wall synthetic complexes by the bacterial morphogenetic proteins MreB and MreD. *Mol. Microbiol.* **2010**, *76*, 616–633. [CrossRef] [PubMed]

50. Stachyra, T.; Dini, C.; Ferrari, P.; Bouhss, A.; van Heijenoort, J.; Mengin-Lecreulx, D.; Blanot, D.; Biton, J.; Le Beller, D. Fluorescence detection-based functional assay for high-throughput screening for MraY. *Antimicrob. Agents Chemother.* **2004**, *48*, 897–902. [CrossRef] [PubMed]

51. Mihalyi, A.; Jamshidi, S.; Slikas, J.; Bugg, T.D.H. Identification of novel inhibitors of phospho-murnac-pentapeptide translocase MraY from library screening: Isoquinoline alkaloid michellamine B and xanthene dye phloxine B. *Bioorg. Med. Chem.* **2014**, *22*, 4566–4571. [CrossRef] [PubMed]

52. Howard, N.I.; Bugg, T.D. Synthesis and activity of 5′-uridinyl dipeptide analogues mimicking the amino terminal peptide chain of nucleoside antibiotic mureidomycin A. *Bioorg. Med. Chem.* **2003**, *11*, 3083–3099. [CrossRef]

53. Mihalyi, A. Screening for novel inhibitors of phospho-murnac-pentapeptide translocase MraY. *Thesis Univ. Warwick* **2014**, *22*, 4566–4571.

54. Branstrom, A.A.; Midha, S.; Longley, C.B.; Han, K.; Baizman, E.R.; Axelrod, H.R. Assay for identification of inhibitors for bacterial MraY translocase or MurG transferase. *Anal. Biochem.* **2000**, *280*, 315–319. [CrossRef] [PubMed]

55. Ravishankar, S.; Kumar, V.P.; Chandrakala, B.; Jha, R.K.; Solapure, S.M.; de Sousa, S.M. Scintillation proximity assay for inhibitors of *Escherichia coli* MurG and, optionally, MraY. *Antimicrob. Agents Chemother.* **2005**, *49*, 1410–1418. [CrossRef] [PubMed]

56. Shapiro, A.B.; Jahic, H.; Gao, N.; Hajec, L.; Rivin, O. A high-throughput, homogeneous, fluorescence resonance energy transfer-based assay for phospho-*N*-acetylmuramoyl-pentapeptide translocase (MraY). *J. Biomol. Screen.* **2012**, *17*, 662–672. [CrossRef] [PubMed]

57. Solapure, S.M.; Raphael, P.; Gayathri, C.N.; Barde, S.P.; Chandrakala, B.; Das, K.S.; de Sousa, S.M. Development of a microplate-based scintillation proximity assay for MraY using a modified substrate. *J. Biomol. Screen.* **2005**, *10*, 149–156. [CrossRef] [PubMed]

58. Hyland, S.A.; Anderson, M.S. A high-throughput solid-phase extraction assay capable of measuring diverse polyprenyl phosphate: Sugar-1-phosphate transferases as exemplified by the WecA, MraY, and MurG proteins. *Anal. Biochem.* **2003**, *317*, 156–165. [CrossRef]

59. Zawadzke, L.E.; Wu, P.; Cook, L.; Fan, L.; Casperson, M.; Kishnani, M.; Calambur, D.; Hofstead, S.J.; Padmanabha, R. Targeting the MraY and MurG bacterial enzymes for antimicrobial therapeutic intervention. *Anal. Biochem.* **2003**, *314*, 243–252. [CrossRef]

60. Dini, C.; Collette, P.; Drochon, N.; Guillot, J.C.; Lemoine, G.; Mauvais, P.; Aszodi, J. Synthesis of the nucleoside moiety of liposidomycins: Elucidation of the pharmacophore of this family of MraY inhibitors. *Bioorg. Med. Chem. Lett.* **2000**, *10*, 1839–1843. [CrossRef]

61. Isono, F.; Katayama, T.; Inukai, M.; Haneishi, T. Mureidomycins A–D, novel peptidylnucleoside antibiotics with spheroplast forming activity. III. Biological properties. *J. Antibiot.* **1989**, *42*, 674–679. [CrossRef] [PubMed]

62. Murakami, R.; Muramatsu, Y.; Minami, E.; Masuda, K.; Sakaida, Y.; Endo, S.; Suzuki, T.; Ishida, O.; Takatsu, T.; Miyakoshi, S.; et al. A novel assay of bacterial peptidoglycan synthesis for natural product screening. *J. Antibiot.* **2009**, *62*, 153–158. [CrossRef] [PubMed]

63. Rodolis, M.T.; Mihalyi, A.; Ducho, C.; Eitel, K.; Gust, B.; Goss, R.J.; Bugg, T.D. Mechanism of action of the uridyl peptide antibiotics: An unexpected link to a protein-protein interaction site in translocase MraY. *Chem. Commun.* **2014**, *50*, 13023–13025. [CrossRef] [PubMed]

64. Rodolis, M.T.; Mihalyi, A.; O'Reilly, A.; Slikas, J.; Roper, D.I.; Hancock, R.E.W.; Bugg, T.D.H. Identification of a novel inhibition site in translocase MraY based upon the site of interaction with lysis protein E from bacteriophage ΦX174. *ChemBioChem* **2014**, *15*, 1300–1308. [CrossRef] [PubMed]

65. Tanino, T.; Al-Dabbagh, B.; Mengin-Lecreulx, D.; Bouhss, A.; Oyama, H.; Ichikawa, S.; Matsuda, A. Mechanistic analysis of muraymycin analogues: A guide to the design of MraY inhibitors. *J. Med. Chem.* **2011**, *54*, 8421–8439. [CrossRef] [PubMed]

66. Takeoka, Y.; Tanino, T.; Sekiguchi, M.; Yonezawa, S.; Sakagami, M.; Takahashi, F.; Togame, H.; Tanaka, Y.; Takemoto, H.; Ichikawa, S.; et al. Expansion of antibacterial spectrum of muraymycins toward *Pseudomonas aeruginosa*. *ACS Med. Chem. Lett.* **2014**, *5*, 556–560. [CrossRef] [PubMed]

67. Wiegmann, D.; Koppermann, S.; Wirth, M.; Niro, G.; Leyerer, K.; Ducho, C. Muraymycin nucleoside-peptide antibiotics: Uridine-derived natural products as lead structures for the development of novel antibacterial agents. *Beilstein J. Org. Chem.* **2016**, *12*, 769–795. [CrossRef] [PubMed]

68. Chung, B.C.; Mashalidis, E.H.; Tanino, T.; Kim, M.; Matsuda, A.; Hong, J.; Ichikawa, S.; Lee, S.Y. Structural insights into inhibition of lipid I production in bacterial cell wall synthesis. *Nature* **2016**, *533*, 557–560. [CrossRef] [PubMed]

69. Dini, C.; Didier-Laurent, S.; Drochon, N.; Feteanu, S.; Guillot, J.C.; Monti, F.; Uridat, E.; Zhang, J.; Aszodi, J. Synthesis of sub-micromolar inhibitors of MraY by exploring the region originally occupied by the diazepanone ring in the liposidomycin structure. *Bioorg. Med. Chem. Lett.* **2002**, *12*, 1209–1213. [CrossRef]

70. Dini, C.; Drochon, N.; Feteanu, S.; Guillot, J.C.; Peixoto, C.; Aszodi, J. Synthesis of analogues of the O-β-D-ribofuranosyl nucleoside moiety of liposidomycins. Part 1: Contribution of the amino group and the uracil moiety upon the inhibition of MraY. *Bioorg. Med. Chem. Lett.* **2001**, *11*, 529–531. [CrossRef]

71. Dini, C.; Drochon, N.; Guillot, J.C.; Mauvais, P.; Walter, P.; Aszodi, J. Synthesis of analogues of the O-β-D-ribofuranosyl nucleoside moiety of liposidomycins. Part 2: Role of the hydroxyl groups upon the inhibition of MraY. *Bioorg. Med. Chem. Lett.* **2001**, *11*, 533–536. [CrossRef]

72. Fer, M.J.; Olatunji, S.; Bouhss, A.; Calvet-Vitale, S.; Gravier-Pelletier, C. Toward analogues of MraY natural inhibitors: Synthesis of 5′-triazole-substituted-aminoribosyl uridines through a Cu-catalyzed azide-alkyne cycloaddition. *J. Org. Chem.* **2013**, *78*, 10088–10105. [CrossRef] [PubMed]

73. Fer, M.J.; Bouhss, A.; Patrao, M.; le Corre, L.; Pietrancosta, N.; Amoroso, A.; Joris, B.; Mengin-Lecreulx, D.; Calvet-Vitale, S.; Gravier-Pelletier, C. 5′-methylene-triazole-substituted-aminoribosyl uridines as MraY inhibitors: Synthesis, biological evaluation and molecular modeling. *Org. Biomol. Chem.* **2015**, *13*, 7193–7222. [CrossRef] [PubMed]

74. Unterreitmeier, S.; Fuchs, A.; Schaffler, T.; Heym, R.G.; Frishman, D.; Langosch, D. Phenylalanine promotes interaction of transmembrane domains via GxxxG motifs. *J. Mol. Biol.* **2007**, *374*, 705–718. [CrossRef] [PubMed]

75. Heifetz, A.; Keenan, R.W.; Elbein, A.D. Mechanism of action of tunicamycin on the UDP-GlcNAc: Dolichyl-phosphate GlcNAc-1-phosphate transferase. *Biochemistry* **1979**, *18*, 2186–2192. [CrossRef] [PubMed]

76. Seres, M.; Cholujova, D.; Bubencikova, T.; Breier, A.; Sulova, Z. Tunicamycin depresses P-glycoprotein glycosylation without an effect on its membrane localization and drug efflux activity in L1210 cells. *Int. J. Mol. Sci.* **2011**, *12*, 7772–7784. [CrossRef] [PubMed]

77. Witte, A.; Blasi, U.; Halfmann, G.; Szostak, M.; Wanner, G.; Lubitz, W. PhiX174 protein e-mediated lysis of *Escherichia coli*. *Biochimie* **1990**, *72*, 191–200. [CrossRef]

78. Bernhardt, T.G.; Roof, W.D.; Young, R. Genetic evidence that the bacteriophage PhiX174 lysis protein inhibits cell wall synthesis. *Proc. Natl. Acad. Sci. USA* **2000**, *97*, 4297–4302. [CrossRef] [PubMed]

79. Halfmann, G.; Gotz, F.; Lubitz, W. Expression of bacteriophage PhiX174 lysis gene E in *Staphylococcus carnosus* TM300. *FEMS Microbiol. Lett.* **1993**, *108*, 139–143. [CrossRef] [PubMed]

80. Bernhardt, T.G.; Struck, D.K.; Young, R. The lysis protein E of PhiX174 is a specific inhibitor of the MraY-catalyzed step in peptidoglycan synthesis. *J. Biol. Chem.* **2001**, *276*, 6093–6097. [CrossRef] [PubMed]

81. Mendel, S.; Holbourn, J.M.; Schouten, J.A.; Bugg, T.D.H. Interaction of the transmembrane domain of lysis protein E from bacteriophage PhiX174 with bacterial translocase MraY and peptidyl-prolyl isomerase SlyD. *Microbiology* **2006**, *152*, 2959–2967. [CrossRef] [PubMed]

82. Tanaka, S.; Clemons, W.M., Jr. Minimal requirements for inhibition of MraY by lysis protein E from bacteriophage PhiX174. *Mol. Microbiol.* **2012**, *85*, 975–985. [CrossRef] [PubMed]

83. Zheng, Y.; Struck, D.K.; Bernhardt, T.G.; Young, R. Genetic analysis of MraY inhibition by the PhiX174 protein E. *Genetics* **2008**, *180*, 1459–1466. [CrossRef] [PubMed]

84. Liu, Y.; Rodrigues, J.P.G.L.M.; Bonvin, A.M.J.J.; Egmond, M.R.; Breukink, E.; Utrecht University, Utrecht, the Netherlands. Docking studies of protein E and bacterial MraY. Unpublished work. 2016.

85. Mohammadi, T.; Karczmarek, A.; Crouvoisier, M.; Bouhss, A.; Mengin-Lecreulx, D.; den Blaauwen, T. The essential peptidoglycan glycosyltransferase MurG forms a complex with proteins involved in lateral envelope growth as well as with proteins involved in cell division in *Escherichia coli*. *Mol. Microbiol.* **2007**, *65*, 1106–1121. [CrossRef] [PubMed]

86. Salmond, G.P.; Lutkenhaus, J.F.; Donachie, W.D. Identification of new genes in a cell envelope-cell division gene cluster of *Escherichia coli*: Cell envelope gene MurG. *J. Bacteriol.* **1980**, *144*, 438–440. [PubMed]

87. Mengin-Lecreulx, D.; Texier, L.; Rousseau, M.; van Heijenoort, J. The MurG gene of *Escherichia coli* codes for the UDP-*N*-acetylglucosamine: *N*-acetylmuramyl-(pentapeptide) pyrophosphoryl-undecaprenol *N*-acetylglucosamine transferase involved in the membrane steps of peptidoglycan synthesis. *J. Bacteriol.* **1991**, *173*, 4625–4636. [PubMed]

88. Chen, L.; Men, H.; Ha, S.; Ye, X.Y.; Brunner, L.; Hu, Y.; Walker, S. Intrinsic lipid preferences and kinetic mechanism of *Escherichia coli* MurG. *Biochemistry* **2002**, *41*, 6824–6833. [CrossRef] [PubMed]

89. Bupp, K.; van Heijenoort, J. The final step of peptidoglycan subunit assembly in *Escherichia coli* occurs in the cytoplasm. *J. Bacteriol.* **1993**, *175*, 1841–1843. [PubMed]

90. Crouvoisier, M.; Mengin-Lecreulx, D.; van Heijenoort, J. UDP-*N*-acetylglucosamine: *N*-acetylmuramoyl-(pentapeptide) pyrophosphoryl undecaprenol *N*-acetylglucosamine transferase from *Escherichia coli*: Overproduction, solubilization, and purification. *FEBS Lett.* **1999**, *449*, 289–292. [CrossRef]

91. Ha, S.; Chang, E.; Lo, M.-C.; Men, H.; Park, P.; Ge, M.; Walker, S. The kinetic characterization of *Escherichia coli* MurG using synthetic substrate analogues. *J. Am. Chem. Soc.* **1999**, *121*, 8415–8426. [CrossRef]

92. Epand, R.M. Role of membrane lipids in modulating the activity of membrane-bound enzyme. In *The Structure of Biological Membranes*, 2nd ed.; Yeagle, P.L., Ed.; CRC Press: Boca Raton, FL, USA, 2004.

93. Van den Brink-van der Laan, E.; Boots, J.W.; Spelbrink, R.E.; Kool, G.M.; Breukink, E.; Killian, J.A.; de Kruijff, B. Membrane interaction of the glycosyltransferase MurG: A special role for cardiolipin. *J. Bacteriol.* **2003**, *185*, 3773–3779. [CrossRef] [PubMed]

94. Liu, H.; Ritter, T.K.; Sadamoto, R.; Sears, P.S.; Wu, M.; Wong, C.H. Acceptor specificity and inhibition of the bacterial cell-wall glycosyltransferase MurG. *ChemBioChem* **2003**, *4*, 603–609. [CrossRef] [PubMed]

95. Ha, S.; Walker, D.; Shi, Y.; Walker, S. The 1.9 Å crystal structure of *Escherichia coli* MurG, a membrane-associated glycosyltransferase involved in peptidoglycan biosynthesis. *Protein Sci.* **2000**, *9*, 1045–1052. [CrossRef] [PubMed]

96. Brakoulias, A.; Jackson, R.M. Towards a structural classification of phosphate binding sites in protein-nucleotide complexes: An automated all-against-all structural comparison using geometric matching. *Proteins* **2004**, *56*, 250–260. [CrossRef] [PubMed]

97. Rosen, M.L.; Edman, M.; Sjostrom, M.; Wieslander, A. Recognition of fold and sugar linkage for glycosyltransferases by multivariate sequence analysis. *J. Biol. Chem.* **2004**, *279*, 38683–38692. [CrossRef] [PubMed]

98. Hu, Y.; Chen, L.; Ha, S.; Gross, B.; Falcone, B.; Walker, D.; Mokhtarzadeh, M.; Walker, S. Crystal structure of the MurG: UDP-GlcNAc complex reveals common structural principles of a superfamily of glycosyltransferases. *Proc. Natl. Acad. Sci. USA* **2003**, *100*, 845–849. [CrossRef] [PubMed]

99. Öhrlein, R. Glycosyltransferase-catalyzed synthesis of non-natural oligosaccharides. In *Biocatalysis—From Discovery to Application*; Fessner, W.-D., Archelas, A., Demirjian, D.C., Furstoss, R., Griengl, H., Jaeger, K.E., Morís-Varas, E., Öhrlein, R., Reetz, M.T., Reymond, J.L., et al., Eds.; Springer: Berlin, Germany, 1999; Volume 200, pp. 227–254.

100. Crouvoisier, M.; Auger, G.; Blanot, D.; Mengin-Lecreulx, D. Role of the amino acid invariants in the active site of MurG as evaluated by site-directed mutagenesis. *Biochimie* **2007**, *89*, 1498–1508. [CrossRef] [PubMed]

101. Brown, K.; Vial, S.C.; Dedi, N.; Westcott, J.; Scally, S.; Bugg, T.D.; Charlton, P.A.; Cheetham, G.M. Crystal structure of the *Pseudomonas aeruginosa* MurG: UDP-GlcNAc substrate complex. *Protein Pept. Lett.* **2013**, *20*, 1002–1008. [CrossRef] [PubMed]

102. Helm, J.S.; Hu, Y.; Chen, L.; Gross, B.; Walker, S. Identification of active-site inhibitors of MurG using a generalizable, high-throughput glycosyltransferase screen. *J. Am. Chem. Soc.* **2003**, *125*, 11168–11169. [CrossRef] [PubMed]

103. Hu, Y.; Helm, J.S.; Chen, L.; Ginsberg, C.; Gross, B.; Kraybill, B.; Tiyanont, K.; Fang, X.; Wu, T.; Walker, S. Identification of selective inhibitors for the glycosyltransferase MurG via high-throughput screening. *Chem. Biol.* **2004**, *11*, 703–711. [CrossRef] [PubMed]

104. Auger, G.; van Heijenoort, J.; Mengin-Lecreulx, D.; Blanot, D. A MurG assay which utilises a synthetic analogue of lipid I. *FEMS Microbiol. Lett.* **2003**, *219*, 115–119. [CrossRef]

105. Terrak, M.; Ghosh, T.K.; van Heijenoort, J.; van Beeumen, J.; Lampilas, M.; Aszodi, J.; Ayala, J.A.; Ghuysen, J.M.; Nguyen-Disteche, M. The catalytic, glycosyl transferase and acyl transferase modules of the cell wall peptidoglycan-polymerizing penicillin-binding protein 1b of *Escherichia coli*. *Mol. Microbiol.* **1999**, *34*, 350–364. [CrossRef] [PubMed]

106. Mann, P.A.; Muller, A.; Xiao, L.; Pereira, P.M.; Yang, C.; Ho Lee, S.; Wang, H.; Trzeciak, J.; Schneeweis, J.; Dos Santos, M.M.; et al. Murgocil is a highly bioactive staphylococcal-specific inhibitor of the peptidoglycan glycosyltransferase enzyme MurG. *ACS Chem. Biol.* **2013**, *8*, 2442–2451. [CrossRef] [PubMed]

107. Mitachi, K.; Siricilla, S.; Klaic, L.; Clemons, W.M., Jr.; Kurosu, M. Chemoenzymatic syntheses of water-soluble lipid I fluorescent probes. *Tetrahedron Lett.* **2015**, *56*, 3441–3446. [CrossRef] [PubMed]

7

Nanosynthesis of Silver-Calcium Glycerophosphate: Promising Association against Oral Pathogens

Gabriela Lopes Fernandes [1], Alberto Carlos Botazzo Delbem [2] [iD], Jackeline Gallo do Amaral [2], Luiz Fernando Gorup [3,4], Renan Aparecido Fernandes [1,5], Francisco Nunes de Souza Neto [3], José Antonio Santos Souza [2], Douglas Roberto Monteiro [6], Alessandra Marçal Agostinho Hunt [7], Emerson Rodrigues Camargo [3] and Debora Barros Barbosa [1,*]

[1] Department of Dental Materials and Prosthodontics, School of Dentistry, Araçatuba, São Paulo State University (UNESP), Araçatuba 16015-050, São Paulo, Brazil; fernandesgabriela@hotmail.com (G.L.F.); renanfernandes@fai.com.br (R.A.F.)

[2] Department of Pediatric Dentistry and Public Health, School of Dentistry, Araçatuba, São Paulo State University (UNESP), Araçatuba 16015-050, São Paulo, Brazil; adelbem@foa.unesp.br (A.C.B.D.); jackelineamaral@gmail.com (J.G.d.A.); joseanonio_249@hotmail.com (J.A.S.S.)

[3] Department of Chemistry, Federal University of São Carlos, São Carlos 13565-905, São Paulo, Brazil; lfgorup@gmail.com (L.F.G.); francisco_nsn@yahoo.com.br (F.N.d.S.N.); camargo@ufscar.br (E.R.C.)

[4] FACET—Department of Chemistry, Federal University of Grande Dourados, Dourados 79804-970, Mato Grosso do Sul, Brazil

[5] Department of Dentistry, University Center of Adamantina (UNIFAI), Adamantina 17800-000, São Paulo, Brazil

[6] Graduate Program in Dentistry (GPD—Master's Degree), University of Western São Paulo (UNOESTE), Presidente Prudente 19050-920, São Paulo, Brazil; douglasmonteiro@hotmail.com

[7] Department of Microbiology and Molecular Genetics, Michigan State University, East Lansing, MI 48823, USA; alehunt@msu.edu

* Correspondence: debora@foa.unesp.br

Abstract: Nanobiomaterials combining remineralization and antimicrobial abilities would bring important benefits to control dental caries. This study aimed to produce nanocompounds containing calcium glycerophosphate (CaGP) and silver nanoparticles (AgNP) by varying the reducing agent of silver nitrate (sodium borohydride (B) or sodium citrate (C)), the concentration of silver (1% or 10%), and the CaGP forms (nano or commercial), and analyze its characterization and antimicrobial activity against ATCC *Candida albicans* (10231) and *Streptococcus mutans* (25175) by the microdilution method. Controls of AgNP were produced and silver ions (Ag^+) were quantified in all of the samples. X-ray diffraction, UV-Vis, and scanning electron microscopy (SEM) analysis demonstrated AgNP associated with CaGP. Ag^+ ions were considerably higher in AgCaGP/C. *C. albicans* was susceptible to nanocompounds produced with both reducing agents, regardless of Ag concentration and CaGP form, being Ag10%CaGP-N/C the most effective compound (19.5–39.0 µg Ag mL^{-1}). While for *S. mutans*, the effectiveness was observed only for AgCaGP reduced by citrate, also presenting Ag10%CaGP-N the highest effectiveness (156.2–312.5 µg Ag mL^{-1}). Notably, CaGP enhanced the silver antimicrobial potential in about two- and eight-fold against *C. albicans* and *S. mutans* when compared with the AgNP controls (from 7.8 to 3.9 and from 250 to 31.2 µg Ag mL^{-1}, respectively). The synthesis that was used in this study promoted the formation of AgNP associated with CaGP, and although the use of sodium borohydride (B) resulted in a pronounced reduction of Ag^+, the composite AgCaGP/B was less effective against the microorganisms that were tested.

Keywords: silver; calcium glycerophosphate; nanoparticles; *Candida albicans*; *Streptococcus mutans*

1. Introduction

The synthesis and study of properties of new biomaterials has been emphasized lately with the improvement of nanotechnology. In this context, the development of nanomaterials has been the focus of many areas of chemistry, physics, and materials science because of the promising characteristics that these materials exhibit [1].

Nanotechnology aims to manipulate particles by creating new structures with favorable properties in many areas, such as medicine and dentistry [2], and new alternatives of treatment for oral pathologies are emerging. Metallic nanoparticles, in particular silver nanoparticles (AgNP), have been studied as an alternative antimicrobial agent against a broad spectrum of species in the control of oral biofilms [3–5]. Although there are several studies where AgNP are used as antimicrobial agents, their mechanism of action is not completely understood. Kim et al. [6] and Besinis et al. [4] related their antimicrobial action to the toxicity resulting from free metal ions dissolution from the surface of the AgNP. In addition, AgNP would lead to oxidative stress through the generation of reactive oxygen species (ROS), interacting with cytoplasmic and nucleic acid components by inhibiting enzymes of the respiratory chain and changing the permeability of the cytoplasmatic bacterial membrane [7–11].

Among oral pathologies, dental caries is one of the most common diseases in humans that relates to genetics, saliva, and diet of the host [9]. *Streptococcus mutans* is the main cariogenic microorganism owing to its ability to produce acids and glucans from sugar metabolism, which exceed the buffering capacity of saliva [9–11] and leads by a localized and irreversible destruction of the tooth structure [9,12]. However, recent evidence indicates the presence of *C. albicans* and *S. mutans* in oral biofilms, suggesting that the interaction between them can lead to the development of caries [9,13,14]. *C. albicans* colonization depends on the presence of the bacteria, which, besides promoting adhesion sites, act as a carbon source for yeast growth. On the other hand, yeasts reduce the levels of oxygen for streptococci [9]. Studies have shown the resistance of many microorganisms to antimicrobial agents currently used [15,16].

Studies since the 1930s [17] have reported the importance of using calcium phosphate derivatives for favouring the remineralization process in dental caries. Calcium glycerophosphate (CaGP) is an organic phosphate salt with anti-caries properties being demonstrated in studies carried out in monkeys [18] and in rats [19]. It is action in dental biofilms may be related to the increase of calcium and phosphate levels [20], buffering capacity [18], and reduction of the mass of the biofilms [21]. Becauses that it seems to interact with dental tissues [22], CaGP has been incorporated in dentifrices [23,24]. Do Amaral et al. [25] and Zaze et al. [26], when associating CaGP (0.25%) in toothpastes with fluoride at low concentrations, found the same efficacy against caries in enamel when compared to dentifrices that were supplemented with a higher concentration of fluoride demonstrating CaGP be an good option for oral products to both prevent caries and avoid fluorose in dental tissues.

The use of a biomaterial containing both an antimicrobial and a compound acting as a source of calcium phosphate for dental remineralization would have a great impact on the prevention and control of dental caries. Therefore, this study aimed to produce nanocompounds containing calcium glycerophosphate (CaGP) and silver nanoparticles (AgNP) by varying the reducing agent of silver nitrate (sodium borohydride or sodium citrate), the concentration of silver (1% or 10%), and the CaGP forms (nano or microparticulated), and analyze its characterization and antimicrobial activity against ATCC strains of *Candida albicans* and *Streptococcus mutans*.

2. Results

2.1. Synthesis and Characterization of Ag-CaGP Nanocomposites

UV-Vis absorption spectroscopy (UV-Vis) showed that Ag-CaGP nanocomposites presented silver in nanosized dimensions in all of the nanocomposites synthesized, regardless of the reducing agent used. It was demonstrated by the presence of an intense absorption peak, denominated plasmonic band, which occurred between 420 and 450 nm (Figure 1a, Figure S1). It characterizes noble metal nanoparticles, with strong absorption band being observed in the visible region [27]. The CaGP did not exhibit absorption peak in the visible region of the electromagnetic spectrum.

X-ray diffraction (XRD) pattern indicated that all of the Ag-CaGP nanocomposites were composed of AgNP and CaGP for confirming the presence of silver in Ag-CaGP nanocomposites through comparison of the nanoparticles and CaGP. The typical powder XRD pattern of the prepared CaGP showed diffraction peaks at $2\theta = 6.30°$, $12.3°$, $26.4°$, $41.1°$, and $44.2°$ (Figure 1b, Figure S2), and the corresponding crystallographic form (PDF No. 1-17) [28]. The typical powder XRD pattern of the silver nanoparticles showed (Figure 1b) diffraction peaks at $2\theta = 38.2°$, $44.4°$, $64.6°$, $77.5°$, and $81.7°$, which can be indexed to (111), (200), (220), (311), and (222) planes of pure silver with face-centered cubic system (PDF No. 04-0783).

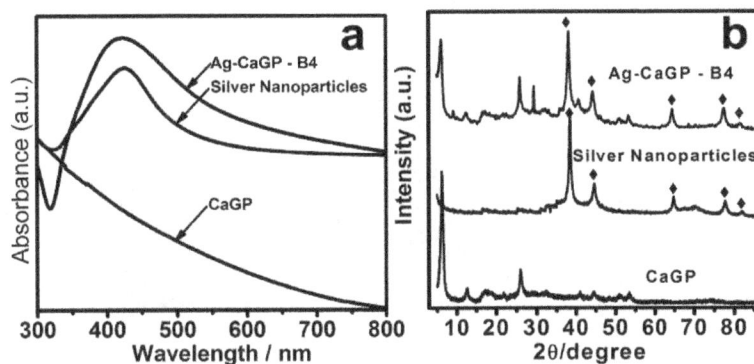

Figure 1. (a) UV-Vis (b) XRD pattern of Ag-CaGP (B4 group) nanocomposite, silver nanoparticles, and CaGP.

Nanostructured materials that exhibit a pattern of small nanoparticles scattered on a larger surface, similar to glass bead embellishments on a Christmas tree, are generally classified as a decorated material. The scanning electron microscopy (SEM) images of Figure 2 show this typical pattern, with spherical silver nanoparticles (indicated by arrows) decorating the surface of the CaGP microparticles in all synthesized nanocomposites containing 10% Ag (B4; B8; C4). In addition, transmission electron microscopy (TEM) was performed for the nanocomposite B4 (Figure S3).

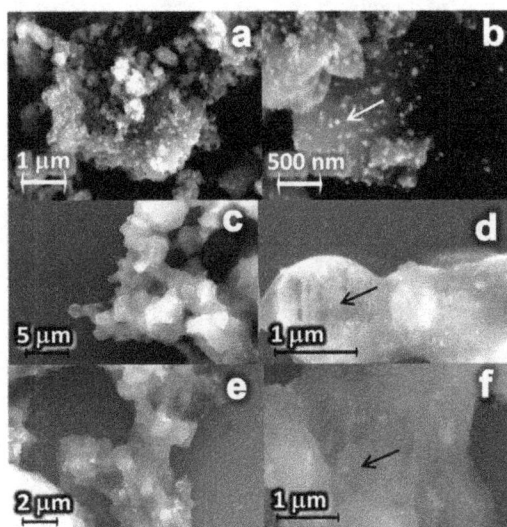

Figure 2. SEM images of the Ag-CaGP nanocomposites: B4 (**a,b**), C4 (**c,d**), and B8 (**e,f**) at different magnifications. The arrows indicate silver nanoparticles on the surface of CaGP in B4 and in the bulk of CaGP in C4 and B8.

The energy-dispersive X-ray sprectroscopy (EDS) clearly showed the outline of Ag-CaGP nanocomposites in all micrographs. Also, Figure 3 (B4), Figure 4 (C4) and Figures S4–S6, the two-dimensional (2D) images were constructed by analyzing the energy released from the issuance Si Kα, O Kα, P Kα, Ca Kα, and Ag Kα, indicating the distribution of these elements on the demarcated area in the micrograph.

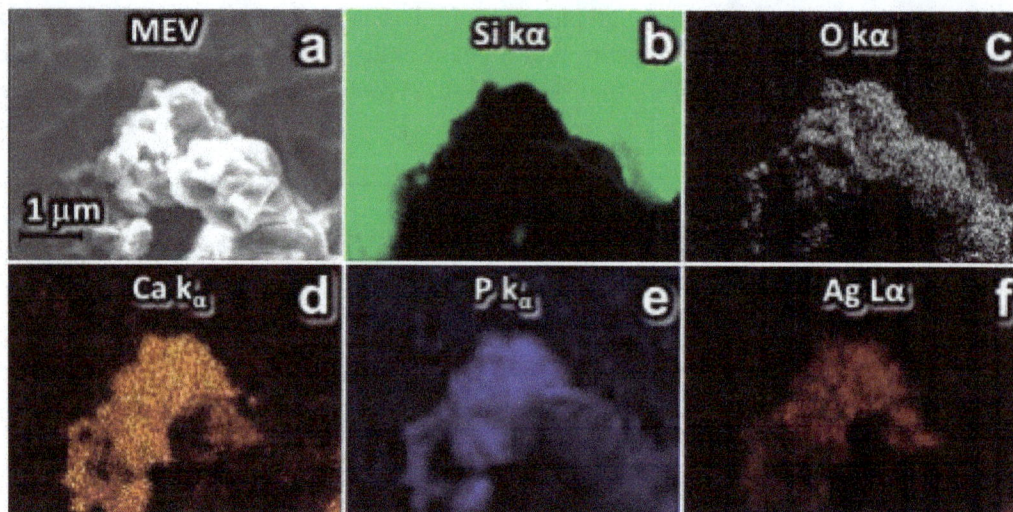

Figure 3. SEM and EDS mapped in 2D elements issuance Si Kα, O Kα, P Kα, Ca Kα, and Ag Kα false color. Analysis of the distribution of silver nanoparticles on the Ag-CaGP for sample B4: (**a**) SEM image; (**b**) chemical mapping of silicon element present in the substrate, where the electron beam was focused directly on the substrate and is showed in green color, and the dark regions the beam was focused in Ag-CaGP nanocomposite B4; (**c–f**) oxygen, calcium, phosphorus, and silver, respectively, demonstrating they are constituents of the Ag-CaGP.

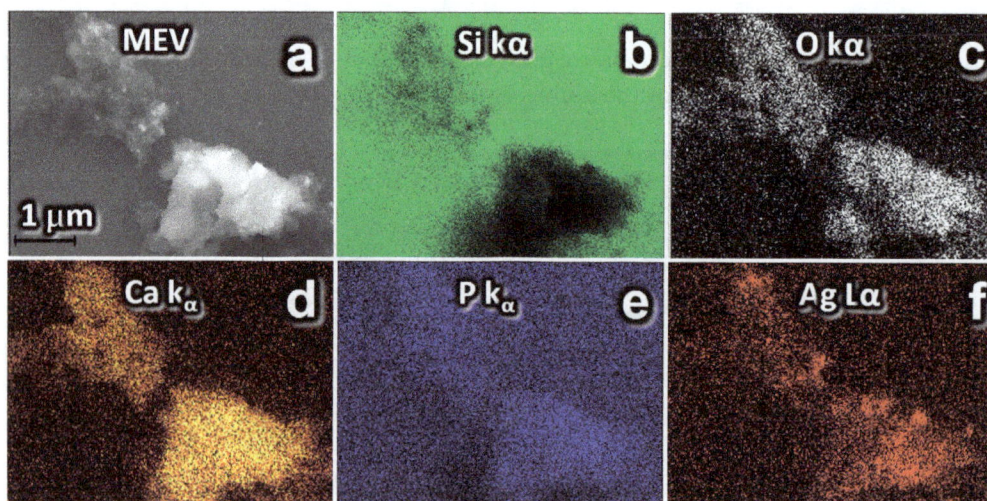

Figure 4. SEM and EDS mapped in 2D elements issuance Si Kα, O Kα, P Kα, Ca Kα, and Ag Kα false color. Analysis of the distribution of silver nanoparticles on the Ag-CaGP for sample C4: (**a**) SEM image; (**b**) chemical mapping of silicon element present in the substrate, where the electron beam was focused directly on the substrate and is showed in green color, and the dark regions the beam was focused in Ag-CaGP nanocomposite C4; and, (**c–f**) oxygen, calcium, phosphorus, and silver, respectively, demonstrating they are constituents of the Ag-CaGP.

2.2. Minimum Inhibitory Concentration

The results showed that the MIC values were related to the synthesis process and the Ag concentration used (Table 1). Nanocomposites that were obtained using $Na_3C_6H_5O_7$ as reducing agent showed the most effective antimicrobial activity against *C. albicans* and *S. mutans*. In these composites, the lowest MIC values were observed for those containing 10% of Ag (C3 and C4), being between 19.05 and 39.05 μg/mL for *C. albicans* and 156.2 and 625 μg/mL for *S. mutans*. The nanocomposites that were synthesized using $NaBH_4$ as reducing agent and isopropanol as solvent showed fungicidal effect varying between 100 and 1600 μg/mL, whilst no effect against *S. mutans* was observed. While the nanocomposites synthesized using the same reducing agent and deionized water as solvent did not show any effect against both microorganisms. In addition to the MICs found for the synthesized compounds, it was carried out the microdilution assay to find the MIC values for the solutions containing only AgNP or CaGP diluted in deionized water, besides the other compounds used in the synthesis reaction as reducing and surfactant agents. These data are showed in Table 2.

Table 1. Values of minimum inhibitory concentration (MIC) of the nanocompounds based on μg of $AgCaGP\ mL^{-1}$ and on μg of $Ag\ mL^{-1}$ in each ones, synthesized using sodium borohydride (Group B) and sodium citrate (Group C), and silver ions concentration (μg Ag^+/mL) in all nanocompounds tested.

GROUP	Ag %/CaGP Form	Solvent	MIC (μg AgCaGP mL⁻¹/μg Ag mL⁻¹)		μg Ag⁺/mL
			C. albicans	S. mutans	
B1	1/M	I	>1600/>16	>1600/>16	2.83
B2	1/N	I	400–1600/0.40–16	>1600/>16	4.46
B3	10/M	I	400–800/40–80	>1600/>16	10.81
B4	10/N	I	100–200/10–20	>1600/>16	63.34
B5	1/M	W	>1600/>16	>1600/>16	0.44
B6	1/N	W	>1600/>16	>1600/>16	2.76
B7	10/M	W	>1600/>16	>1600/>16	5.97
B8	10/N	W	>1600/>16	>1600/>16	15.63
C1	1/M	W	156.2–312.5/1.56–3.12	1250/12.5	305.43
C2	1/N	W	156.2–312.5/1.56–3.12	1250/12.5	168.14
C3	10/M	W	39.0/3.9	312.5–625/31.2–62.5	506.73
C4	10/N	W	19.5–39.0/1.9–3.9	156.2–312.5/15.6–31.2	487.95

Table 2. Values of minimum inhibitory concentrations (MIC) (μg/mL) and silver ions (Ag^+) (μg Ag^+/mL) of the control solutions: AgNP reduced by sodium citrate ($Na_3C_6H_5O_7$), and by sodium borohydride ($NaBH_4$); silver nitrate ($AgNO_3$); nanoparticulated CaGP (CaGP-nano), and CaGP in commercial form (CaGP-commercial); sodium citrate and surfactant ($Na_3C_6H_5O_7$+NH-PM), and sodium borohydride and surfactant ($NaBH_4$+NH-PM).

Controls	MIC		Ag⁺
	C. albicans	S. mutans	
AgNP ($Na_3C_6H_5O_7$)	7.8	250	107.2
AgNP ($NaBH_4$)	62.5	125	576.2
$AgNO_3$	5.3	21.2	-
CaGP-nano	>5000	>5000	-
CaGP-commercial	>5000	>5000	-
$Na_3C_6H_5O_7$+NH-PM	>400	>400	-
$NaBH_4$+NH-PM	>1500	>1500	-

2.3. Determination of Ag^+ Concentration

The Ag^+ concentration of all the nanocomposites containing Ag (AgNP and Ag-CaGP) is showed in Table 1. For samples that were obtained through $NaBH_4$ route (B1–B8), a reduction of ionic silver higher than 98% was observed, when considering the total amount of ionic silver added to the reaction was 500 µg Ag$^+$/mL for B1, B2, B5, B6, and 5000 µg Ag$^+$/mL for B3, B4, B7, and B8. While for the compounds that were synthesized using $Na_3C_6H_5O_7$ as reducing agent, the ionic silver remaining was higher and reached about 10% in those samples that were produced using initially 5000 µg Ag$^+$/mL in the reaction process (C3 and C4). C1 and C2 presented 61.1% and 33.3%, respectively, of ionic silver in samples as the total Ag$^+$ added in the reaction was 500 µg Ag$^+$/mL. For AgNP with no CaGP added to the reaction (Table 2) obtained by $Na_3C_6H_5O_7$ route (nanoAg($Na_3C_6H_5O_7$)) the Ag$^+$ concentration was 107.25 µg/mL, whereas for AgNP produced through $NaBH_4$ (nanoAg($NaBH_4$)) the Ag$^+$ concentration was 576.19 µg/mL.

3. Discussion

In the present study, both of the synthesis methods proposed using sodium citrate or sodium borohydride as reducing agents, led to the anchorage between the silver nanoparticles and calcium glycerophosphate (Figure 2). Besides, in general, the nanocomposites (AgCaGP) were effective against reference strains of *Candida albicans* and *Streptococcus mutans*. Notably, CaGP substantively increased the antimicrobial effectiveness of silver in the AgCaGP, reducing up to a quarter their minimum inhibitory concentration when compared to the respective AgNP controls (Tables 1 and 2).

Although the CaGP has been previously nanoparticulated before the Ag-CaGP synthesis, in our study it was not characterized as being in nanoparticulated form when associated with silver. It might be happen due to the poor solubility of calcium at pH = 7 [29], even when using the same dispersant (NH-PM), as preconized by Miranda et al., whom synthesized AgNP with hydroxyapatite. A pastier bulk was particularly noted in micrographics of Ag-CaGP when water was used as solvent instead of isopropanol (Figure 2c–f), regardless of the reducing agent that was used in the reaction. Although there has not been difference between micro and nanoparticulated-CaGP in the SEM images, its form influenced the amount of silver ions in the compounds (Table 1). In addition, our results showed the antimicrobial effectiveness against *C. albicans* and *S. mutans* for the samples of group C, and it could be explained by the highest amount of silver ions that are present in those compounds [4,30–35].

This expressive difference in the quantity of silver ions between groups B and C would be related to the characteristics of the reducing agents used, being sodium borohydride considered a stronger reducing agent than sodium citrate [33]. Although silver ions are effective to kill several pathogenic microorganisms, they are easily dispersed, which quickly decreases its local concentration to levels of low effectivity. Moreover, ambient light reduces ionic silver forming typical black spots on skin or on any surface of contact [36]. This process causes aesthetic problems and it has potential to injure healthy living tissues. Silver nanoparticles, contrary to ionic silver, induce the production of reactive oxygen species (ROS), which is the primary antimicrobial mechanism [37]. However, AgNP tend to form aggregates in the absence of any support, reducing their efficacy. Therefore, substrates decorated with immobilized AgNP exhibits enhanced antimicrobial activity for longer periods, reducing the undesirable secondary effects that are associated to free ionic silver [38]. Although the difficult to separate the impact of free ionic silver from the AgNP antimicrobial action, differences that were observed in minimum inhibitory concentrations (MIC), as shown in Table 1, for *C. albicans* and *S. mutans* suggests the influence of their respective metabolism on the efficacy of silver against each microorganism.

Furthermore, other factors may influence the antimicrobial potential of AgNP [34]. For instance, how the compound containing silver interacts with the microorganisms would dependent on the characteristics of the AgNP formed, as well as the chemical and physical changes that may occur when they are added to the medium of interest [33]. In general, for the synthesis of AgNP, $AgNO_3$ is used as source of silver, water or ethanol as solvent, and sodium borohydride or sodium citrate as reducing agent [39]. Fabricated under similar conditions, the AgNP would have a negative surface charge [33,40], and this fact is noteworthy to elucidate the lower effectiveness of the compounds against *S. mutans*. Bacteria have a negative outer membrane charge [41] and the electrostatic attraction may have been hampered, and hence the action of the AgNP associated or not with CaGP on the *S. mutans* was diminished. On the other hand, apart from fungi present a neutral surface charge [41] and might enhance the attraction of AgNP, the presence of phospholipid components, which contain phosphate groups, may have improved the antimicrobial activity of silver by targeting these sites [42,43]. Indeed, the control of AgNP reduced by sodium citrate showed a lower amount of ions (107.2 µg Ag^+/mL) than the control that was produced using sodium borohydride (576.2 µg Ag^+/mL), and it was more effective against *C. albicans*, suggesting an antifungal potential of AgNP by itself, which may have afforded the disruption of the *C. albicans* cell membrane by damaging the inner layers of the cell wall, increasing their permeabilization and then allowing for the passage of these particles to into the cell.

On the contrary, against *S. mutans* plaktonic cells, Ag^+ may have played a preponderant role, particularly in view of the MIC values that are found for $AgNO_3$ (21.2 µg/mL) when compared to those for AgNP, regardless of the reducing agent that is used in the reaction (250 and 125 µg/mL, respectively, for AgNP ($Na_3C_6H_5O_7$) and AgNP ($NaBH_4$)). Noteworthy was the effect that was produced against *S. mutans* when CaGP was associated with AgNP (Table 1). CaGP afforded an increment in the silver activity and it could be related to the acidogenic and acidic characteristic of *S. mutans*, acting CaGP probably as a buffer, and hence might have prevented the proliferation of the cells in the medium [44–46]. So that, the CaGP buffer activity and the highest amount of Ag^+ ions could account for the better effectiveness of the samples of C group against that gram positive bacteria tested.

4. Materials and Methods

4.1. Synthesis of Silver-Calcium Glycerophosphate (Ag/CaGP) Nanocomposites

Ag/CaGP nanocomposites were synthesized at the Interdisciplinary Laboratory of Electrochemistry and Ceramics of the Chemistry Department in Federal University of São Carlos. Initially, the commercial form of calcium glycerophosphate (80% β-isomer and 20% rac-α-isomer, CAS 58409-70-4, Sigma-Aldrich Chemical Co., St. Louis, MO, USA) was acquired and was nanoparticulated using a ball mill for 24 h at 120 rpm, obtaining nanoparticles of approximately 10 nm. Then, two chemistry methods were employed for the synthesis. The first method was employed using sodium borohydride as reducing agent ($NaBH_4$, Sigma-Aldrich Chemical Co., St. Louis, MO, USA) and was based on the methodology that was proposed by Miranda et al. [29]. The synthesis was carried out in an alcoholic medium (isopropanol) or deionized water. For this, suspensions containing 5 g of CaGP and silver nitrate ($AgNO_3$ Merck KGaA, Darmstadt, Hessen, Germany) at 0.85 or 0.085 g were prepared in the presence of 0.5 mL of a surfactant (ammonium salt of polymethacrylic acid (NH-PM), Polysciences Inc., Warrington, PA, USA) (Table 1). Then, $NaBH_4$ (0.015 g) was added to each suspension, which caused the reduction of Ag^+ to metallic silver nanoparticles in the presence of CaGP. The molar stoichiometric ratio between Ag^+ and $NaBH_4$ was 1:1.26, respectively. The second method was based on that proposed by Turkevich et al. [47] and Gorup et al. [48] (2011, p. 355). The reducing agent of $AgNO_3$ was sodium citrate ($Na_3C_6H_5O_7$, Merck KGaA) and the stoichiometric ratio of each compound was, respectively, 1:3. Thus, in a flask containing 100 mL of deionized H_2O 5 g of CaGP was added following of 0.5 mL NH-PM and 1.4 g of $Na_3C_6H_5O_7$. This mixture was kept under magnetic stirring and heating. After reaching 95 °C temperature, $AgNO_3$ was added and this suspension was maintained stirring for 30 min until occurring the color change, which qualitatively indicated the formation of AgNP. Controls containing only the reducing agents and surfactant, and AgNP produced by both reducing were also prepared.

4.2. Characterization of Ag-CaGP Nanocomposites

In order to demonstrate the presence of AgNP and CaGP in the compounds, the UV-Vis absorption spectroscopy was employed. The measure is based on the phenomenon of plasmon resonance band, as observed in metallic nanoparticles. Thus, UV-Vis spectra of Ag-CaGP nanocomposites were obtained from aqueous solutions poured out in a commercial quartz cuvette with 1 cm optical path using a spectrophotometer (Shimadzu MultSpec-1501 spectrophotometer; Shimadzu Corporation, Tokyo, Japan) at 300 to 800 nm. Water was used as blank.

After a drying step, the resulting powder, Ag-CaGP, was subjected to X-ray diffraction (XRD) phase characterization using Cu Kα radiation (λ = 1.5406 Å), generated at a voltage of 30 kV and a current of 30 mA with continuous sweep in the range of $5° < 2θ < 80°$, at a scan rate of 2°/min (Diffractometer Rigaku DMax-2000PC, Rigaku Corporation, Tokyo, Japan). The particles morphology was also characterized by scanning electron microscopy (SEM) on a Zeiss Supra 35VP microscope (S-360 Microscope, Leo, Cambridge, MA, USA), with field emission gun electron effect (FEG-SEM) operating at 10 kV. A drop of each sample were added with a micropipette and deposited on silicon metal plate (111) and dried at 40 °C for 2 h. With this technique, we can identify in the synthesized biomaterials the presence of silver, oxygen, silicon, phosphate, and calcium, which were artificially colored (Figures 3 and 4).

4.3. Minimum Inhibitory Concentration (MIC)

The MIC values for each sample were determined through the microdilution method and followed the Clinical Laboratory Standards Institute guidelines (CLSI, documents M27-A2 and M07-A9). *Candida albicans* (ATCC 10231) was cultivated on Sabouraud Dextrose Agar (SDA, Difco, Le Pont de Claix, France) and *S. mutans* (ATCC 25175) on Brain Heart Infusion Agar (BHI, Difco, Le Pont de Claix, France). Inocula from 24 h cultures on the respective media were adjusted to a turbidity equivalent to a 0.5 McFarland standard in saline solution (0.85% NaCl). This suspension was diluted (1:5) in saline solution, and afterwards diluted (1:20) in RPMI 1640 or BHI. Initially, the Ag-CaGP nanocomposite was diluted in deionized water in a geometric progression, from 2 to 1024 times. Afterwards, each Ag-CaGP nanocomposite concentration obtained previously was diluted (1:5) in RPMI 1640 medium (Sigma-Aldrich) for *C. albicans* and in BHI for *S. mutans*. The final concentrations of Ag-CaGP nanocomposite in the dispersion ranged from 5 to 0.01 mg/mL. Each inoculum (100 μL) was added to the respective well of microtiter plates containing 100 μL of each specific concentration of the Ag-CaGP nanocomposite solution. The microtiter plates were incubated at 37 °C, and the MIC values were determined visually as the lowest concentration of Ag-CaGP with no microorganism growth after 48 h for *C. albicans* and 24 h for *S. mutans*. All of the assays were repeated in triplicate on three different occasions.

4.4. Determination of Ag+ Concentration

The evaluation of Ag+ concentration in Ag-CaGP and AgNP, as obtained by both reducing agents, was determined by a specific electrode 9616 BNWP (Thermo Scientific, Beverly, MA, USA) coupled to an ion analyzer (Orion 720 A+, Thermo Scientific, Beverly, MA, USA). A 1000 μg/mL silver standard was prepared placing 1.57 g of dried $AgNO_3$ into a 1 L volumetric flask containing deionized water. This solution was stored in an opaque bottle in a dark location and diluted in deionized water at the moment of dosage in order to achieve the standard concentrations used. Thus, the combined electrode was calibrated with standards containing 6.25 to 100 μg Ag/mL at the same conditions of samples. A silver ionic strength adjuster solution (ISA, Cat. No. 940011) that provides a constant background ionic strength was used (1 mL of each sample/standard: 0.02 mL ISA).

5. Conclusions

In conclusion, the synthesis that is proposed in this study promoted the anchorage of AgNP with the CaGP, and the nanocomposites produced using sodium citrate as reducing agent were effective against both of the microorganisms tested. Also, the highlight of our study was that the addition of CaGP to AgNP expressively reduced the MIC values when it was compared with the MIC values of AgNP by itself. These promising results strongly encourage further studies with the purpose of producing biomaterials with antimicrobial and remineralizing functions in the near future, particularly in the dental field.

Supplementary Materials: The following are available online at http://www.mdpi.com/2079-6382/7/3/52/s1, Figure S1: UV–Visible spectrum of Ag-CaGP nanocomposites, Figure S2: X-ray diffraction pattern of Ag-CaGP nanocomposites, Figure S3: TEM images of B4 Ag-CaGP nanocomposite, Figure S4: SEM images and energy-dispersive X-ray sprectroscopy (EDS) mapping in 2D elements issuance Si Kα, O Kα, P Kα,Ca Kα and Ag Kα false color. Analysis of the distribution of silver nanoparticles in the Ag-CaGP nanocomposites B1, B2 and B3, Figure S5: SEM images and EDS mapping in 2D elements issuance Si Kα, O Kα, P Kα,Ca Kα and AgKα false color. Analysis of the distribution of silver in the Ag-CaGP nanocomposites B5, B6 and B7, Figure S6: SEM images and EDS mapping in 2D elements issuance Si Kα, O Kα, P Kα,Ca Kα and Ag Kα false color. Analysis of the distribution of silver nanoparticles in the Ag-CaGP nanocomposites C1, C2 and C3.

Author Contributions: G.L.F., D.B.B., A.C.B.D. conceived and designed the experiments; G.L.F., R.A.F., J.G.d.A., J.A.S.S. performed the experiments; G.L.F., D.B.B., A.C.B.D., D.R.M. analyzed the data; F.N.d.S.N., L.F.G., E.R.C. contributed reagents/materials/analysis tools; G.L.F., D.B.B., A.M.A.H. wrote the paper.

Funding: This study was supported by: São Paulo Research Foundation (FAPESP, Processes 2013/24200-9 and 2014/08648-2), Brazil; and Coordination for the Improvement of Higher Education Personnel (Capes, Process 88881.030445/2013-01), Brazil.

References

1. De Oliveira, J.F.; Cardoso, M.B. Partial aggregation of silver nanoparticles induced by capping and reducing agents competition. *Langmuir ACS J. Surf. Colloids* **2014**, *30*, 4879–4886. [CrossRef] [PubMed]

2. Zandparsa, R. Latest biomaterials and technology in dentistry. *Dent. Clin. N. Am.* **2014**, *58*, 113–134. [CrossRef] [PubMed]

3. Perez-Diaz, M.A.; Boegli, L.; James, G.; Velasquillo, C.; Sanchez-Sanchez, R.; Martinez-Martinez, R.E.; Martinez-Castanon, G.A.; Martinez-Gutierrez, F. Silver nanoparticles with antimicrobial activities against *Streptococcus mutans* and their cytotoxic effect. *Mater. Sci. Eng. C Mater. Biol. Appl.* **2015**, *55*, 360–366. [CrossRef] [PubMed]

4. Besinis, A.; De Peralta, T.; Handy, R.D. The antibacterial effects of silver, titanium dioxide and silica dioxide nanoparticles compared to the dental disinfectant chlorhexidine on *Streptococcus mutans* using a suite of bioassays. *Nanotoxicology* **2014**, *8*, 1–16. [CrossRef] [PubMed]

5. Li, Q.; Mahendra, S.; Lyon, D.Y.; Brunet, L.; Liga, M.V.; Li, D.; Alvarez, P.J. Antimicrobial nanomaterials for water disinfection and microbial control: Potential applications and implications. *Water Res.* **2008**, *42*, 4591–4602. [CrossRef] [PubMed]

6. Kim, K.J.; Sung, W.S.; Suh, B.K.; Moon, S.K.; Choi, J.S.; Kim, J.G.; Lee, D.G. Antifungal activity and mode of action of silver nano-particles on *Candida albicans*. *Biomet. Int. J. Role Met. Ions Biol. Biochem. Med.* **2009**, *22*, 235–242. [CrossRef] [PubMed]

7. Kim, J.S.; Kuk, E.; Yu, K.N.; Kim, J.H.; Park, S.J.; Lee, H.J.; Kim, S.H.; Park, Y.K.; Park, Y.H.; Hwang, C.Y.; et al. Antimicrobial effects of silver nanoparticles. *Nanomedicine* **2007**, *3*, 95–101. [CrossRef] [PubMed]

8. Monteiro, D.R.; Silva, S.; Negri, M.; Gorup, L.F.; de Camargo, E.R.; Oliveira, R.; Barbosa, D.B.; Henriques, M. Silver nanoparticles: Influence of stabilizing agent and diameter on antifungal activity against *Candida albicans* and *Candida glabrata* biofilms. *Lett. Appl. Microbiol.* **2012**, *54*, 383–391. [CrossRef] [PubMed]

9. Metwalli, K.H.; Khan, S.A.; Krom, B.P.; Jabra-Rizk, M.A. *Streptococcus mutans*, *Candida albicans*, and the human mouth: A sticky situation. *PLoS Pathog.* **2013**, *9*, e1003616. [CrossRef] [PubMed]

10. Lemos, J.A.; Quivey, R.G., Jr.; Koo, H.; Abranches, J. *Streptococcus mutans*: A new Gram-positive paradigm? *Microbiology* **2013**, *159*, 436–445. [CrossRef] [PubMed]

11. Falsetta, M.L.; Klein, M.I.; Lemos, J.A.; Silva, B.B.; Agidi, S.; Scott-Anne, K.K.; Koo, H. Novel antibiofilm chemotherapy targets exopolysaccharide synthesis and stress tolerance in *Streptococcus mutans* to modulate virulence expression in vivo. *Antimicrob. Agents Chemother.* **2012**, *56*, 6201–6211. [CrossRef] [PubMed]

12. Rouabhia, M.; Chmielewski, W. Diseases Associated with Oral Polymicrobial Biofilms. *Open Mycol. J.* **2012**, *6*, 27–32.

13. Barbieri, D.S.V.; Vicente, V.A.; Fraiz, F.C.; Lavoranti, O.J.; Svidzinski, T.I.E.; Pinheiro, R.L. Analysis of the in vitro adherence of *Streptococcus mutans* and *Candida albicans*. *Braz. J. Microbiol.* **2007**, *38*, 624–631. [CrossRef]

14. Jarosz, L.M.; Deng, D.M.; van der Mei, H.C.; Crielaard, W.; Krom, B.P. *Streptococcus mutans* competence-stimulating peptide inhibits *Candida albicans* hypha formation. *Eukaryot. Cell* **2009**, *8*, 1658–1664. [CrossRef] [PubMed]

15. Monteiro, D.R.; Gorup, L.F.; Silva, S.; Negri, M.; de Camargo, E.R.; Oliveira, R.; Barbosa, D.B.; Henriques, M. Silver colloidal nanoparticles: Antifungal effect against adhered cells and biofilms of *Candida albicans* and *Candida glabrata*. *Biofouling* **2011**, *27*, 711–719. [CrossRef] [PubMed]

16. Monteiro, D.R.; Gorup, L.F.; Takamiya, A.S.; Ruvollo-Filho, A.C.; de Camargo, E.R.; Barbosa, D.B. The growing importance of materials that prevent microbial adhesion: Antimicrobial effect of medical devices containing silver. *Int. J. Antimicrob. Agents* **2009**, *34*, 103–110. [CrossRef] [PubMed]

17. Lynch, R.J.; ten Cate, J.M. Effect of calcium glycerophosphate on demineralization in an in vitro biofilm model. *Caries Res.* **2006**, *40*, 142–147. [CrossRef] [PubMed]

18. Bowen, W.H. The cariostatic effect of calcium glycerophosphate in monkeys. *Caries Res.* **1972**, *6*, 43–51. [CrossRef] [PubMed]

19. Grenby, T.H. Trials of 3 organic phosphorus-containing compounds as protective agents against dental caries in rats. *J. Dent. Res.* **1973**, *52*, 454–461. [CrossRef] [PubMed]

20. Duke, S.A.; Rees, D.A.; Forward, G.C. Increased plaque calcium and phosphorus concentrations after using a calcium carbonate toothpaste containing calcium glycerophosphate and sodium monofluorophosphate. Pilot study. *Caries Res.* **1979**, *13*, 57–59. [CrossRef] [PubMed]

21. Nordbo, H.; Rolla, G. Desorption of salivary proteins from hydroxyapatite by phytic acid and glycerophosphate and the plaque-inhibiting effect of the two compounds in vivo. *J. Dent. Res.* **1972**, *51*, 800–811. [CrossRef] [PubMed]

22. Grenby, T.H.; Bull, J.M. Use of high-performance liquid chromatography techniques to study the protection of hydroxylapatite by fluoride and glycerophosphate against demineralization in vitro. *Caries Res.* **1980**, *14*, 221–232. [CrossRef] [PubMed]

23. Naylor, M.N.; Glass, R.L. A three-year clinical trial of a calcium carbonate dentifrice containing calcium glycerophosphate and sodium monofluorophosphate. *Caries Res.* **1979**, *13*, 39–46. [CrossRef] [PubMed]

24. Mainwaring, P.J.; Naylor, M.N. A four-year clinical study to determine the caries-inhibiting effect of calcium glycerophosphate and sodium fluoride in calcium carbonate base dentifrices containing sodium monofluorophosphate. *Caries Res.* **1983**, *17*, 267–276. [CrossRef] [PubMed]

25. do Amaral, J.G.; Sassaki, K.T.; Martinhon, C.C.; Delbem, A.C. Effect of low-fluoride dentifrices supplemented with calcium glycerophosphate on enamel demineralization in situ. *Am. J. Dent.* **2013**, *26*, 75–80. [PubMed]

26. Zaze, A.C.; Dias, A.P.; Amaral, J.G.; Miyasaki, M.L.; Sassaki, K.T.; Delbem, A.C. In situ evaluation of low-fluoride toothpastes associated to calcium glycerophosphate on enamel remineralization. *J. Dent.* **2014**, *42*, 1621–1625. [CrossRef] [PubMed]

27. Ghosh, S.K.; Pal, T. Interparticle coupling effect on the surface plasmon resonance of gold nanoparticles: From theory to applications. *Chem. Rev.* **2007**, *107*, 4797–4862. [CrossRef] [PubMed]

28. Inoue, M.; In, Y.; Ishida, T. Calcium binding to phospholipid: Structural study of calcium glycerophosphate. *J. Lipid Res.* **1992**, *33*, 985–994. [PubMed]

29. Miranda, M.; Fernandez, A.; Lopez-Esteban, S.; Malpartida, F.; Moya, J.S.; Torrecillas, R. Ceramic/metal biocidal nanocomposites for bone-related applications. *J. Mater. Sci. Mater. Med.* **2012**, *23*, 1655–1662. [CrossRef] [PubMed]

30. Pal, S.; Tak, Y.K.; Song, J.M. Does the antibacterial activity of silver nanoparticles depend on the shape of the nanoparticle? A study of the Gram-negative bacterium *Escherichia coli*. *Appl. Environ. Microbiol.* **2007**, *73*, 1712–1720. [CrossRef] [PubMed]

31. Bradford, A.; Handy, R.D.; Readman, J.W.; Atfield, A.; Mühling, M. Impact of silver nanoparticle contamination on the genetic diversity of natural bacterial assemblages in estuarine sediments. *Environ. Sci. Technol.* **2009**, *43*, 4530–4536. [CrossRef] [PubMed]

32. Duran, N.; Duran, M.; de Jesus, M.B.; Seabra, A.B.; Favaro, W.J.; Nakazato, G. Silver nanoparticles: A new view on mechanistic aspects on antimicrobial activity. *Nanomedicine* **2016**, *12*, 789–799. [CrossRef] [PubMed]

33. Le Ouay, B.; Stellacci, F. Antibacterial activity of silver nanoparticles: A surface science insight. *Nanotoday* **2015**, *10*, 339–354. [CrossRef]

34. Lok, C.N.; Zou, T.; Zhang, J.J.; Lin, I.W.; Che, C.M. Controlled-release systems for metal-based nanomedicine: Encapsulated/self-assembled nanoparticles of anticancer gold(III)/platinum(II) complexes and antimicrobial silver nanoparticles. *Adv. Mater.* **2014**, *26*, 5550–5557. [CrossRef] [PubMed]

35. Lok, C.N.; Ho, C.M.; Chen, R.; He, Q.Y.; Yu, W.Y.; Sun, H.; Tam, P.K.; Chiu, J.F.; Che, C.M. Proteomic analysis of the mode of antibacterial action of silver nanoparticles. *J. Proteom. Res.* **2006**, *5*, 916–924. [CrossRef] [PubMed]

36. Hou, W.C.; Stuart, B.; Howes, R.; Zepp, R.G. Sunlight-driven reduction of silver ions by natural organic matter: Formation and transformation of silver nanoparticles. *Environ. Sci. Technol.* **2013**, *47*, 7713–7721. [CrossRef] [PubMed]

37. Onodera, A.; Nishiumi, F.; Kakiguchi, K.; Tanaka, A.; Tanabe, N.; Honma, A.; Yayama, K.; Yoshioka, Y.; Nakahira, K.; Yonemura, S.; et al. Short-term changes in intracellular ROS localisation after the silver nanoparticles exposure depending on particle size. *Toxicol. Rep.* **2015**, *2*, 574–579. [CrossRef] [PubMed]

38. Agnihotri, S.; Mukherji, S.; Mukherji, S. Immobilized silver nanoparticles enhance contact killing and show highest efficacy: Elucidation of the mechanism of bactericidal action of silver. *Nanoscale* **2013**, *5*, 7328–7340. [CrossRef] [PubMed]

39. Tolaymat, T.M.; El Badawy, A.M.; Genaidy, A.; Scheckel, K.G.; Luxton, T.P.; Suidan, M. An evidence-based environmental perspective of manufactured silver nanoparticle in syntheses and applications: A systematic review and critical appraisal of peer-reviewed scientific papers. *Sci. Total Environ.* **2010**, *408*, 999–1006. [CrossRef] [PubMed]

40. Solomon, S.D.; Bahadory, M.; Jeyarajasingam, A.V.; Rutkowsky, S.A.; Boritz, C. Synthesis and Study of Silver Nanoparticles. *J. Chem. Educ.* **2007**, *84*, 322–325.

41. Malanovic, N.; Lohner, K. Gram-positive bacterial cell envelopes: The impact on the activity of antimicrobial peptides. *Biochim. Biophys. Acta* **2016**, *1858*, 936–946. [CrossRef] [PubMed]

42. Loffler, J.; Einsele, H.; Hebart, H.; Schumacher, U.; Hrastnik, C.; Daum, G. Phospholipid and sterol analysis of plasma membranes of azole-resistant *Candida albicans* strains. *FEMS Microbiol. Lett.* **2000**, *185*, 59–63. [CrossRef]

43. Lara, H.H.; Romero-Urbina, D.G.; Pierce, C.; Lopez-Ribot, J.L.; Arellano-Jimenez, M.J.; Jose-Yacaman, M. Effect of silver nanoparticles on *Candida albicans* biofilms: An ultrastructural study. *J. Nanobiotechnol.* **2015**, *13*, 91. [CrossRef] [PubMed]

44. Stoimenov, P.K.; Klinger, R.L.; Marchin, G.L.; Klabunde, K.J. Metal Oxide Nanoparticles as Bactericidal Agents. *Langmuir ACS J. Surf. Colloids* **2002**, *18*, 6679–6686. [CrossRef]

45. Hamouda, T.; Baker, J.R., Jr. Antimicrobial mechanism of action of surfactant lipid preparations in enteric Gram-negative bacilli. *J. Appl. Microbiol.* **2000**, *89*, 397–403. [CrossRef] [PubMed]

46. Lynch, R.J. Calcium glycerophosphate and caries: A review of the literature. *Int. Dent. J.* **2004**, *54*, 310–314. [CrossRef] [PubMed]

47. Turkevich, J.; Stevenson, P.C.; Hillier, J. A study of the nucleation and growth processes in the synthesis of colloidal gold. *Discuss. Faraday Soc.* **1951**, *11*, 55–75. [CrossRef]

48. Gorup, L.F.; Longo, E.; Leite, E.R.; Camargo, E.R. Moderating effect of ammonia on particle growth and stability of quasi-monodisperse silver nanoparticles synthesized by the Turkevich method. *J. Colloid Interface Sci.* **2011**, *360*, 355–358. [CrossRef] [PubMed]

8

Protein Expression Modifications in Phage-Resistant Mutants of *Aeromonas salmonicida* after AS-A Phage Treatment

Catarina Moreirinha [1,†] [ID], Nádia Osório [2,†], Carla Pereira [1,†], Sara Simões [2], Ivonne Delgadillo [3] and Adelaide Almeida [1,*] [ID]

1   Departament of Biology & CESAM, Campus Universitário de Santiago, Universidade de Aveiro, 3810-193 Aveiro, Portugal; anacatarinafernandes@gmail.com (C.M.); csgp@ua.pt (C.P.)
2   Escola Superior de Tecnologia da Saúde, Rua 5 de Outubro, SM Bispo. Instituto Politécnico de Coimbra, Apartado 7006, 3046-854 Coimbra, Portugal; nadia.osorio@estescoimbra.pt (N.O.); sarajmsimoes@hotmail.com (S.S.)
3   Departament of Chemistry, QOPNA, University of Aveiro, Campus Universitário de Santiago, 3810-193 Aveiro, Portugal; ivonne@ua.pt
*   Correspondence: aalmeida@ua.pt
†   These authors contributed equally to this work.

Abstract: The occurrence of infections by pathogenic bacteria is one of the main sources of financial loss for the aquaculture industry. This problem often cannot be solved with antibiotic treatment or vaccination. Phage therapy seems to be an alternative environmentally-friendly strategy to control infections. Recognizing the cellular modifications that bacteriophage therapy may cause to the host is essential in order to confirm microbial inactivation, while understanding the mechanisms that drive the development of phage-resistant strains. The aim of this work was to detect cellular modifications that occur after phage AS-A treatment in *A. salmonicida*, an important fish pathogen. Phage-resistant and susceptible cells were subjected to five successive streak-plating steps and analysed with infrared spectroscopy, a fast and powerful tool for cell study. The spectral differences of both populations were investigated and compared with a phage sensitivity profile, obtained through the spot test and efficiency of plating. Changes in protein associated peaks were found, and these results were corroborated by 1-D electrophoresis of intracellular proteins analysis and by phage sensitivity profiles. Phage AS-A treatment before the first streaking-plate step clearly affected the intracellular proteins expression levels of phage-resistant clones, altering the expression of distinct proteins during the subsequent five successive streak-plating steps, making these clones recover and be phenotypically more similar to the sensitive cells.

Keywords: phage therapy; *Aeromonas salmonicida*; furunculosis; phage-resistant mutants; proteins; infrared spectroscopy

1. Introduction

Aquaculture produces around 30% of the seafood for human consumption, being an increasingly important food fish source worldwide [1]. Generally, fish aquaculture is subjected to greater stress than wild conspecifics, which affects their natural immune system and often favours bacterial infection, especially during early life stages. This happens because of the high organic content and low concentration of dissolved oxygen often recorded in culture water, as well as the proximity of cultured individuals. Thus, opportunistic infections can easily emerge, causing significant economic losses to producers [2].

The Food and Agriculture Organization (FAO) and most aquaculture organizations recommend a decrease, or even the avoidance, of antibiotics in aquaculture, though they are still often used by the industry worldwide [1]. This can lead to the development of resistant bacteria and dispersal of antibiotic resistance in the environment, indirectly affecting bacterial species that are not associated with disease (non-target), allowing resistant strains to enter the human food chain [3,4].

Although vaccination is considered the best approach for the prevention of fish infections, it is practically impossible to employ during fish early life stages, due to their small size and low capacity to develop immunity [5,6]. Consequently, the development and application of innovative treatment technologies are demanded by the fish farming industry in order to increase the efficacy of aquaculture production, by lowering production costs and fish mortality, with reduced environmental impacts.

Aeromonas salmonicida, the causative agent of furunculosis, is a significant fish pathogen in aquaculture. This disease causes high mortality and morbidity in a broad variety of fish, with important economic losses in aquaculture worldwide [7]. The chronic skin ulcers in weakened old fish make them unsuitable for human consumption [8]. The acute form is more common in juveniles and, usually, leads to septicaemia, being fatal in two to three days [9,10].

Phage therapy is an alternative approach to treat fish bacterial infections, being based on the use of bacteriophages (viruses that infect bacteria) to inactivate pathogenic bacteria. Compared to conventional methods such as antibiotics and vaccination, it presents several advantages: (a) phages are target specific; (b) serious or irreversible side effects of phage addition are not known; (c) phage therapy is an environmentally friendly strategy; (d) phages are resistant to various environmental conditions; (e) phage therapy is a flexible, fast and inexpensive technology [11,12]. Consequently, phage therapy appears to be a promising and environmentally friendly methodology to control bacterial infection. However, there are some studies reporting the development of phage-resistance by some bacteria [13–16]. This resistance may be due to the modification or loss of the bacterial cell surface receptors, blocking of the receptors by the bacterial extracellular matrix, production of modified restriction endonucleases that degrade the phage DNA, and inhibition of phage DNA penetration [17]. Additional causes for the development of resistance again bacteriophages are genetic mutations affecting phage receptors, restriction modification or abortive infection associated with the presence of clustered regularly interspaced short palindromic repeats (CRISPRs) in the bacterial genome [17,18]. Apart from genetic, resistance may also be phenotypic, which has been mostly disregarded in the literature [12,19,20]. It has been previously hypothesized that some of the reasons for phenotypic resistance may be: (i) induced, the products of phage-lysed bacteria result in a change in uninfected bacterial gene expression, thus reducing adsorption; (ii) intrinsic, reduced adsorption is due to a physiological or gene expression state that happens prior to the phage introduction; and (ii) dynamic, degradation or blocking of bacterial receptors by phage proteins released during cell lysis [19]. As very little is known about the effects of the phage infection in the bacterial cells, it is important to understand the inactivation mechanisms and the modifications that are induced by bacteriophages in the host cell, in order to obtain knowledge and a solution to the problem of phage-resistant bacteria.

Infrared spectroscopy (IR) has been a valuable method for detection and differentiation of microbial cells. It has also been successfully used to detect modification in proteins and lipids extracted from bacteria after exposure to a stress [21], and to study DNA structure [22]. Another advantage is the possibility of studying the whole cell, without the need to extract cellular components [23,24]. This methodology has already been used to discriminate phage-resistant from phage-susceptible bacteria [15]. The infrared absorbance spectrum represents a "fingerprint" that is characteristic of a chemical or biological substance. The main reasons for the wide acceptance of this method are the speed with which samples can be characterized with almost no handling, the flexibility of the equipment, the minimum sample amount required and the low cost of the analysis [25]. The analytical information from the spectra can be interpreted using a multivariate analysis that relates the spectra obtained with the properties of the object of study, thus facilitating data interpretation [26].

The main objective of this study was to understand the cellular modifications that occur in host targets after phage therapy, using the causative agent of furunculosis, *A. salmonicida*, and its specific phage AS-A as a model.

2. Results

2.1. Detection of Host Sensitivity to Phages after Phage Contact

Firstly, five phage resistant colonies that grew inside a clear spot-test were selected for use in the subsequent steps. These colonies were smaller than the sensitive ones and took three times longer to appear on the petri plates. These colonies were subjected to five successive streak-plating steps. It was observed that the spot-tests were negative (Figure 1A) until the fourth streak-plating step, when the spot tests became positive (Figure 1B). However, efficiency of plating (EOP) results indicated that even after the fourth streak-plating step, phages neither form lysis plaques nor adsorb and replicate in the presence of the phage-resistant clones.

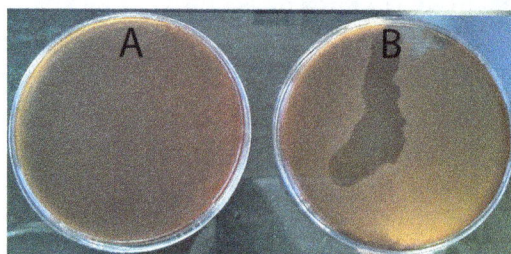

Figure 1. Spot test results using a phage-resistant mutant of phage AS-A and phage AS-A after first (**A**) and fifth streak-plating steps (**B**).

2.2. Infrared Spectroscopy of Whole Cells

The phage resistant clones from the five streaking-steps were analysed by IR spectroscopy in order to understand if there were any detectable differences in cellular components between these clones.

Principal component analysis (Figure 2) of the whole bacterial cells shows two distinct groups. It is visible a good discrimination between control phage-sensitive colonies and resistant colonies after the fourth and fifth streak-plating steps (negative PC1) and colonies from earlier streaking steps, corresponding to days 1, 2 and 3 (positive PC1).

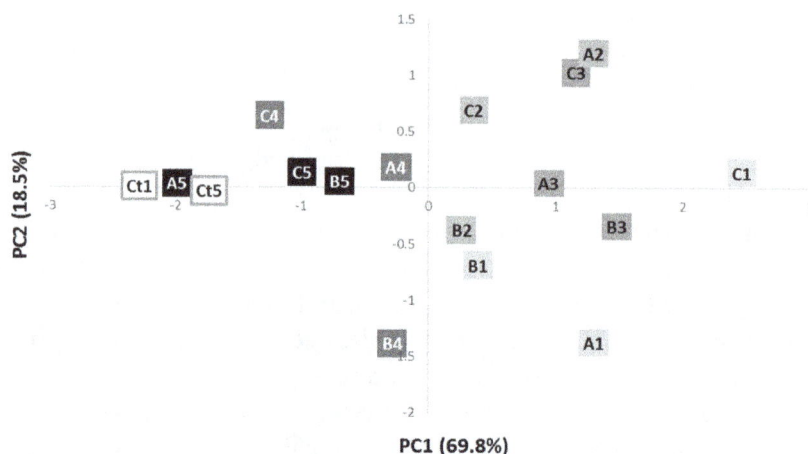

Figure 2. Scores scatter plot of the IR spectra of phage-resistant colonies A, B and C, along the 5 streak plating steps, and control phage sensitive colonies after 1 (Ct1) and 5 (Ct5) streaking steps. The letters correspond to the different colonies (A is colony A; B is colony B; C is colony C) and the numbers to the streaking-plate days (1 is day 1; 2 is day 2; 3 is day 3; 4 is day 4; 5 is day 5).

Analysing the loadings plot profile (Figure 3), there are various peaks that are contributing to the distribution of the samples according to the principal component analysis (PCA). The samples that are located in negative PC1, that is, the later streaking days and the controls that are sensitive to phage are characterized by peaks at 1510 cm^{-1}, 1440 cm^{-1}, 1380 cm^{-1}, 1150 cm^{-1}, 1070 cm^{-1}, 1025 cm^{-1} and 980 cm^{-1}. The samples corresponding to the early streaking steps (1, 2 and 3), located in positive PC1, are characterized by peaks at 1695 cm^{-1}, 1650 cm^{-1}, 1590 cm^{-1}, 1570 cm^{-1}, 1560 cm^{-1}, 1250 cm^{-1} and 1175 cm^{-1}. Table 1 summarizes the infrared spectra peak assignments. It was found that the proteins were the most affected cellular component between phage-sensitive bacteria and phage-resistant bacteria. Taking into account these results, we decided to verify if there was also differential expression of the intracellular proteins in these cases. Phage-resistant clones of day 1, i.e., after one streak-plating step, and phage-resistant clones of day 5, i.e., after five streak-plating steps were chosen to perform protein analysis.

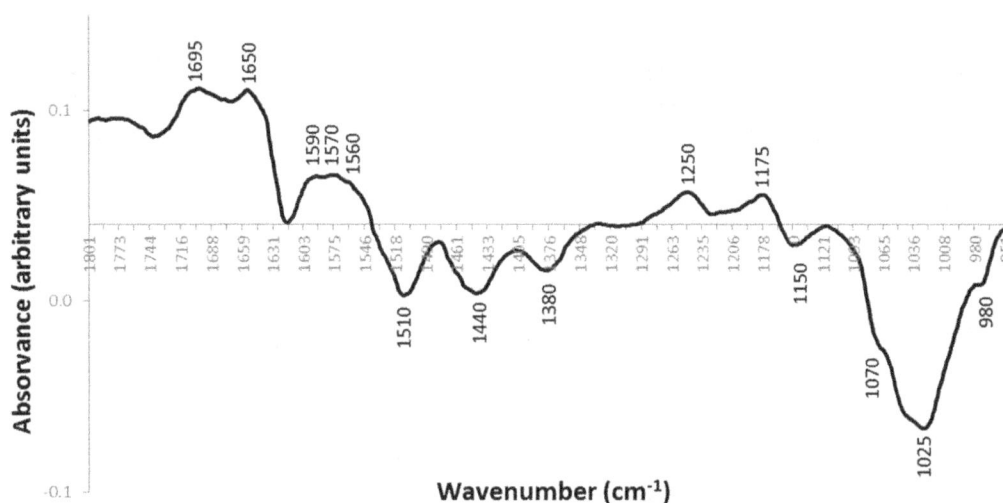

Figure 3. Loadings plot profile of PC1 corresponding to the IR spectra of the phage-resistant colonies A, B and C, along the 5 streak-plating steps, and control phage sensitive colonies.

Table 1. Peaks/regions assignments (wavenumber) from principal component analysis (PCA) loadings plot profile of spectra from colonies of *A. salmonicida* sensitive and resistant to phage AS-A.

PC1 − (cm^{-1})	PC1 + (cm^{-1})	Assignment	Reference
	1695	Amide I—proteins (β-sheet)	[27]
	1650	Amide I—proteins (α-helix)	[23,27]
	1590, 1570, 1560	Amide II—proteins	[27]
1510		Amide II—proteins	[27]
1440		CH$_3$ bending—proteins (methyl groups)	[28]
1380		COO$^-$—acids and methyl groups from proteins/CO bonds or deformation of C-H or N-H bonds of proteins	[28,29]
	1250	Amide III—proteins/PO$_2$$^-$—phospholipids	[30,31]
	1175	C-O—proteins and glycomaterials	[32,33]
1150		C-O carbohydrates	[33]
1070		PO$_2$$^-$—nucleotides	[34]
1025		Carbohydrates	[35]
980		OCH$_3$—polysaccharides	[36]

2.3. Differential Expression of the Proteins of the Phage-Resistant Clones (First Streak-Plating and Fifth Streak-Plating)

In order to try to understand why phage-sensitive bacteria (control) and clones after five streak-plating steps were different from clones after one streak-plating step, 1D SDS-PAGE gels were performed, comparing control and first streak-plating clones (Figure 4A), and comparing control and fifth streak-plating clones (Figure 5A).

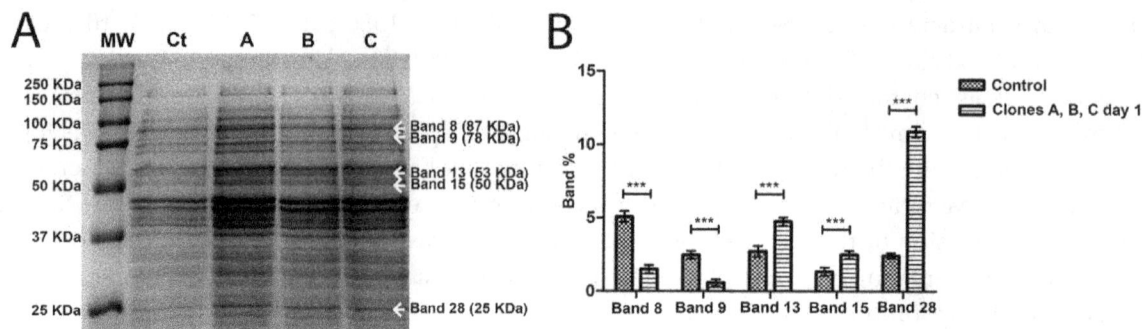

Figure 4. (**A**) SDS PAGE gel of the intracellular proteins of *A. salmonicida* on first streak-plating. MW, molecular weight marker; Ct, control phage-sensitive *A. salmonicida*; A is Colony A of the phage-resistant *A. salmonicida* mutant; B is Colony B of the phage-resistant *A. salmonicida* mutant; C is Colony C of the phage-resistant *A. salmonicida* mutant. The marked bands are the ones that showed differential expression between control and clones A, B and C. Band weight is expressed in kilodalton (KDa). (**B**) Differential expression of the bands, in percentage, comparing Control (phage-sensitive *A. salmonicida*) with clones A, B and C (phage-resistant *A. salmonicida*) after 1 streak-plating steps. *** $p < 0.001$.

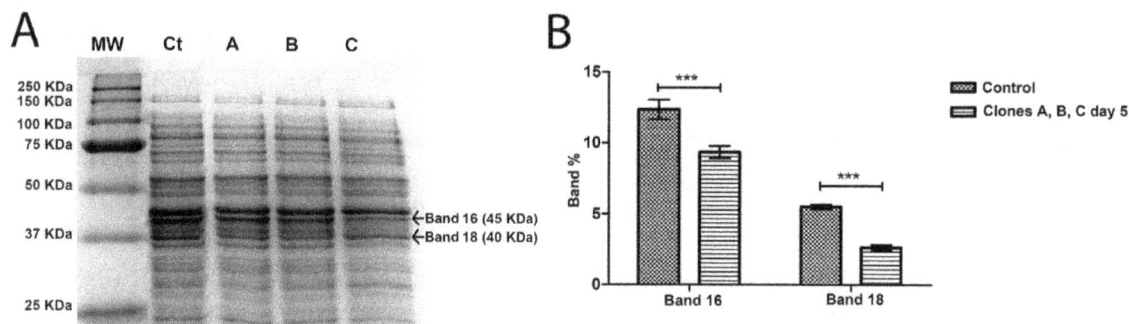

Figure 5. (**A**) SDS PAGE gel of the intracellular proteins of *A. salmonicida* on fifth streak plating. MW, molecular weight marker; Ct, control phage-sensitive *A. salmonicida*; A is Colony A of the phage-resistant *A. salmonicida* mutant; B is Colony B of the phage-resistant *A. salmonicida* mutant; C is Colony C of the phage-resistant *A. salmonicida* mutant. The marked bands are the ones that showed differential expression between control and clones A, B and C. Band weight is expressed in kilodalton (KDa). (**B**) Differential expression of the bands, in percentage, comparing Control (phage-sensitive *A. salmonicida*) with clones A, B and C (phage-resistant *A. salmonicida*) after 5 streak-plating steps. *** $p < 0.001$.

In total, 39 bands were detected and compared, in the control and *A. salmonicida* clones, both in first streak-plating and fifth streak-plating clones. When compared to the control, the bands that were significantly differentially expressed on first streak-plating clones were bands 8, 9, 13, 15 and 28 (Figure 4B). The expression patterns of the bands 8 and 9 in *A. salmonicida* first streak-plating clones tend to be less when compared to the control. However, the 13, 15 and 28 bands tend to have an increased expression compared to the control (Figure 4B). On fifth streak-plating clones, the differentially expressed bands were band 16 and 18 (Figure 5B). All of the bands with differential expression decreased between the control and fifth streak-plating clones.

By using the homology of the molecular weight of the bands with differential expression, consulting the databases referred to in the Section 4, presumptive identification of the proteins was made (Table 2).

Table 2. Presumptive band identification of the 1-D electrophoresis gel of intracellular proteins, associated proteins and their molecular functions.

Band	MW (KDa)	Protein/Gene	Molecular Function
Band 8	87	Phage transcriptional protein (ASA_3866)	Interacts selectively and non-covalently with the DNA with a specific nucleotide composition or with a specific sequence motif or type of DNA.
Band 9	78	Phage shock protein B (pspB, ASA_2424)	Response of the bacteria to a variety of stimuli, including phage infection. It is involved in bacterial protection mechanisms.
Band 13	53	Sec-independent protein translocase proteinTatA (tatA, ASA_3970)	Biological process: controlled liberation of proteins from a cell.
Band 15	50	ASA_P5G151	Unknown function.
Band 16	45	Transposase (VO70_17345, VO70_21745)	Facilitates the transference of genetic material between organisms.
Band 18	40	Toxin-antitoxin system, toxin component (VO68_18510, VO70_09250)	Plasmid maintenance, stress regulation and adaptation, growth control and programmed cellular death.
Band 28	25	Q70WF0, Q70WF0_AERSA	Unknown function.

3. Discussion

The emergence of phage-resistant mutants during phage infection has been reported in many studies [12,37–41], but the mechanisms of bacteria resistance to phages are not yet completely understood. A previous study by our group [41] showed that the agent of furunculosis can be efficiently inactivated by the phage AS-A (reduction of 4 Log CFU·mL^{-1} after 8 h of treatment). However, some bacteria survived the infection by the phage due to the development of phage-resistance [41]. Nevertheless, the frequency of resistance, with a value of 2.24×10^{-4} Log CFU·mL^{-1}, was limited as already reported in previous studies [14,42,43].

So, in our previous study [41] we verified that although a specific phage against the agent of furunculosis can efficiently control the bacterial growth, some phage-resistant bacteria emerge after treatment. In the present study, we observed that the resistant colonies after the fourth and fifth streak-plating steps are clearly distinct from those of the earlier streaking steps (steps 1, 2 and 3). A significant modification in the expression of intracellular proteins was observed when compared with the phage-sensitive bacteria. Moreover, these modifications affect distinct proteins after the first and the fifth streak-plating steps, allowing "lysis from without" (positive spot test) after the forth streak-plating step, contrary to that observed for bacteria from the first, second and third streak-plating steps.

It has been stated in the literature that resistance to phages can be overcome by the phage itself because it evolves along with the host [44]. Moreover, it has also been asserted that resistance to phages entails great costs to the bacteria [45]. In fact, as observed for other phages, colonies of AS-A phage-resistant mutants were smaller than colonies formed by the non-phage added control [14]. These results suggest that the remaining bacterial mutants (forming small size colonies) maintained their viability in the presence of phages but their phenotypes were affected. The decrease in the bacterial size after phage exposure could be a fitness cost, which might contribute to their elimination from the environment faster than their wild-type parents.

In this study, as already observed for other phages [15,16], it was detected that phage-resistant bacteria also mutate after successive streak-plating steps. Although the spot tests showed negative results until the fourth streak-plating step, at the fourth and fifth steps, the spot test was positive, as also observed in other studies [15,16]. These results were confirmed by infrared spectroscopy data of the whole cells. Infrared spectroscopy results show that the spectra obtained from the fourth and fifth streak-plating colonies are similar to ones from phage-sensitive control colonies, suggesting that these colonies are more similar to control phage-sensitive bacteria than the colonies from streak-plating steps 1, 2 and 3. It seems that the resistant bacteria somehow "recovered", being more similar to control bacterial populations, which are sensitive to the phage infection. The infrared peaks that contributed to these results were found to be especially associated with proteins. Taking this into account, we focused further studies on protein analysis with 1D SDS PAGE gels.

Regarding the presumptively identified proteins with differential expression on first streak-plating phage-resistant clones, a decrease in band 8 is noticeable when compared to the control, being the band associated with a phage transcriptional protein with regulation function in the transcription of phage genes [46]. This may be a response by the bacteria to the viral infection, preventing the transcription of the viral genome. Similarly, the expression of the protein corresponding to band 9 in first streak-plating clones decreased when compared to the control. This protein, phage-shock B protein, is involved in a regulation system that responds to aggression, habitually to phage secretins, promoting the defensive response of the bacteria [47]. This protein has been previously detected in the response of other bacteria, however, this response mechanism is not yet completely understood [47,48]. In our case, this protein is less expressed in the phage-resistant clones, which seems contradictory. Nevertheless, it was stated that bacteria synthesise phage shock proteins after being infected with phage, that, in the case of the resistant clones could not happen [49]. Contrarily, the protein associated to band 13, TatA, increased in *A. salmonicida* first streak-plating clones. This protein belongs to the Tat system (twin-arginine translocation) which is responsible for the transport of various substances at the membrane level, against the concentration gradient of the cytoplasm to the extracellular space, namely proteins, being associated with the bacterial pathogenicity in the secretion of virulence factors [50,51]. This increase suggests that these first streak-plating clones could be more virulent than control bacteria. However, some studies have shown that phage-resistant clones are less pathogenic than phage sensitive bacteria [20,52]. This suggests that the increase in the expression of this protein could be associated with other mechanisms not related with pathogenicity.

Regarding the proteins with differential expression on phage-resistant clones in the fifth streak-plating, that have a positive spot-test, band 16 suggests the expression of a transposase that is decreased in these clones when compared to control phage-sensitive bacteria. These type of enzymes facilitates the transference of the genetic material between organisms [53]. The bacteria may have decreased the expression of this protein as a defence mechanism in order to prevent the phage replication. Band 18, corresponds to a toxin-antitoxin system, which is implied in the maintenance of plasmids, stress regulation and adaptation, as well as in growth control and programmed cellular death [54,55]. This system requires the dual activity of a toxin and an antagonistic antitoxin [56]. A decrease in this band in the clones of the fifth streak-plating was found when compared to the control. As this protein decreased in this study, this suggests that in the fifth streak-plating clones, the stress caused by the phage decreased. In fact, the efficiency of plating (EOP) results indicate that the fifth streak-plating clones do not replicate the phage. Other authors [57] have obtained similar results, designating this situation by "lysis from without". The spot test lysis when the phage is not replicated by the host (EOP is zero) has been described as a plausible mechanism which happens when an overload of phage simultaneously infects a bacterium leading to lysis, either from the action of phage lysins or from rapid depletion of the cell resources [58]. As in the spot test the same volume of phage suspension was used and lysis was only observed for the clones of the fourth and fifth streak-plating, so, the hypothesis of rapid depletion of the cells resources does not seems plausible. As stated before, the lysis can be due to the presence of phage lysins. However, it is difficult to understand why the spot test was only positive for the clones of the fourth and fifth streak-plating and not for the clones of the first, second and third streak-plating. However, modifications in the bacterial proteins along the successive streak-plating could allow the clones to recover the sensitivity to the phage lysins. This is in agreement with the infrared spectroscopy results which showed that the fourth and fifth streak-plating clones were similar to the phage-sensitive bacteria (control), but clearly different from those of the first, second and third streak-plating steps. In order to test this hypothesis, further studies are needed.

It would be interesting, for example, to try to correlate IR spectra with the regaining of sensitivity to phage lysins to extract more information from the spectra.

We noticed that the different analysed clones present significant modifications in intracellular proteins related to phage infection, both in the first and fifth streak-plating steps. However, there are more proteins that are differentially expressed in clones of the first streak-plating than in clones of the fifth streak-plating, which is in accordance with infrared spectroscopy results. The fact that the phage-sensitive control bacteria have infrared spectra that are more similar to the fourth and fifth streak-plating clones may be because the cellular envelope, used by the phages to infect the bacteria, became more similar in these cases. This may be related to the fact that the spot test turns positive again for the fourth and fifth streak-plating clones, which might be due to phenotypical similarities in the cell envelope. In our study, phenotypic resistance may have been acquired by phage-resistant cells, showing less pronounced cell modifications than genetic resistance, which would be more definitive. In order to better understand this, more experiments should be done, such as serial dilution spot-tests and EOP tests with varying multiplicity of infection (MOI). In order to confirm these results, the presumptively identified proteins and the non-identified proteins that show differential expression between the clones should be confirmed/identified by methods such as mass spectrometry. In future experiments, it would also be interesting to include the whole cell proteins, which would provide more information. Moreover, since there are some indications of which proteins seem to alter their expression, molecular assays using specific primers for these proteins would be a reliable method to use in order to explore and elucidate the whole process of the clone expression pattern.

4. Materials and Methods

4.1. Bacteria and Phage

The bacteria *A. salmonicida* CECT 894 was used in this study. Fresh plate bacterial cultures were maintained in solid Tryptic Soy Agar medium (TSA; Liofilchem, Roseto degli Abruzzi, Italy) at 4 °C. Before each assay, one isolated colony was aseptically transferred to 10 mL of Tryptic Soy Broth medium (TSB; Liofilchem, Roseto degli Abruzzi, Italy) and was grown overnight at 25 °C. An aliquot of this culture (100 μL) was aseptically transferred to 10 mL of fresh TSB medium (Liofilchem, Roseto degli Abruzzi, Italy) and grown overnight at 25 °C to reach an optical density (O.D. 600) of 0.8, corresponding to about 10^9 cells·mL^{-1}.

Phage AS-A was isolated from sewage water from a lift station of the sewage network of Aveiro, Portugal (station EEIS9 of SIMRIA Multi Sanitation System of Ria de Aveiro) using *A. salmonicida* as host, according to [41]. The phage stocks were stored at 4 °C and 1% chloroform (final volume) (Scharlau, Sentmenat, Spain) was added. The phage suspension titre was determined by the double-layer agar method using TSA (Liofilchem, Roseto degli Abruzzi, Italy) as the culture medium [59]. The plates were incubated at 25 °C for 12 h and the number of lysis plaques was counted. The results were expressed as plaque forming units per millilitre (PFU·mL^{-1}).

4.2. Isolation of A. salmonicida Phage-Resistant Mutants

Only bacterial colonies that were resistant to the phage were used (bacteria that developed inside phage plates). For this, bacteria *A. salmonicida* and phage AS-A were plated by the double layer agar method and the plates were incubated for 24 h at 25 °C. After that, several colonies that grew inside the phage plates, thus, resistant to phage infection, were visible. Three individualized colonies (A, B and C) were chosen and used in the subsequent assays.

4.3. Detection of Bacteria Sensitivity to the Phage after One Cycle of Phage Contact

The phage resistant colonies obtained in Section 4.2 were used. The colonies were inoculated in TSB medium for 24 h at 25 °C. After that, the culture was used to perform a spot test and was also plated in TSA medium. This procedure was done 4 more times, making a total of 5 streak plating steps. This procedure was done for the 3 selected colonies.

4.4. Efficiency of Plating (EOP)

The efficiency of plating was determined for bacteria that shown positive spot tests (clear lysis area), i.e., for the bacteria from the fourth and fifth streak-plating steps, according to Pereira et al. [15] using the double-agar method [59]. The EOP was calculated (average PFU on target bacteria/average PFU on host bacteria), three independent assays were performed.

4.5. Phage Adsorption

The determination of phage adsorption was performed according to Pereira et al. [15]. Briefly, ten microliters of phage suspension of about 10^6 PFU/mL were added to 10 mL of *A. salmonicida* culture of about 10^9 CFU/mL (corresponding to an optical density (600 nm) of 0.8) [60] and incubated at 25 °C. Aliquots of this culture were collected after 0, 5, 10, 15, 20, 25, 30, 40, 50, 60 and 70 min of incubation and chloroform was added to a final concentration of 1%. The mixture was centrifuged at $12,000 \times g$ for 5 min, after that the supernatants were filtered using 0.2 µL membranes (Millipore, Bedford, VA, USA). The filtrates containing unadsorbed phages were then diluted and titrated. The plates were then incubated at 25 °C and observed after 8 h for plaque formation. The values were calculated as the decrease of phage titre in supernatant (percentage) compared with time zero. Three independent assays were performed.

4.6. Infrared Spectroscopy

In order to access the spectral differences of sensitive *A. salmonicida* colonies and phage resistant mutant colonies, mid-infrared spectroscopy was used, as it was previously described [15,24]. They were used for the *A. salmonicida* phage resistant colonies A, B and C (from Section 4.3).

To analyse the whole cells, colonies A, B and C were analysed during the 5 days of streaking (Section 4.3), as well as control sensitive colonies Ct1 and Ct5 (after the 1 and 5 streak plating steps). The colonies were collected with a loop and placed in the crystal of a horizontal single reflection ATR accessory. The colonies were gently air dried and the spectra were acquired.

Spectra were done in a MIR (Bruker ALPHA FTIR spectrometer, Germany) with a resolution of 4 cm^{-1} and 32 scans, in the infrared region (4000 to 600 cm^{-1}). At least 5 replicate spectra were performed for each colony. Mid-infrared spectra were obtained in OPUS format (OPUS 6.5, Bruker, Germany) and transferred via JCAMP.DX format for use in a house-developed data analysis software (CATS build 97). The spectra were SNV (standard normal deviate) corrected previous to multivariate analysis. Principal component analysis (PCA) was done in order to find the major sources of variability in the spectra and to detect groups.

4.7. Extraction and Quantification of Intracellular Proteins from Phage-Sensitive and Phage-Resistant Bacteria

The proteins extracts were obtained from the growth until the late exponential phase of the strains (OD 0.9 at 550 nm) in Luria Bertani Broth (Merck, Darmstadt, Germany). The cells were separated from the supernatant by centrifugation at $8000 \times g$ for 10 min at 4 °C. The protein extractions were made in three independent experiments per each strain and the protein quantification was performed in triplicate.

The cell pellets were washed three times in 10 mM phosphate buffered saline pH 7.4. After that they were resuspended in 1 mL of lysis and protein solubilisation buffer solution (7 M urea, 2 M thiourea, 4% cholamidopropyl dimethylammonio-1-propanesulfonate (CHAPS), 30 mM Tris base, pH 8.5). Crude cell-free extracts were obtained by sonication in ice to minimize protein damage, during a 2 min period, using a 30% duty cycle, 2 s pulses with intervening periods of 3 s. The intracellular protein solution was incubated with 1 mg·mL^{-1} of Dnase I (GE Healthcare, Uppsala, Sweden) and 10 mM of protease inhibitor mix (GE Healthcare, Uppsala, Sweden) for 1 h at 15 °C. The final solution was collected by centrifugation at $20,000 \times g$ for 40 min at 4 °C and then, the protein concentration was measured using the 2-D Quant Kit (GE Healthcare, Uppsala, Sweden), following the manufacturer's instructions. The procedure was performed in triplicate.

4.8. Protein Separation by 1-D Electrophoresis

Proteins were separated by 12.5% SDS-PAGE [61], in a Mini-PROTEAN 3 Cell (Bio-Rad, Hercules, CA, USA), for 50 min at 150 V. 5 μg/mL of each protein sample were used in this assay. Proteins were visualized by colloidal Coomassie Brilliant BlueG-250 (CBB) staining [62]. Gel images were acquired using the Gel DocTM XR+ (Bio-Rad, Hercules, CA, USA). The comparative analysis of the acquired images was performed in Image Lab v3.0 software (Biorad, Hercules, CA, USA) and based on the optical density measurement of each band. To minimize possible differences in the quantity of the proteins loaded, the results were normalized and expressed as a band percentage, resulting from the value of the optical density of a given band in the total of the bands per lane $\times$ 100. The comparison of the differential expression of the intracellular proteins of the different tested *A. salmonicida* clones in the different analysis times was made through a two-way ANOVA, using GraphPad Prism software v7 (USA). The differences were considered statistically significant when $p < 0.05$.

4.9. Presumptive Identification of the Proteins in Differentially Expressed Bands

The molecular weight of the bands that were differentially expressed between control and *A. salmonicida* clones on day 1 and between control and day 5, using the databases UniProtKB (www.uniprot.org) and NCBI (www.ncbi.nlm.nih.gov/pubmed) allowed us to presumptively identify the proteins and their respective function, based on the deposited genome of *Aeromonas salmonicida* A449.

5. Conclusions

A single cycle of phage treatment causes a significant modification in the expression of intracellular proteins of phage-resistant bacterial clones relative to the phage sensitive bacteria, but after successive streaking-plate steps these clones recover and are phenotypically more similar to the sensitive cells. Taking this information into account, this study paves the way for future experiments in order to better understand the bacterial resistance mechanisms to phages.

Acknowledgments: This work was supported by FEDER through COMPETE—Programa Operacional Factores de Competitividade, and by National funding through Fundação para a Ciência e Tecnologia (FCT), within the research projects FCOMP-01-0124-FEDER-013934 and ENV/ES/001048. Financial support was provided to Catarina Moreirinha in the form of a Postdoctoral grant (ENV/ES/001048), and Carla Pereira in the form of a PhD grant (SFRH/BD/76414/2011).

Author Contributions: Catarina Moreirinha, Nádia Osório, Carla Pereira and Sara Simões performed the experiments. Catarina Moreirinha wrote the paper and Nádia Osório and Carla Pereira also contributed to the writing. Ivonne Delgadillo and Adelaide Almeida supervised the work, revised the paper and contributed with reagents and analysis tools.

References

1. FAO. *The State of World Fisheries and Aquaculture*; FAO: Rome, Italy, 2014.
2. Iwama, G.K.; Pickering, A.D.; Sumpter, J.P.; Schreck, C.B. *Fish Stress and Health in Aquaculture*; Cambridge University Press: Cambridge, UK, 2011; Volume 62, p. 279.
3. Furushita, M.; Shiba, T.; Maeda, T.; Yahata, M.; Kaneoka, A.; Takahashi, Y.; Torii, K.; Hasegawa, T.; Ohta, M. Similarity of Tetracycline Resistance Genes Isolated from Fish Farm Bacteria to Those from Clinical Isolates. *Appl. Environ. Microbiol.* **2003**, *69*, 5336–5342. [CrossRef] [PubMed]
4. World Health Organization (WHO). *Use of Antimicrobials Outside Medicine and Resultant Antimicrobial Resistance in Humans*; WHO: Geneva, Switzerland, 2002; Volume 268, p. 2.
5. Duckworth, D.H.; Gulig, P.A. Bacteriophages. *BioDrugs* **2002**, *16*, 57–62. [CrossRef] [PubMed]

6.   Vadstein, O. The use of immunostimulation in marine larviculture: Possibilities and challenges. *Aquaculture* **1997**, *155*, 401–417. [CrossRef]

7.   Wiklund, T.; Dalsgaard, I. Occurrence and significance of atypical Aeromonas salmonicida in non-salmonid and salmonid fish species: A review. *Dis. Aquat. Organ.* **1998**, *32*, 49–69. [CrossRef] [PubMed]

8.   Uhland, F.C.; Martineau, D.; Mikaelian, I.; Canada, S.-L.V. *Maladies des Poissons D'eau Douce du Québec: Guide de Diagnostic*; University Press of Montreal: Montreal, QC, Canada, 2000; ISBN 2760617785.

9.   Boyd, J.; Williams, J.; Curtis, B.; Kozera, C.; Singh, R.; Reith, M. Three small, cryptic plasmids from Aeromonas salmonicida subsp. *salmonicida A449. Plasmid* **2003**, *50*, 131–144. [CrossRef]

10. Burr, S.E.; Pugovkin, D.; Wahli, T.; Segner, H.; Frey, J. Attenuated virulence of an Aeromonas salmonicida subsp. *salmonicida type III secretion mutant in a rainbow trout model. Microbiology* **2005**, *151*, 2111–2118.

11. Almeida, A.; Cunha, A.; Gomes, N.C.M.; Alves, E.; Costa, L.; Faustino, M.A.F. Phage therapy and photodynamic therapy: Low environmental impact approaches to inactivate microorganisms in fish farming plants. *Mar. Drugs* **2009**, *7*, 268–313. [CrossRef] [PubMed]

12. Vieira, A.; Silva, Y.J.; Cunha, A.; Gomes, N.C.M.; Ackermann, H.-W.W.; Almeida, A.; Cunha, A.; Gomes, N.C.M.; Ackermann, H.-W.W.; Almeida, A. Phage therapy to control multidrug-resistant Pseudomonas aeruginosa skin infections: In vitro and ex vivo experiments. *Eur. J. Clin. Microbiol. Infect. Dis.* **2012**, *31*, 3241–3249. [CrossRef] [PubMed]

13. Gill, J.; Hyman, P. Phage Choice, Isolation, and Preparation for Phage Therapy. *Curr. Pharm. Biotechnol.* **2010**, *11*, 2–14. [CrossRef] [PubMed]

14. Silva, Y.J.; Costa, L.; Pereira, C.; Mateus, C.; Cunha, A.; Calado, R.; Gomes, N.C.M.; Pardo, M.A.; Hernandez, I.; Almeida, A. Phage Therapy as an Approach to Prevent Vibrio anguillarum Infections in Fish Larvae Production. *PLoS ONE* **2014**, *9*, e114197. [CrossRef] [PubMed]

15. Pereira, C.; Moreirinha, C.; Lewickab, M.; Almeida, P.; Clemente, C.; Delgadillo, I.; Romalde, J.L.; Nunes, M.L.; Lewicka, M.; Almeida, P.; et al. Bacteriophages with potential to inactivate Salmonella Typhimurium: Use of single phage suspensions and phage cocktails. *Virus Res.* **2016**, *220*, 179–192. [CrossRef] [PubMed]

16. Pereira, C.; Moreirinha, C.; Lewicka, M.; Almeida, P.; Clemente, C.; Romalde, J.L.; Nunes, M.; Almeida, A. Characterization and in vitro evaluation of new bacteriophages for the biocontrol of Escherichia coli. *Virus Res.* **2017**, *227*, 171–182. [CrossRef] [PubMed]

17. Labrie, S.J.; Samson, J.E.; Moineau, S. Bacteriophage resistance mechanisms. *Nat. Rev. Microbiol.* **2010**, *8*, 317–327. [CrossRef] [PubMed]

18. Heller, K.J. Molecular interaction between bacteriophage and the gram-negative cell envelope. *Arch. Microbiol.* **1992**, *158*, 235–248. [CrossRef] [PubMed]

19. Bull, J.J.; Vegge, C.S.; Schmerer, M.; Chaudhry, W.N.; Levin, B.R. Phenotypic Resistance and the Dynamics of Bacterial Escape from Phage Control. *PLoS ONE* **2014**, *9*, e94690. [CrossRef] [PubMed]

20. Laanto, E.; Bamford, J.J.K.H.; Laakso, J.; Sundberg, L.L.-R. Phage-driven loss of virulence in a fish pathogenic bacterium. *PLoS ONE* **2012**, *7*, e53157. [CrossRef] [PubMed]

21. Santos, A.L.; Moreirinha, C.; Lopes, D.; Esteves, A.C.; Henriques, I.; Almeida, A.; Domingues, M.R.M.; Delgadillo, I.; Correia, A.; Cunha, A.; et al. Effects of UV Radiation on the Lipids and Proteins of Bacteria Studied by Mid-Infrared Spectroscopy. *Environ. Sci. Technol.* **2013**, *47*, 6306–6315. [CrossRef] [PubMed]

22. Taillandier, E.; Liquier, J. *DNA Structures Part A: Synthesis and Physical Analysis of DNA*; Methods in Enzymology; Elsevier: Amsterdam, The Netherlands, 1992; Volume 211, ISBN 9780121821128.

23. Helm, D.; Naumann, D. Identification of some bacterial cell components by FT-IR spectroscopy. *FEMS Microbiol. Lett.* **1995**, *126*, 75–79. [CrossRef]

24. Moreirinha, C.; Nunes, A.; Barros, A.A.; Almeida, A.; Delgadillo, I. Evaluation of the potential of Mid-infrared spectroscopy to assess the microbiological quality of ham. *J. Food Saf.* **2015**, *35*, 270–275. [CrossRef]

25. Blanco, M.; Villarroya, I. NIR spectroscopy: A rapid-response analytical tool. *TrAC Trends Anal. Chem.* **2002**, *21*, 240–250. [CrossRef]

26. Brereton, R. *Chemometrics: Data Analysis for the Laboratoty and Chemical Plant*; Wiley: London, UK, 2003.

27. Barth, A. Infrared spectroscopy of proteins. *Biochim. Biophys. Acta* **2007**, *1767*, 1073–1101. [CrossRef] [PubMed]

28. Alves, E.; Moreirinha, C.; Faustino, M.A.; Cunha, Â.; Delgadillo, I.; Neves, M.G.; Almeida, A. Overall biochemical changes in bacteria photosensitized with cationic porphyrins monitored by infrared spectroscopy. *Future Med. Chem.* **2016**, *8*, 613–628. [CrossRef] [PubMed]

29. Pudziuvyte, B.; Bakiene, E.; Bonnett, R.; Shatunov, P.A.; Magaraggia, M.; Jori, G. Alterations of Escherichia coli envelope as a consequence of photosensitization with tetrakis(N-ethylpyridinium-4-yl)porphyrin tetratosylate. *Photochem. Photobiol. Sci.* **2011**, *10*, 1046. [CrossRef] [PubMed]

30. Naumann, D. Infrared and NIR Raman Spectroscopy in Medical Microbiology. *Proc. SPIE* **1998**, *3257*. [CrossRef]

31. Dovbeshko, G.I.; Gridina, N.Y.; Kruglova, E.B.; Pashchuk, O.P. FTIR spectroscopy studies of nucleic acid damage. In *Talanta*; Elsevier: Amsterdam, The Netherlands, 2000; Volume 53, pp. 233–246.

32. Gasper, R.; Dewelle, J.; Kiss, R.; Mijatovic, T.; Goormaghtigh, E. IR spectroscopy as a new tool for evidencing antitumor drug signatures. *Biochim. Biophys. Acta Biomembr.* **2009**, *1788*, 1263–1270. [CrossRef] [PubMed]

33. Smith, B.C. *Infrared Spectral Interpretation: A Systematic Approach*; CRC Press: Boca Raton, FL, USA, 1999; ISBN 9780849324635.

34. Huffman, S.W.; Lukasiewicz, K.; Geldart, S.; Elliott, S.; Sperry, J.F.; Brown, C.W. Analysis of Microbial Components Using LC-IR. *Anal. Chem.* **2003**, *75*, 4606–4611. [CrossRef] [PubMed]

35. Salzer, R.; Siesler, H.W. *Infrared and Raman Spectroscopic Imaging*; Wiley-VCH: Weinheim, Germany, 2014; ISBN 3527336524.

36. Stuart, B. *Infrared Spectroscopy: Fundamentals and Applications*, 2nd ed.; John Wiley & Sons, Ltd.: Chichester, UK, 2004.

37. Kudva, I.T.; Jelacic, S.; Tarr, P.I.; Hovde, C.J.; Youderian, P. Biocontrol of Escherichia coli O157 with Biocontrol of Escherichia coli O157 with O157-Specific Bacteriophages. *Appl. Environ. Microbiol.* **1999**, *65*, 3767–3773. [PubMed]

38. Tomat, D.; Mercanti, D.; Balague, C.; Quiberoni, A. Phage biocontrol of enteropathogenic and shiga toxin-producing escherichia coli during milk fermentation. *Lett. Appl. Microbiol.* **2013**, *57*, 3–10. [CrossRef] [PubMed]

39. Park, S.; Nakai, T. Bacteriophage control of Pseudomonas plecoglossicida infection in ayu. *Dis. Aquat. Organ.* **2003**, *53*, 33–39. [CrossRef] [PubMed]

40. O'Flynn, G.; Coffey, A.; Fitzgerald, G.; Ross, R. The newly isolated lytic bacteriophages st104a and st104b are highly virulent against Salmonella enterica. *J. Appl. Microbiol.* **2006**, *101*, 251–259. [CrossRef] [PubMed]

41. Silva, Y.J.; Moreirinha, C.; Pereira, C.; Costa, L.; Rocha, R.J.M.; Cunha, Â.; Gomes, N.C.M.; Calado, R.; Almeida, A. Biological control of Aeromonas salmonicida infection in juvenile Senegalese sole (Solea senegalensis) with Phage AS-A. *Aquaculture* **2016**, *450*, 225–233. [CrossRef]

42. Filippov, A.A.; Sergueev, K.V.; He, Y.; Huang, X.-Z.; Gnade, B.T.; Mueller, A.J.; Fernandez-Prada, C.M.; Nikolich, M.P. Bacteriophage-resistant mutants in Yersinia pestis: Identification of phage receptors and attenuation for mice. *PLoS ONE* **2011**, *6*, e25486. [CrossRef] [PubMed]

43. Levin, B.R.; Bull, J.J. Population and evolutionary dynamics of phage therapy. *Nat. Rev. Microbiol.* **2004**, *2*, 166–173. [CrossRef] [PubMed]

44. Koskella, B.; Brockhurst, M.A. Bacteria-phage coevolution as a driver of ecological and evolutionary processes in microbial communities. *FEMS Microbiol. Rev.* **2014**, *38*, 916–931. [CrossRef] [PubMed]

45. Scanlan, P.D.; Buckling, A.; Hall, A.R. Experimental evolution and bacterial resistance: (Co)evolutionary costs and trade-offs as opportunities in phage therapy research. *Bacteriophage* **2015**, *5*, e1050153. [CrossRef] [PubMed]

46. Joly, N.; Schumacher, J.; Buck, M. Heterogeneous Nucleotide Occupancy Stimulates Functionality of Phage Shock Protein F, an AAA+ Transcriptional Activator. *J. Biol. Chem.* **2006**, *281*, 34997–35007. [CrossRef] [PubMed]

47. Lloyd, L.J.; Jones, S.E.; Jovanovic, G.; Gyaneshwar, P.; Rolfe, M.D.; Thompson, A.; Hinton, J.C.; Buck, M. Identification of a New Member of the Phage Shock Protein Response in Escherichia coli, the Phage Shock Protein G (PspG). *J. Biol. Chem.* **2004**, *279*, 55707–55714. [CrossRef] [PubMed]

48. Darwin, A.J. The phage-shock-protein response. *Mol. Microbiol.* **2005**, *57*, 621–628. [CrossRef] [PubMed]

49. Brissette, J.L.; Russel, M.; Weiner, L.; Model, P. Phage shock protein, a stress protein of Escherichia coli. *Proc. Natl. Acad. Sci. USA* **1990**, *87*, 862–866. [CrossRef] [PubMed]

50. Fröbel, J.; Rose, P.; Müller, M. Early Contacts between Substrate Proteins and TatA Translocase Component in Twin-arginine Translocation. *J. Biol. Chem.* **2011**, *286*, 43679–43689. [CrossRef] [PubMed]

51. Bageshwar, U.K.; VerPlank, L.; Baker, D.; Dong, W.; Hamsanathan, S.; Whitaker, N.; Sacchettini, J.C.; Musser, S.M. High Throughput Screen for Escherichia coli Twin Arginine Translocation (Tat) Inhibitors. *PLoS ONE* **2016**, *11*, e0149659. [CrossRef] [PubMed]

52. Friman, V.-P.; Hiltunen, T.; Jalasvuori, M.; Lindstedt, C.; Laanto, E.; Örmälä, A.-M.; Laakso, J.; Mappes, J.; Bamford, J.K.H. High Temperature and Bacteriophages Can Indirectly Select for Bacterial Pathogenicity in Environmental Reservoirs. *PLoS ONE* **2011**, *6*, e17651. [CrossRef] [PubMed]

53. Domingues, S.; Harms, K.; Fricke, W.F.; Johnsen, P.J.; da Silva, G.J.; Nielsen, K.M. Natural Transformation Facilitates Transfer of Transposons, Integrons and Gene Cassettes between Bacterial Species. *PLoS Pathog.* **2012**, *8*, e1002837. [CrossRef] [PubMed]

54. Schuster, C.F.; Mechler, L.; Nolle, N.; Krismer, B.; Zelder, M.-E.; Götz, F.; Bertram, R. The MazEF Toxin-Antitoxin System Alters the β-Lactam Susceptibility of Staphylococcus aureus. *PLoS ONE* **2015**, *10*, e0126118. [CrossRef] [PubMed]

55. Magnuson, R.D. Hypothetical functions of toxin-antitoxin systems. *J. Bacteriol.* **2007**, *189*, 6089–6092. [CrossRef] [PubMed]

56. Dy, R.L.; Przybilski, R.; Semeijn, K.; Salmond, G.P.C.; Fineran, P.C. A widespread bacteriophage abortive infection system functions through a Type IV toxin-antitoxin mechanism. *Nucleic Acids Res.* **2014**, *42*, 4590–4605. [CrossRef] [PubMed]

57. Mirzaei, K.M.; Nilsson, A.S. Isolation of Phages for Phage Therapy: A Comparison of Spot Tests and Efficiency of Plating Analyses for Determination of Host Range and Efficacy. *PLoS ONE* **2015**, *10*, e0118557. [CrossRef] [PubMed]

58. Abedon, S.T. Lysis from without. *Bacteriophage* **2011**, *1*, 46–49. [CrossRef] [PubMed]

59. Adams, M.H. *Bacteriophages*; John Wiley and Sons Inc.: New York, NY, USA, 1959.

60. Stuer-Lauridsen, B.; Janzen, T.; Schnabl, J.; Johansen, E. Identification of the host determinant of two prolate-headed phages infecting lactococcus lactis. *Virology* **2003**, *309*, 10–17. [CrossRef]

61. Laemli, U.K. Cleavage of Structural Proteins during the Assembly of the Head of Bacteriophage T4. *Nature* **1970**, *227*, 680–685. [CrossRef]

62. Neuhoff, V.; Arold, N.; Taube, D.; Ehrhardt, W. Improved staining of proteins in polyacrylamide gels including isoelectric focusing gels with clear background at nanogram sensitivity using Coomassie Brilliant Blue G-250 and R-250. *Electrophoresis* **1988**, *9*, 255–262. [CrossRef] [PubMed]

9

Identification of Essential Oils with Strong Activity against Stationary Phase *Borrelia burgdorferi*

Jie Feng [1], Wanliang Shi [1], Judith Miklossy [2], Genevieve M. Tauxe [1], Conor J. McMeniman [1] and Ying Zhang [1,*]

[1]   Department of Molecular Microbiology and Immunology, Bloomberg School of Public Health, Johns Hopkins University, Baltimore, MD 21205, USA; jfeng16@jhu.edu (J.F.); wshi3@jhu.edu (W.S.); gtauxe1@jhu.edu (G.M.T.); cmcmeni1@jhu.edu (C.J.M.)
[2]   International Alzheimer Research Centre, Prevention Alzheimer International Foundation, Martigny-Croix CP 16 1921, Switzerland; judithmiklossy@bluewin.ch
*   Correspondence: yzhang@jhsph.edu

Abstract: Lyme disease is the most common vector borne-disease in the United States (US). While the majority of the Lyme disease patients can be cured with 2–4 weeks antibiotic treatment, about 10–20% of patients continue to suffer from persisting symptoms. While the cause of this condition is unclear, persistent infection was proposed as one possibility. It has recently been shown that *B. burgdorferi* develops dormant persisters in stationary phase cultures that are not killed by the current Lyme antibiotics, and there is interest in identifying novel drug candidates that more effectively kill such forms. We previously identified some highly active essential oils with excellent activity against biofilm and stationary phase *B. burgdorferi*. Here, we screened another 35 essential oils and found 10 essential oils (*Allium sativum* L. bulbs, *Pimenta officinalis* Lindl. berries, *Cuminum cyminum* L. seeds, *Cymbopogon martini* var. *motia* Bruno grass, *Commiphora myrrha* (T. Nees) Engl. resin, *Hedychium spicatum* Buch.-Ham. ex Sm. flowers, *Amyris balsamifera* L. wood, *Thymus vulgaris* L. leaves, *Litsea cubeba* (Lour.) Pers. fruits, *Eucalyptus citriodora* Hook. leaves) and the active component of cinnamon bark cinnamaldehyde (CA) at a low concentration of 0.1% have strong activity against stationary phase *B. burgdorferi*. At a lower concentration of 0.05%, essential oils of *Allium sativum* L. bulbs, *Pimenta officinalis* Lindl. berries, *Cymbopogon martini* var. *motia* Bruno grass and CA still exhibited strong activity against the stationary phase *B. burgdorferi*. CA also showed strong activity against replicating *B. burgdorferi*, with a MIC of 0.02% (or 0.2 µg/mL). In subculture studies, the top five essential oil hits *Allium sativum* L. bulbs, *Pimenta officinalis* Lindl. berries, *Commiphora myrrha* (T. Nees) Engl. resin, *Hedychium spicatum* Buch.-Ham. ex Sm. flowers, and *Litsea cubeba* (Lour.) Pers. fruits completely eradicated all *B. burgdorferi* stationary phase cells at 0.1%, while *Cymbopogon martini* var. *motia* Bruno grass, *Eucalyptus citriodora* Hook. leaves, *Amyris balsamifera* L. wood, *Cuminum cyminum* L. seeds, and *Thymus vulgaris* L. leaves failed to do so as shown by visible spirochetal growth after 21-day subculture. At concentration of 0.05%, only *Allium sativum* L. bulbs essential oil and CA sterilized the *B. burgdorferi* stationary phase culture, as shown by no regrowth during subculture, while *Pimenta officinalis* Lindl. berries, *Commiphora myrrha* (T. Nees) Engl. resin, *Hedychium spicatum* Buch.-Ham. ex Sm. flowers and *Litsea cubeba* (Lour.) Pers. fruits essential oils all had visible growth during subculture. Future studies are needed to determine if these highly active essential oils could eradicate persistent *B. burgdorferi* infection in vivo.

Keywords: *Borrelia burgdorferi*; persisters; biofilm; antimicrobial activity; essential oils

1. Introduction

Lyme disease, which is caused by the spirochetal organism *Borrelia burgdorferi,* is the most common vector borne-disease in the United States (US) with about 300,000 cases a year [1]. While the majority of the Lyme disease patients can be cured with the standard 2–4 weeks antibiotic monotherapy with doxycycline or amoxicillin or cefuroxime [2], about 36% of patients continue to suffer from persisting symptoms of fatigue, joint, or musculoskeletal pain, and neuropsychiatric symptoms, even six months after taking the standard antibiotic therapy [3]. These latter patients suffer from a poorly understood condition, called post-treatment Lyme disease (PTLDS) syndrome. While the cause for PTLDS is unclear and is likely multifactorial, the following factors may be involved: autoimmunity [4], host response to dead debris of *Borrelia* organism [5], tissue damage caused during the infection, and persistent infection. There have been various anecdotal reports demonstrating persistence of the organism despite standard antibiotic treatment [6–8]. For example, culture of *B. burgdorferi* bacteria from patients despite treatment has been reported as infrequent case reports [9]. In addition, in animal studies with mice, dogs and monkeys, it has been shown that the current Lyme antibiotic treatment with doxycycline, cefuroxime, or ceftriaxone is unable to completely eradicate the *Borrelia* organism, as detected by xenodiagnosis and PCR [6–8,10], but viable organism cannot be cultured in the conventional sense as in other persistent bacterial infections, like tuberculosis after treatment [11,12].

Recently, it has been demonstrated that *B. burgdorferi* can form various dormant non-growing persisters in stationary phase cultures that are tolerant or not killed by the current antibiotics that are used to treat Lyme disease [13–16]. Thus, while the current Lyme antibiotics are good at killing the growing *B. burgdorferi* they have poor activity against the non-growing persisters enriched in stationary phase culture [14,16,17]. Therefore, there is interest to identify drugs that are more active against the *B. burgdorferi* persisters than the current Lyme antibiotics. We used the stationary phase culture of *B. burgdorferi* as a persister model and performed high throughput screens and identified a range of drug candidates such as daptomycin, clofazimine, sulfa drugs, daunomycin, etc., which have strong activity against *B. burgdorferi* persisters. These persister active drugs act differently from the current Lyme antibiotics, as they seem to preferentially target the membrane. We found that the variant persister forms such as round bodies, microcolonies, and biofilms with increasing degree of persistence in vitro, cannot be killed by the current Lyme antibiotics or even persister drugs like daptomycin alone, and that they can only be killed by a combination of drugs that kill persisters and drugs that kill the growing forms [14]. These observations provide a possible explanation in support of persistent infection despite antibiotic treatment in vivo.

Although daptomycin has good anti-persister activity, it is expensive and is an intravenous drug and difficult to administer and adopt in clinical setting and it has limited penetration through blood brain barrier (BBB). Thus, there is interest to identify alternative drug candidates with high anti-persister activity. We recently screened a panel of 34 essential oils and found the top three candidates oregano oil and its active component carvacrol, cinnamon bark, and clove bud as having even better anti-persister activity than daptomycin at 40 μM [18]. To identify more essential oils with strong activity against *B. burgdorferi* persisters, in this study, we screened an additional 35 different essential oils and found 10 essential oils (garlic, allspice, cumin, palmarosa, myrrh, hydacheim, amyris, thyme white, *Litsea cubeba*, lemon eucalyptus) and the active component of cinnamon bark cinnamaldehyde as having strong activity in the stationary phase *B. burgdorferi* persister model.

2. Materials and Methods

2.1. Organism and Culture Conditions

A low passaged strain *B. burgdorferi* B31 5A19 was kindly provided by Dr. Monica Embers [15]. Firstly, we prepared the *B. burgdorferi* B31 culture in BSK-H medium (HiMedia Laboratories, Mumbai, India), supplemented with 6% rabbit serum (Sigma-Aldrich, St. Louis, MO, USA) without antibiotics. After incubation for seven days in microaerophilic incubator (33 °C, 5% CO_2), the *B. burgdorferi* culture went into stationary phase ($\sim 10^7$ spirochetes/mL), followed by evaluating potential anti-persister activity of essential oils in a 96-well plate (see below).

2.2. Essential Oils and Drugs

We purchased a panel of essential oils (Plant Guru, Plainfield, NJ, USA) and cinnamaldehyde (CA) (Sigma-Aldrich, St. Louis, MO, USA). The essential oils from Plant Guru company are tested by third party laboratory using GC/MS, and the GC/MS report can be found on their website [19]. Dimethyl sulfoxide (DMSO)-soluble essential oils were prepared at 10% (v/v) in DMSO as stock solution, which was then added with seven-day old stationary phase cultures at ration of 1:50 to achieve 0.2% of essential oils in the mixture. The 0.2% essential oils were further diluted to the stationary phase culture to get the desired concentration for evaluating anti-borrelia activity. DMSO-insoluble essential oils were directly added to *B. burgdorferi* cultures, then vortexed to form aqueous suspension, followed by immediate transfer of essential oil aqueous suspension in serial dilutions to desired concentrations and then added to *B. burgdorferi* cultures. Doxycycline (Dox), cefuroxime (CefU), (Sigma-Aldrich, St. Louis, MO, USA), and daptomycin (Dap) (AK Scientific, Union City, CA, USA) were prepared at a concentration of 5 mg/mL in suitable solvents [20,21], then filter-sterilized by 0.2 μm filter and stored at $-20\,^{\circ}$C as stock solutions.

2.3. Microscopy

Treated *B. burgdorferi* cell suspensions were checked with BZ-X710 All-in-One fluorescence microscope (KEYENCE, Itasca, IL, USA). The bacterial viability was evaluated by SYBR Green I/PI assay, which was performed by calculating the ratio of green/red fluorescence after dying to determine the ratio of live and dead cells, as described previously [16,22]. The residual cell viability reading was obtained by analyzing three representative images of the same bacterial cell suspension taken by fluorescence microscopy. To quantitatively determine the bacterial viability from microscope images, software of BZ-X Analyzer and Image Pro-Plus were employed to evaluate fluorescence intensity, as we described previously [14].

2.4. Evaluation of Essential Oils for Their Activities Against B. Burgdorferi Stationary Phase Cultures

To evaluate the possible activity of the essential oils against stationary phase *B. burgdorferi*, 10% DMSO-soluble essential oils or aqueous suspension of DMSO-insoluble essential oils were added to 100 μL of the seven-day old stationary phase *B. burgdorferi* culture in 96-well plate to obtain the desired concentrations. In the primary screen, each essential oil was assayed with final concentrations of 0.2% and 0.1% (v/v) in 96-well plates. Drugs of daptomycin, doxycycline, and cefuroxime were used as control with final concentration of 40 μM. The active hits were checked further with lower concentrations of 0.1% and 0.05%; all of the tests mentioned above were run in triplicate. All of the plates were sealed and incubated at 33 $^{\circ}$C without shaking for seven days, and 5% CO_2 were maintained in the incubator.

2.5. Essential Oil and Drug Susceptibility Testing

The live and dead cells after seven-day treatment with essential oils or antibiotics were evaluated using the SYBR Green I/PI assay combined with fluorescence microscopy, as described [16,22]. Briefly, the ratio of live and dead cells was reflected by the ratio of green/red fluorescence, which was calculated through the regression equation and regression curve with least-square fitting analysis.

To determine the Minimum inhibitory concentration (MIC) of cinnamaldehyde on growth of *B. burgdorferi*, the standard microdilution method was used and the growth inhibition was assessed by microscopy. 10% cinnamaldehyde DMSO stock was added to *B. burgdorferi* cultures (1×10^4 spirochetes/mL) to get an initial suspension with 0.5% of cinnamaldehyde, and then a series of suspension was prepared by two-fold dilutions, with cinnamaldehyde concentrations ranging from 0.5% (=5 μg/mL) to 0.004% (=0.04 μg/mL). All of the experiments were carried out in triplicate.

The *B. burgdorferi* cultures after treatment in 96-well microplate were incubated at 33 °C for seven days. Cell proliferation was assessed by the SYBR Green I/PI assay combined with BZ-X710 All-in-One fluorescence microscope.

2.6. Subculture Studies to Assess Viability of Essential Oil-Treated B. Burgdorferi Organisms

Essential oils or control drugs were added into 1 mL of seven-day old *B. burgdorferi* stationary phase culture in 1.5 mL Eppendorf tubes, incubated for seven days at 33 °C without shaking. Next, cells were centrifuged and cell pellets were washed with fresh BSK-H medium (1 mL) followed by resuspension in 500 μL of the same medium without antibiotics. Then, 50 μL of cell suspension was inoculated into 1 mL of fresh BSK-H medium, incubated at 33 °C for 20 days for subculture. Cell growth was assessed using SYBR Green I/PI assay and fluorescence microscopy, as described above.

3. Results

3.1. Evaluating Activity of Essential Oils Against Stationary Phase B. Burgdorferi

In this study, we explored activity of another panel of 35 new essential oils together with control drugs against a seven-day old *B. burgdorferi* stationary phase culture in 96-well plates incubated for seven days. Our previous study discovered that cinnamon bark essential oil showed very strong activity against *B. burgdorferi* culture at stationary phase even at 0.05% concentration [18]. To identify the active components of cinnamon bark essential oil, we also added cinnamaldehyde (CA), the major ingredient of cinnamon bark, in this screen. Table 1 outlines the activity of the 35 essential oils and CA against *B. burgdorferi* culture at stationary phase. Although the *Litsea cubeba* essential oil showed too strong autofluorescence to determine its activity at 0.2% concentration, all the other essential oil candidates, except parsley seed, showed significantly stronger activity ($p < 0.05$) than the doxycycline control (Table 1) at 0.2% concentration with SYBR Green I/PI assay. Among them, 16 essential oils and CA at 0.2% concentration were found to have strong activity against *B. burgdorferi* culture at stationary phase as compared to the control antibiotics doxycycline, cefuroxime, and daptomycin (Table 1). As previously described [23], we calculated the ratio of residual live cells and dead cells of microscope images using Image Pro-Plus software, which could eliminate the autofluorescence of the background. Using fluorescence microscopy, we confirmed that, at 0.2% concentration, the 16 essential oils and CA could eradicate all live cells with only dead and aggregated cells left as shown in Table 1 and Figure 1. At concentration of 0.1%, 10 essential oils (garlic, allspice, cumin, palmarosa, myrrh, hydacheim, amyris, thyme white, *Litsea cubeba*, lemon eucalyptus), and CA still exhibited significant activity ($p < 0.05$) over the current clinically used doxycycline (Table 1; Figure 2). Among them, the most active essential oils were garlic, allspice, cumin, palmarosa, myrrh, and hydacheim because of their remarkable activity even at 0.1%, as shown by totally red (dead) cells with SYBR Green I/PI assay and fluorescence microscope tests (Figure 1). CA also showed very strong activity at 0.1% concentration. Although the plate reader data showed carrot seed and deep muscle essential oils had a significant activity ($p < 0.05$) compared with the doxycycline control, the microscope result did not confirm it due to high residual viability (60% and 68%, $p > 0.05$) (Table 1). For the other six essential oils (cornmint, fennel sweet, ho wood, birch, petitgrain, and head ease), which showed strong activity at 0.2% concentration, we did not find them to have higher activity than the doxycycline control at 0.1% concentration (Table 1, Figure 2). In addition, although essential oils of birch and *Litsea cubeba* have autofluorescence, which showed false high residual viability and interfered with the SYBR Green I/PI plate reader assay, they both exhibited strong activity against the stationary phase *B. burgdorferi*, as confirmed by SYBR Green I/PI fluorescence microscopy.

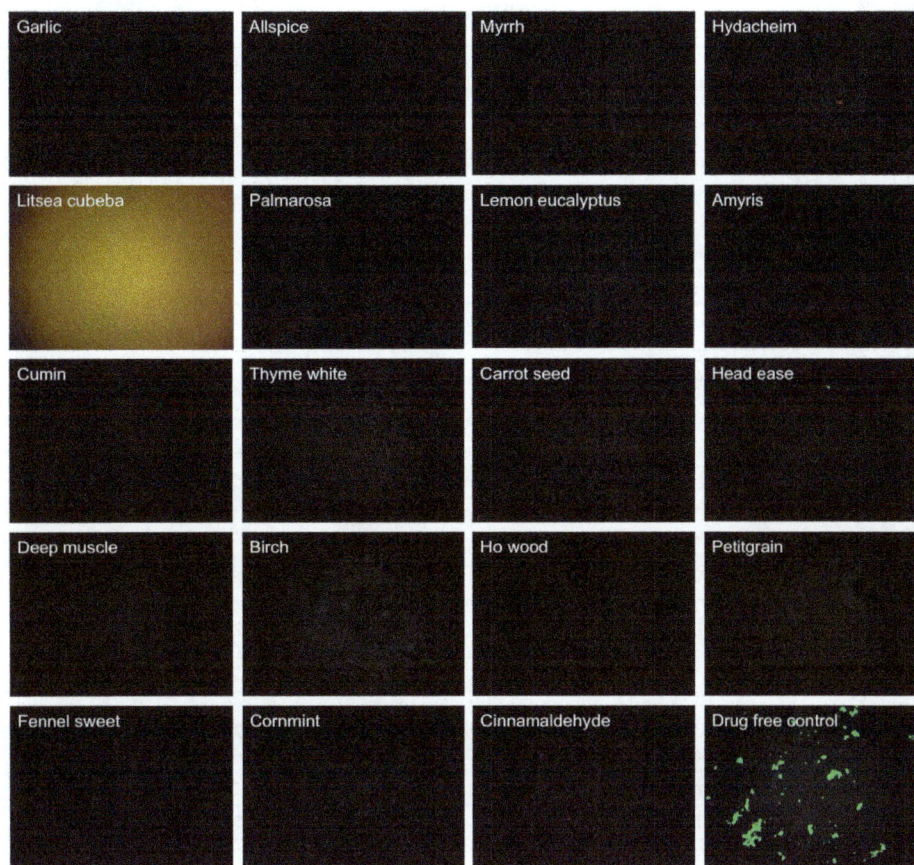

Figure 1. Effect of 0.2% essential oils on the viability of stationary phase *B. burgdorferi*. A 7-day old *B. burgdorferi* stationary phase culture was treated with 0.2% (*v/v*) essential oils for seven days followed by staining with SYBR Green I/PI viability assay and fluorescence microscopy.

Table 1. Effect of essential oils on a seven-day old stationary phase *B. burgdorferi* [a].

Essential Oils and Control Drugs	Plant and Extracted Part	Residual Viability (%) after 0.2% EO or 40 µM Antibiotic Treatment			Residual Viability (%) after 0.1% EO Treatment		
		Plate Reader [b]	Microscope [c]	*p*-Value [e]	Plate Reader [b]	Microscope [c]	*p*-Value [e]
Doxycycline	–	73 ± 4	66 ± 2	1.000	–	–	–
Cefuroxime	–	58 ± 3	55 ± 3	0.0016	–	–	–
Daptomycin	–	28 ± 5	21 ± 1	0.0004	–	–	–
Cinnamaldehyde	–	26 ± 5	0	0.0002	54 ± 2	28	0.0016
Garlic	*Allium sativum* L. (syn. *Porrum sativum* (L.) Rchb.), bulbs	25 ± 4	0	0.0001	24 ± 6	18 ± 2	0.0002
Allspice	*Pimenta officinalis* Lindl., berries	21 ± 4	0	0.0001	30 ± 6	25 ± 3	0.0005
Myrrh	*Commiphora myrrha* (T. Nees) Engl. (syn. *Balsamea myrrha* (T. Nees) Oken), resin	32 ± 3	0	0.0001	35 ± 6	25 ± 2	0.0009
Hydacheim	*Hedychium spicatum* Thymus (syn. *Gandasulium spicatum* (Buch.-Ham. ex Sm.) Kuntze), flowers	34 ± 4	23 ± 2	0.0002	38 ± 7	26 ± 1	0.0017
Litsea cubeba	*Litsea cubeba* (Lour.) Pers. (syn. *Benzoin cubeba* (Lour.) Hatus., *Persea cubeba* (Lour.) Spreng.), fruits	98 ± 4	ND [d]	–	77 ± 4	27 ± 3	(0.00004)

Table 1. *Cont.*

Essential Oils and Control Drugs	Plant and Extracted Part	Residual Viability (%) after 0.2% EO or 40 µM Antibiotic Treatment			Residual Viability (%) after 0.1% EO Treatment		
		Plate Reader [b]	Microscope [c]	*p*-Value [e]	Plate Reader [b]	Microscope [c]	*p*-Value [e]
Palmarosa	*Cymbopogon martini* var. *motia* Bruno, grass	26 ± 5	0	0.0002	35 ± 5	29 ± 2	0.0004
Lemon eucalyptus	*Eucalyptus citriodora* Hook. (syn. *Corymbia citriodora* (Hook.) K.D. Hill & L.A.S. Johnson), leaves	35 ± 6	0	0.0006	39 ± 7	29 ± 4	0.0015
Amyris	*Amyris balsamifera* L. (syn. *Elemifera balsamifera* (L.) Kuntze), wood	32 ± 3	4 ± 2	0.0001	38 ± 5	29 ± 3	0.0006
Cumin	*Cuminum cyminum* L., seeds	31 ± 3	0	0.0001	31 ± 6	30 ± 1	0.0005
Thyme white	*Thymus vulgaris* L. (syn. *Origanum thymus* (L.) Kuntze), leaves	37 ± 2	26 ± 2	0.0001	36 ± 1	30 ± 2	0.0001
Carrot seed	*Daucus carota* L., seeds	38 ± 4	5 ± 3	0.0004	40 ± 3	60 ± 2	0.0003 (0.0705)
Head ease	Synergy blend	41 ± 3	25 ± 3	0.0003	74 ± 4	65 ± 1	0.8008
Deep muscle	Synergy blend	42 ± 4	3 ± 2	0.0004	56 ± 4	68 ± 4	0.0060 (0.3911)
Birch	*Betula lenta* L., bark	86 ± 5	22 ± 2	(0.00001)	91 ± 4	69 ± 2	–
Ho wood	*Cinnamomum camphora* (L.) J. Presl (syn. *Cinnamomum camphora* (L.) Nees & Eberm., *Cinnamomum camphora* (L.) Siebold), twigs and bark	36 ± 4	3 ± 2	0.0004	69 ± 5	70 ± 3	0.3078
Petitgrain	*Citrus aurantium* L, trees and leaves	38 ± 3	19 ± 2	0.0002	71 ± 4	70 ± 3	0.4743
Fennel sweet	*Foeniculum vulgare* Mill., seeds	40 ± 5	2 ± 1	0.0006	72 ± 3	75 ± 4	0.6235
Cornmint	*Mentha arvensis*, leaf	35 ± 5	0	0.0004	68 ± 4	85 ± 1	0.1359
Citrus blast	Synergy blend	51 ± 5	>70	0.0039	71 ± 5	>70	0.5865
Nutmeg	*Myristica fragrans* Houtt., seeds	43 ± 4	>70	0.0008	71 ± 4	>70	0.6533
Alive	Synergy blend	40 ± 4	>70	0.0004	71 ± 3	>70	0.5228
New beginning	Synergy blend	48 ± 4	>70	0.0013	75 ± 4	>70	0.5107
Happy	Synergy blend	47 ± 4	>70	0.0009	78 ± 2	>70	–
Meditation	Synergy blend	55 ± 4	>70	0.0041	79 ± 4	>70	–
Deep forest	Synergy blend	61 ± 1	>70	0.0039	79 ± 3	>70	–
Copaiba	*Copaifera officinalis* (Jacq.) L., balsm	51 ± 2	>70	0.0007	79 ± 2	>70	–
Balsam fir	*Abies balsamea* (L.) Mill. (syn. *Peuce balsamea* (L.) Rich.), needles	57 ± 5	>70	0.0124	80 ± 1	>70	–
Juniper Berry	*Juniperus communis* L., berries	56 ± 5	>70	0.0086	82 ± 3	>70	–
Camphor	*Cinnamomum camphora* (L.) J. Presl (syn. *Cinnamomum camphora* (L.) Nees & Eberm., *Cinnamomum camphora* (L.) Siebold), wood	58 ± 3	>70	0.0047	82 ± 3	>70	–
Vetiver	*Vetiveria zizanioides* (L.) Nash (syn. *Phalaris zizanioides* L.), root	41 ± 3	>70	0.0003	82 ± 5	>70	–
Fir needle	*Abies sibirica* Ledeb. (syn. *Pinus sibirica* (Ledeb.) Turcz.), needles	60 ± 3	>70	0.0109	83 ± 5	>70	–
Sleep tight	Synergy blend	57 ± 5	>70	0.0130	85 ± 6	>70	–
Turmeric	*Curcuma longa* L. (syn. *Kua domestica* (L.) Medik.), root	50 ± 2	>70	0.0007	93 ± 3	>70	–
Elemi	*Canarium luzonicum* (Blume) A. Gray (syn. *Pimela luzonica* Blume), resin	58 ± 3	>70	0.0059	95 ± 2	>70	–
Parsley seed	*Petroselinum sativum* Hoffm., seeds	64 ± 5	>70	0.0645	97 ± 3	>70	–

[a] A seven-day old *B. burgdorferi* stationary phase culture was treated with essential oils or control drugs for 7 days. Bold type indicates the essential oils that had better or similar activity compared with 40 µM daptomycin used as the positive persister-drug control. [b] Residual viable (mean ± SD) *B. burgdorferi* was calculated according to the regression equation and ratios of Green/Red fluorescence obtained by SYBR Green I/PI assay [22]. [c] Residual viability (mean ± SD) calculated by fluorescence microscope measurements. [d] Autofluorescence of essential oil is too strong to be observed under fluorescence microscope. [e] *p*-value of the standard *t*-test for the 0.1% essential oil treated group versus doxycycline treated control group was calculated by data of the plate reader or microscope test (shown in the brackets). The essential oil groups with higher residual viability than control group were not included in the standard *t*-test.

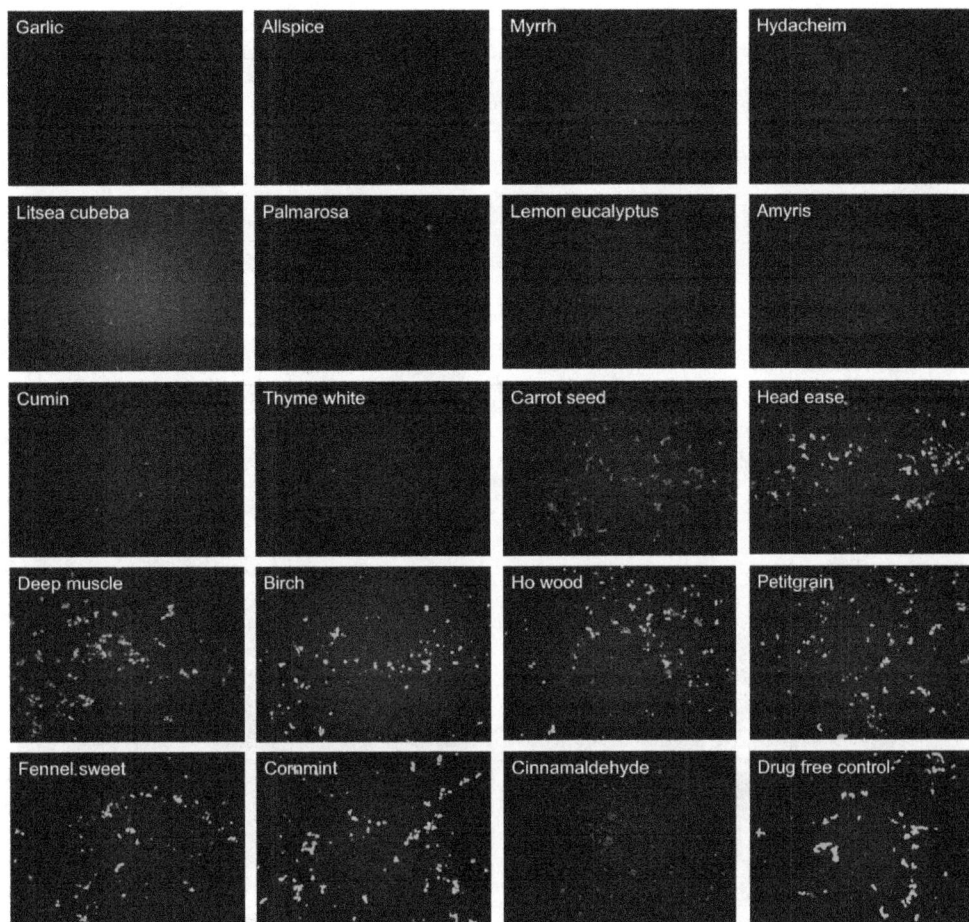

Figure 2. Effect of 0.1% essential oils on the viability of stationary phase *B. burgdorferi*. A seven-day old *B. burgdorferi* stationary phase culture was treated with 0.1% (*v/v*) essential oils for seven days followed by staining with SYBR Green I/PI viability assay and fluorescence microscopy.

The top 10 essential oils and CA (residual viability lower 60%) were chosen to evaluate their activities and explore their potential to eradicate *B. burgdorferi* cultures at stationary phase that harbor large numbers of persisters using lower essential oil concentrations (0.1% and 0.05%). We did the confirmation tests with 1 mL stationary phase *B. burgdorferi* in 1.5 mL Eppendorf tubes. At 0.1% concentration, the tube tests confirmed the active hits from the previous 96-well plate screen, although the activity of all essential oils decreased slightly in the tube tests when compared to the 96-well plate tests (Table 2, Figure 3). At a very low concentration of 0.05%, we noticed that garlic, allspice, palmarosa, and CA still exhibited strong activity against the stationary phase *B. burgdorferi*, approved by few residual green aggregated cells shown in Table 2 and Figure 3. Meanwhile, we also found CA showed strong activity against replicating *B. burgdorferi*, with an MIC of 0.02% (equal to 0.2 µg/mL).

Table 2. Comparison of top 10 essential oil activities against stationary phase *B. burgdorferi* with 0.1% and 0.05% (*v/v*) treatment and subculture [a].

Essential Oil Treatment	Residual Viability after 0.1% Essential Oil Treatment		Residual Viability after 0.05% Essential Oil Treatment	
	Treatment [b]	Subculture [c]	Treatment [b]	Subculture [c]
Drug free control	93%	+	93%	+
Daptomycin+Doxycycline+Cefuroxime [d]	18%[d]	− [d]	N/A	N/A
Garlic	30%	−	33%	−
Allspice	34%	−	48%	+
Myrrh	42%	−	41%	+

Table 2. *Cont.*

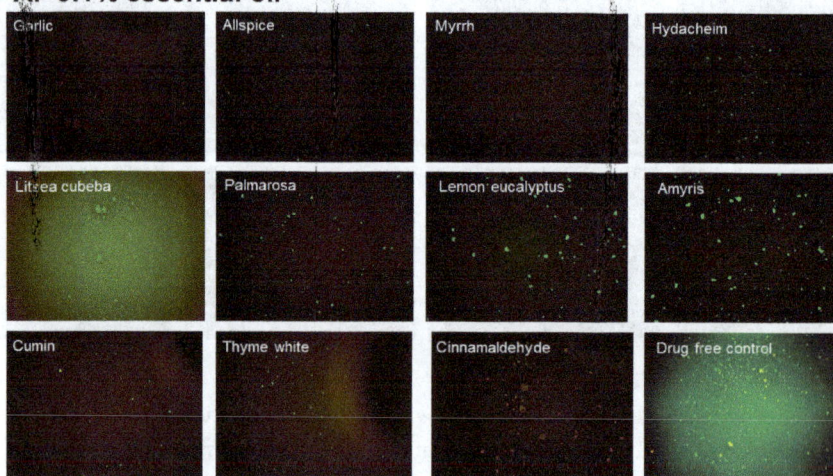

Essential Oil Treatment	Residual Viability after 0.1% Essential Oil Treatment		Residual Viability after 0.05% Essential Oil Treatment	
	Treatment [b]	Subculture [c]	Treatment [b]	Subculture [c]
Hydacheim	44%	−	61%	+
Litsea cubeba	68%	−	69%	+
Palmarosa	39%	+	67%	+
Lemon eucalyptus	46%	+	79%	+
Amyris	48%	+	71%	+
Cumin	42%	+	60%	+
Thyme white	40%	+	76%	+
Cinnamaldehyde	34%	−	56%	−

[a] A 7-day old stationary phase *B. burgdorferi* was treated with 0.05% or 0.1% essential oils for seven days when the viability of the residual organisms was assessed by subculture. [b] Residual viable percentage of *B. burgdorferi* was calculated according to the regression equation and ratio of Green/Red fluorescence obtained by SYBR Green I/PI assay as described [22]. Viabilities are the average of three replicates. [c] "+" indicates growth in subculture; "−" indicates no growth in subculture. [d] Activity was tested with 5 µg/mL of each antibiotic in combination.

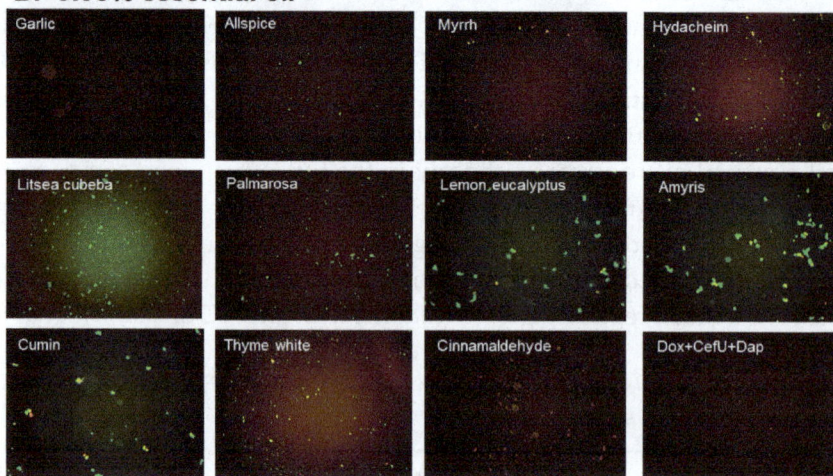

Figure 3. Effect of active essential oils on stationary phase *B. burgdorferi*. A 1 mL *B. burgdorferi* stationary phase culture (seven-day old) was treated with 0.1% (**A**) or 0.05% (**B**) essential oils (labeled on the image) in 1.5 mL Eppendorf tubes for 7 days followed by staining with SYBR Green I/PI viability assay and fluorescence microscopy.

3.2. Subculture Studies to Evaluate the Activity of Essential Oils Against Stationary Phase B. burgdorferi

To validate the capability of the essential oils in eradicating *B. burgdorferi* cells at stationary phase, we performed subculture studies by incubating essential oils treated cells in fresh BSK medium after the removal of the drugs with washing, as previously described [14]. We picked the top 10 active essential oils (garlic, allspice, myrrh, hydacheim, *Litsea cubeba*, palmarosa, lemon eucalyptus, amyris, cumin, and thyme white) to further confirm whether they could eradicate the stationary phase *B. burgdorferi* cells at 0.1% or 0.05% concentration by subculture experiments after the essential oil exposure (Table 2). At 0.1% concentration, we did not find any regrowth in samples of the top five hits, including garlic, allspice, myrrh, hydacheim, and *Litsea cubeba* (Table 2, Figure 4A). However, palmarosa, lemon eucalyptus, amyris, cumin and thyme white could not eradicate *B. burgdorferi* cells at stationary phase as many spirochetes were still visible after 21 days' subculture (Figure 4A). The subculture study also confirmed the strong activity of CA by showing no growth of spirochete after treatment with 0.1% CA. At concentration of 0.05%, we did not observe spirochetal regrowth in the garlic essential oil treated samples that were subcultured for 21 days (Figure 4B), which indicates that garlic essential oil could completely kill all *B. burgdorferi* forms even at 0.05% concentration. On the other hand, the other four active essential oils (allspice, myrrh, hydacheim and *Litsea cubeba*) at a concentration of 0.05% could not sterilize the *B. burgdorferi* culture at stationary phase, since spirochetes were visible after 21 days subculture (Figure 4B). Similar to the previous subculture result of cinnamon bark essential oil [18], 0.05% cinnamaldehyde sterilized the *B. burgdorferi* stationary phase culture as shown by no regrowth after 21 days subculture (Figure 4B), indicating that the active component of cinnamon bark essential oil is attributable to cinnamaldehyde.

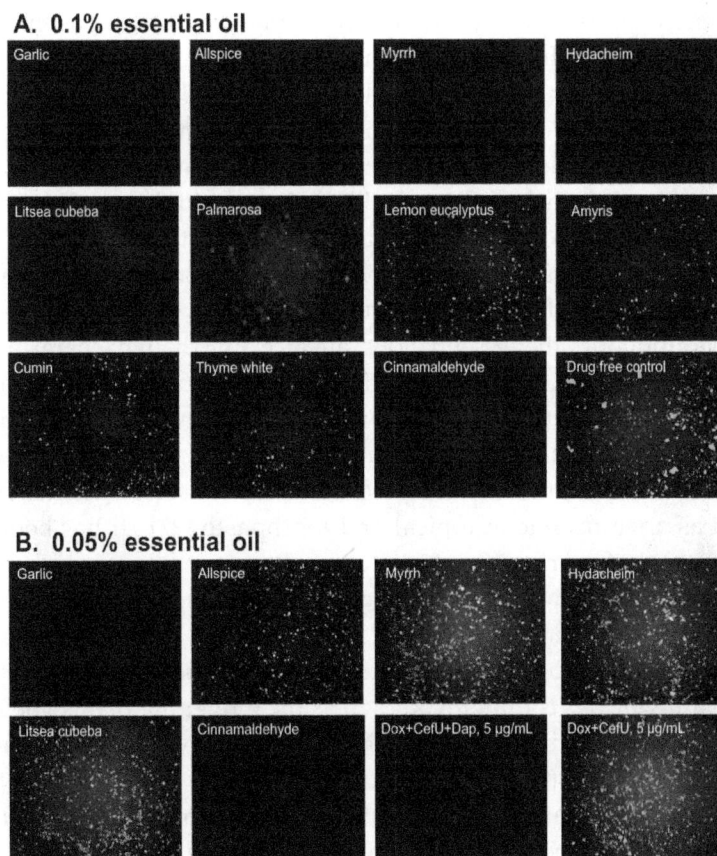

Figure 4. Subculture of *B. burgdorferi* after treatment with essential oils. A *B. burgdorferi* stationary phase culture (seven-day old) was treated with the indicated essential oils at 0.1% (**A**) or 0.05% (**B**) for seven days followed by washing and resuspension in fresh BSK-H medium and subculture for 21 days. The viability of the subculture was examined by SYBR Green I/PI stain and fluorescence microscopy.

4. Discussion

We recently found that many essential oils have better activity against *B. burgdorferi* cells at stationary phase than the current clinically used antibiotics for treating Lyme disease [18]. Here, we screened another panel of 35 new essential oils using *B. burgdorferi* culture at stationary phase as a persister model [16]. Previously, we found that 23 essential oils had strong activity at 1% concentration, but only five of them showed good activity at a lower concentration of 0.25% [18]. To identify the essential oils that have activity against *B. burgdorferi* persisters at low concentrations, we performed the screen at 0.2% and 0.1% concentrations in this study. Some essential oils, such as *Litsea cubeba* oil, showed high autofluorescence after SYBR Green I/PI stain, which significantly interfered with the SYBR Green I/PI assay (Table 1, Figure 1). However, using lower concentration (0.1%) and fluorescence microscopy, we were able to verify the results from the SYBR Green I/PI assay and eliminate the problem of autofluorescence with some essential oils. Another limitation of the SYBR Green/PI assay is that not all cells turning red are dead, and further subculture studies are needed to verify whether the PI- stained red cells are indeed dead after drug exposure. In this study, we identified 18 essential oils (at 0.2% concentration) that are more active than 40 µM daptomycin (a persister drug control that could eradicate *B. burgdorferi* stationary phase cells), from which 10 essential oils stand out as having a remarkable activity even at 0.1% concentration (Table 1). Among them, garlic essential oil exhibited the best activity as shown by the lowest residual viability of *B. burgdorferi* at 0.1%. In the subsequent comparison studies, the garlic essential oil highlighted itself as showing a sterilizing activity even at a lower concentration of 0.05%, because no *Borrelia* cells grew up in the subculture study (Table 2). Garlic as a common spice has been used throughout history as an antimicrobial, and a variety of garlic supplements have been commercialized as tablets and capsules. The antibacterial activity of garlic was described by ancient Chinese, and in more recent times, by Louis Pasteur in 1858. Although allicin, an antibacterial compound from garlic, is shown to have antibacterial activity against multiple bacterial species [24,25], it has not been well studied on *B. burgdorferi*, especially the non-growing stationary phase organism, despite its anecdotal clinical use by some patients with Lyme disease (http://www.natural-homeremedies.com/blog/best-home-remedies-for-lyme-disease/; http://lymebook.com/blog/supplements/garlic-allimax-allimed-alli-c-allicin/). In this study, garlic essential oil was identified as the most potent candidate having activity against stationary phase *B. burgdorferi*, and its activity is equivalent to that of oregano and cinnamon bark essential oils, the two most active essential oils against *B. burgdorferi* we identified in our previous study [18].

Additionally, we found four other essential oils, allspice, myrrh, hydacheim, and *Litsea cubeba* that showed excellent activity against *B. burgdorferi* at the stationary phase, though the extracts or essential oils of these four plants were reported to possess antibacterial activity on other bacteria. Allspice is a commonly used flavoring agent in food processing and is known to have antibacterial activities on many organisms [26]. Myrrh as a traditional medicine has been used since ancient times. In modern times, myrrh is used as an antiseptic in topical and toothpaste [27]. It has been shown that some sesquiterpene components of myrrh, including furanodien-6-one, methoxyfuranoguai-9-en-8-one possess in vitro bactericidal, and fungicidal activity against multiple pathogenic bacteria, including *E. coli*, *S. aureus*, *P. aeruginosa*, and *C. albicans* [28], but these two most active compounds were not detected in our samples [19] (Table 3). Hydacheim essential oil is extracted from the flower of *Hedychium spicatum* plant which is commonly known as the ginger lily plant. The methanol extract of *H. spicatum* is reported to have antimicrobial activity against many bacteria, including *Shigella boydii*, *E. coli*, *S. aureus*, *P. aeruginosa*, and *K. pneumoniae* [29]. *Litsea cubeba* is also used in traditional Chinese medicine for a long time. Its essential oils from stem, alabastrum, leaf, flower, root, fruit parts are also reported to exhibit antibacterial activity on *B. subtilis*, *E. coli*, *E. faecalis*, *S. aureus*, *P. aeruginosa*, and *M. albicans* [30]. Based on these studies and application of allspice, myrrh, hydacheim, and *Litsea cubeba*, it would be of interest to develop effective regimens to fight against Lyme disease in the future.

Table 3. The top five major compositions of the three most active essential oils.

Essential Oil	Components	Content [a]
Garlic *Allium sativum* bulbs	Diallyl disulfide	19%
	(E)-1-Allyl-2-(prop-1-en-1-yl) disulfane	15%
	Disulfide, methyl 2-propenyl	6%
	2-Vinyl-4H-1,3-dithiine	6%
	(E)-methyl 1-propenyl sulfide	4%
Allspice *Pimenta officinalis* berries	Eugenol	82%
	β-Caryophyllene	6%
	Methyleugenol	5%
	α-Humulene	1%
	α-Selinene	0.47%
Myrrh *Commiphora myrrha* resin	Curzerene	38%
	Furanoeudesma-1,3-diene	24%
	β-Elemene	7%
	Lindestrene	7%
	E-Elemene	3%

[a] The content of components were calculated according to the GC-MS analysis in our lab (Garlic essential oil) and PhytoChemia Laboratories reports on Plant Guru company website (Allspice and Myrrh) [19].

Although the active essential oils we identified have strong activity against stationary phase cells of *B. burgdorferi* in vitro, their activity in vivo is unknown at this time. In future studies, we will use GC-Mass Spectrometry to identify the active ingredients of the active essential oils and confirm their activity against growing and non-growing *B. burgdorferi*. Once we identify the active components of active essential oils drug combination studies can be performed to enhance activity against persister bacteria. In addition, we will study the mechanism of action of the active compounds in the near future. The pharmacokinetic (PK) profile of the active compounds in these active essential oils will be assessed and their effective dosage and toxicity will be determined in vivo. In our previous study, we found that the cinnamon bark essential oil showed excellent activity against stationary phase *B. burgdorferi* [18], here we found CA is an active component of cinnamon bark essential oil. CA could eradicate the stationary phase *B. burgdorferi* at 0.05% concentration as no regrowth occurred in subculture (Table 2). This indicates that CA possess similar activity against stationary phase *B. burgdorferi* as carvacrol, which is the one of the most active compounds against non-growing *B. burgdorferi* we identified from natural products [18]. Furthermore, CA is observed to be very active against growing *B. burgdorferi* cells with an MIC of 0.2 μg/mL. The antibacterial activity of CA was also reported on some other bacteria. The mechanism of the antibacterial activity of CA has been studied on different microorganisms, which suggests that its antibacterial action is mainly through interaction with the cell membrane [31]. CA as a common favoring agent in food processing is also used as food preservative to protect animal feeds and human food from pathogenic bacteria [31]. CA is considered as a safe compound for mammals, as the median lethal dose LD_{50} of CA is 1850 ± 37 mg/kg by oral administration in the acute toxicity study with oral administration rat model [32]. These findings suggest that CA could be a good drug candidate for further evaluation against *B. burgdorferi* in future studies. We also want to point out that the safety of using essential oils and their components needs more thorough research; for example, the intravenous toxicity of carvacrol is considerably higher than oral toxicity [33]. Thus, appropriate animal studies are necessary to confirm the safety and activity of CA and other active essential oils in animal models before human studies.

This study used *B. burgdorferi* stationary phase cultures enriched in persisters as a persister model for essential oil screens. The reason we used this model is that studies with tuberculosis persister drug pyrazinamide (PZA), which is more active against stationary phase cells and persisters than against log phase growing cells and shortens the therapy [34,35], suggest that drugs active against stationary phase cells/persisters will be more effective at curing persistent infections than drugs active against growing cultures. This has been shown in the case of colistin as a persister drug for *E. coli* when being used together with quinolone or nitrofuran could more effectively eradicate urinary tract infection in mice [36]. Future studies are needed to determine if the essential oils active against non-growing stationary phase *B. burgdorferi* cultures enriched in persisters are more effective in eradicating persistent *B. burgdorferi* infections in animal models than the current Lyme antibiotics which are mainly active against growing *Borrelia*.

5. Conclusions

In summary, we identified some additional essential oils that have strong activity against stationary-phase cells of *B. burgdorferi*. The most active essential oils include garlic, allspice, myrrh, hydacheim, and *Litsea cubeba*. Among them, garlic oil could completely eradicate stationary phase *B. burgdorferi* with no regrowth at 0.05%, and the others could reach the same activity at 0.1%. Additionally, cinnamaldehyde is identified to be an active ingredient of cinnamon bark oil with very strong activity against *B. burgdorferi* stationary phase cells. Future studies will be carried out to identify the active components in the candidate essential oils, and to determine their in vitro activity alone or in combination with other active essential oils or antibiotics against *B. burgdorferi* sensu lato strains, including *B. burgdorferi*, *B. garinii* and *B. afzelii*, and assess their safety and efficacy against *B. burgdorferi* in animal models before human trials.

Author Contributions: Conceptualization, Y.Z. and J.M.; Methodology, J.F., W.S., G.M.T. and C.J.M.; Validation, J.F., W.S., G.M.T. and C.J.M.; Formal Analysis, J.F. and W.S.; Writing-Original Draft Preparation, J.F. and Y.Z.; Writing-Review & Editing, Y.Z., J.M.; Supervision, Y.Z.; Funding Acquisition, Y.Z.

Funding: This research was funded in part by Global Lyme Alliance, LivLyme Foundation, NatCapLyme, and the Einstein-Sim Family Charitable Fund.

Acknowledgments: We acknowledge the support by Global Lyme Alliance, LivLyme Foundation, NatCapLyme, and the Einstein-Sim Family Charitable Fund.

References

1.   CDC. Lyme Disease. Available online: http://www.cdc.gov/lyme/ (accessed on 7 March 2018).
2.   Wormser, G.P.; Dattwyler, R.J.; Shapiro, E.D.; Halperin, J.J.; Steere, A.C.; Klempner, M.S.; Krause, P.J.; Bakken, J.S.; Strle, F.; Stanek, G.; et al. The clinical assessment, treatment, and prevention of lyme disease, human granulocytic anaplasmosis, and babesiosis: Clinical practice guidelines by the infectious diseases society of America. *Clin. Infect. Dis.* **2006**, *43*, 1089–1134. [CrossRef] [PubMed]
3.   Aucott, J.N.; Rebman, A.W.; Crowder, L.A.; Kortte, K.B. Post-treatment Lyme disease syndrome symptomatology and the impact on life functioning: Is there something there? *Qual. Life Res.* **2013**, *22*, 75. [CrossRef] [PubMed]
4.   Steere, A.C.; Gross, D.; Meyer, A.L.; Huber, B.T. Autoimmune mechanisms in antibiotic treatment-resistant Lyme arthritis. *J. Autoimmun.* **2001**, *16*, 263–268. [CrossRef] [PubMed]
5.   Bockenstedt, L.K.; Gonzalez, D.G.; Haberman, A.M.; Belperron, A.A. Spirochete antigens persist near cartilage after murine Lyme borreliosis therapy. *J. Clin. Investig.* **2012**, *122*, 2652–2660. [CrossRef] [PubMed]
6.   Hodzic, E.; Imai, D.; Feng, S.; Barthold, S.W. Resurgence of Persisting Non-Cultivable *Borrelia burgdorferi* following Antibiotic Treatment in Mice. *PLoS ONE* **2014**, *9*, e86907. [CrossRef] [PubMed]
7.   Embers, M.E.; Barthold, S.W.; Borda, J.T.; Bowers, L.; Doyle, L.; Hodzic, E.; Jacobs, M.B.; Hasenkampf, N.R.; Martin, D.S.; Narasimhan, S.; et al. Persistence of *Borrelia burgdorferi* in rhesus macaques following antibiotic treatment of disseminated infection. *PLoS ONE* **2012**, *7*, e29914. [CrossRef]
8.   Hodzic, E.; Feng, S.; Holden, K.; Freet, K.J.; Barthold, S.W. Persistence of *Borrelia burgdorferi* following antibiotic treatment in mice. *Antimicrob. Agents Chemother.* **2008**, *52*, 1728–1736. [CrossRef] [PubMed]
9.   Marques, A.; Telford, S.R., 3rd; Turk, S.P.; Chung, E.; Williams, C.; Dardick, K.; Krause, P.J.; Brandeburg, C.; Crowder, C.D.; Carolan, H.E.; et al. Xenodiagnosis to detect *Borrelia burgdorferi* infection: A first-in-human study. *Clin. Infect. Dis.* **2014**, *58*, 937–945. [CrossRef] [PubMed]
10. Straubinger, R.K.; Summers, B.A.; Chang, Y.F.; Appel, M.J. Persistence of *Borrelia burgdorferi* in experimentally infected dogs after antibiotic treatment. *J. Clin. Microbiol.* **1997**, *35*, 111–116. [PubMed]

11. Zhang, Y. Persistent and dormant tubercle bacilli and latent tuberculosis. *Front. Biosci.* **2004**, *9*, 1136–1156. [CrossRef] [PubMed]

12. Zhang, Y.; Yew, W.W.; Barer, M.R. Targeting persisters for tuberculosis control. *Antimicrob. Agents Chemother.* **2012**, *56*, 2223–2230. [CrossRef] [PubMed]

13. Sharma, B.; Brown, A.V.; Matluck, N.E.; Hu, L.T.; Lewis, K. *Borrelia burgdorferi*, the causative agent of Lyme disease, forms drug-tolerant persister cells. *Antimicrob. Agents Chemother.* **2015**, *59*, 4616–4624. [CrossRef] [PubMed]

14. Feng, J.; Auwaerter, P.G.; Zhang, Y. Drug Combinations against *Borrelia burgdorferi* persisters in vitro: Eradication achieved by using daptomycin, cefoperazone and doxycycline. *PLoS ONE* **2015**, *10*, e0117207. [CrossRef] [PubMed]

15. Caskey, J.R.; Embers, M.E. Persister development by *Borrelia burgdorferi* populations in vitro. *Antimicrob. Agents Chemother.* **2015**, *59*, 6288–6295. [CrossRef] [PubMed]

16. Feng, J.; Wang, T.; Shi, W.; Zhang, S.; Sullivan, D.; Auwaerter, P.G.; Zhang, Y. Identification of novel activity against *Borrelia burgdorferi* persisters using an FDA approved drug library. *Emerg. Microbes Infect.* **2014**, *3*, e49. [CrossRef] [PubMed]

17. Feng, J.; Zhang, S.; Shi, W.; Zhang, Y. Ceftriaxone pulse dosing fails to eradicate biofilm-like microcolony *B. burgdorferi* persisters which are sterilized by daptomycin/doxycycline/cefuroxime without pulse dosing. *Front. Microbiol.* **2016**, *7*, 1744. [CrossRef] [PubMed]

18. Feng, J.; Zhang, S.; Shi, W.; Zubcevik, N.; Miklossy, J.; Zhang, Y. Selective Essential oils from spice or culinary herbs have high activity against stationary phase and biofilm *Borrelia burgdorferi*. *Front. Med.* **2017**, *4*, 169. [CrossRef] [PubMed]

19. GC/MS TESTING. Available online: https://www.theplantguru.com/gc-ms-testing (accessed on 13 September 2018).

20. Wikler, M.A.; National Committee for Clinical Laboratory. *Performance Standards for Antimicrobial Susceptibility Testing: Fifteenth Informational Supplement*; Clinical and Laboratory Standards Institute: Wayne, PA, USA, 2005.

21. The United States Pharmacopeial Convention. *The United States Pharmacopeia*, 24th ed.; The United States Pharmacopeial Convention: Philadelphia, PA, USA, 2000.

22. Feng, J.; Wang, T.; Zhang, S.; Shi, W.; Zhang, Y. An Optimized SYBR Green I/PI Assay for Rapid Viability Assessment and Antibiotic Susceptibility Testing for *Borrelia burgdorferi*. *PLoS ONE* **2014**, *9*, e111809. [CrossRef] [PubMed]

23. Feng, J.; Shi, W.; Zhang, S.; Zhang, Y. Identification of new compounds with high activity against stationary phase *Borrelia burgdorferi* from the NCI compound collection. *Emerg. Microbes Infect.* **2015**, *4*, e31. [CrossRef] [PubMed]

24. Lawson, L.D. Garlic: A Review of Its Medicinal Effects and Indicated Active Compounds. In *Phytomedicines of Europe*; American Chemical Society: Washington, DC, USA, 1998; pp. 176–209.

25. Petrovska, B.B.; Cekovska, S. Extracts from the history and medical properties of garlic. *Pharmacogn. Rev.* **2010**, *4*, 106–110. [CrossRef] [PubMed]

26. Shelef, L.A.; Naglik, O.A.; Bogen, D.W. Sensitivity of some common food-borne bacteria to the spices sage, rosemary, and allspice. *J. Food Sci.* **1980**, *45*, 1042–1044. [CrossRef]

27. Lisa, E.L.; Carac, G.; Barbu, V.; Robu, S. The synergistic antioxidant effect and antimicrobial efficacity of propolis, myrrh and chlorhexidine as beneficial toothpaste components. *Rev. Chim.-Buchar.* **2017**, *68*, 2060–2065.

28. Dolara, P.; Corte, B.; Ghelardini, C.; Pugliese, A.M.; Cerbai, E.; Menichetti, S.; Lo Nostro, A. Local anaesthetic, antibacterial and antifungal properties of sesquiterpenes from myrrh. *Planta Med.* **2000**, *66*, 356–358. [CrossRef] [PubMed]

29. Ritu, A.; Avijit, M. Phytochemical screening and antimicrobial activity of rhizomes of hedychium spicatum. *Phcog. J.* **2017**, *9*. [CrossRef]

30. Wang, H.; Liu, Y. Chemical composition and antibacterial activity of essential oils from different parts of Litsea cubeba. *Chem. Biodivers.* **2010**, *7*, 229–235. [CrossRef] [PubMed]

31. Friedman, M. Chemistry, antimicrobial mechanisms, and antibiotic activities of cinnamaldehyde against pathogenic bacteria in animal feeds and human foods. *J. Agric. Food Chem.* **2017**, *65*, 10406–10423. [CrossRef] [PubMed]

32. Subash Babu, P.; Prabuseenivasan, S.; Ignacimuthu, S. Cinnamaldehyde—A potential antidiabetic agent. *Phytomedicine* **2007**, *14*, 15–22. [CrossRef] [PubMed]

33. Feketa, V.V.; Marrelli, S.P. Systemic Administration of the TRPV3 Ion Channel Agonist Carvacrol Induces Hypothermia in Conscious Rodents. *PLoS ONE* **2015**, *10*, e0141994. [CrossRef] [PubMed]

34. Zhang, Y.; Shi, W.; Zhang, W.; Mitchison, D. Mechanisms of Pyrazinamide Action and Resistance. *Microbiol. Spectr.* **2013**, *2*, 1–12. [CrossRef] [PubMed]

35. Zhang, Y.; Permar, S.; Sun, Z. Conditions that may affect the results of susceptibility testing of Mycobacterium tuberculosis to pyrazinamide. *J. Med. Microbiol.* **2002**, *51*, 42–49. [CrossRef] [PubMed]

36. Cui, P.; Niu, H.; Shi, W.; Zhang, S.; Zhang, H.; Margolick, J.; Zhang, W.; Zhang, Y. Disruption of membrane by colistin kills uropathogenic *Escherichia coli* persisters and enhances killing of other antibiotics. *Antimicrob. Agents Chemother.* **2016**, *60*, 6867–6871. [CrossRef] [PubMed]

10

Evidence for Anti-*Pseudogymnoascus destructans* (*Pd*) Activity of Propolis

Soumya Ghosh [1,†], Robyn McArthur [1,†], Zhi Chao Guo [1], Rory McKerchar [1], Kingsley Donkor [1], Jianping Xu [2] (ID) and Naowarat Cheeptham [1,*] (ID)

[1] Department of Biological Sciences, Thompson Rivers University, Kamloops, BC V2C 0C8, Canada; sghosh@tru.ca (S.G.); rmcarthur645@gmail.com (R.M.); michelle8472@hotmail.com (Z.C.G.); rory-mckerchar@hotmail.com (R.M.); kdonkor@tru.ca (K.D.)

[2] Department of Biology, McMaster University, Hamilton, ON L8S 4K1, Canada; jpxu@mcmaster.ca

* Correspondence: ncheeptham@tru.ca

† Equally contributed author.

Academic Editor: Leonard Amaral

Abstract: White-nose syndrome (WNS) in bats, caused by *Pseudogymnoascus destructans* (*Pd*), is a cutaneous infection that has devastated North American bat populations since 2007. At present, there is no effective method for controlling this disease. Here, we evaluated the effect of propolis against *Pd* in vitro. Using Sabouraud dextrose agar (SDA) medium, approximately 1.7×10^7 conidia spores of the *Pd* strain M3906-2/mL were spread on each plate and grown to form a consistent lawn. A Kirby–Bauer disk diffusion assay was employed using different concentrations of propolis (1%, 2%, 3%, 4%, 5%, 10%, 15%, 20%, 25%), in plates incubated at 8 °C and 15 °C. At 8 °C and 15 °C, as the concentration of propolis increased, there was an increasing zone of inhibition (ZOI), reaching the highest degree at 10% and 25% concentrations, respectively. A germule suppression assay showed a similar effect on *Pd* conidia germination. A MALDI-TOF-MS analysis of propolis revealed multiple constituents with a potential anti-*Pd* activity, including cinnamic acid, p-coumaric acid, and dihydrochalcones, which could be further tested for their individual effects. Our study suggests that propolis or its individual constituents might be suitable products against *Pd*.

Keywords: propolis; white-nose syndrome; *Pseudogymnoascus destructans*; anti-*Pd* activities; anti-fungal; fungal infection in bats

1. Introduction

White-nose syndrome (WNS) has devastated many eastern North American bat populations since 2007, killing more than six million bats [1]. Since the first observations of mortality at a cave near Albany, New York in 2007, WNS has spread to 31 US states and 5 eastern Canadian provinces [2], most recently appearing in 2017 in the states of Mississippi, Texas, and Washington, USA [2]. The etiological agent of WNS is *Pseudogymnoascus destructans* (*Pd*), a psychrophilic fungus that grows optimally on hibernating bats at temperatures between 12–16 °C [3].

Pseudogymnoascus destructans (*Pd*) preferentially infects thinly haired regions on the skin of hibernating bats, and is able to degrade collagen and invade living tissues [4]. Hibernating bats lower their body temperature to near-ambient temperature during torpor bouts [5]. During hibernation, bats generally seek microclimates that remain above freezing and can be as warm as 15 °C or more for some species [5–7], and are relatively high in humidity. Bats generally adapt to the temperature of their surroundings to maximize their energy budget [8]. The similarity between the preferred hibernating environment of bats and the optimal growth condition of the *Pd* pathogen is a major contributor to the WNS epidemic. *Pd* infection disrupts the normal torpor and arousal cycles of hibernating bats [9], causing premature depletion of fat reserves, in addition to electrolyte imbalances and dehydration, resulting in mortality [10]. Bats are essential components of both the natural, agricultural, and other human ecosystems [11]. They play important roles in maintaining ecosystem stability, consume insects that are human or animal pests, and redistribute nutrients through their guano [11,12]. To reduce bat mortality and eliminate the likelihood of species extinction by *Pd*, it is essential to identify effective methods to control *Pd*.

In regard to investigations of anti-*Pd* agents, several recent studies have identified putative anti-*Pd* agents, including (i) volatile compounds produced by the bacteria *Rhodococcus rhodochrous* DAP96253 [13] and by *Pseudomonas spp.* isolated from bat wings [14]; (ii) cold-pressed, terpeneless orange oil (CPT) [15]; and (iii) sesquiterpene trans, trans-farnesol (*Candida albicans* quorum-sensing compound) [13]. Our goal was to identify alternative or additional potent treatments against *Pd* using substances likely to be unharmful to cave environments and to bats.

Propolis is a resinous substance produced by honey bees in beehives throughout the year [16,17]. Stingless bees are widely spread, especially in the tropical and subtropical areas of the world. Propolis produced from such bees possesses therapeutic properties [18], including antimicrobial, antitumor [18], antioxidant [19], anti-stimulant [20], anti-inflammatory [21–24], antiulcer [22–25], and anti-HIV activities [25]. For instance, two compounds, cardanol and cardol, isolated from a Thai propolis, possessed antiproliferation and cytotoxicity against carcinomas originated from the lungs, the liver, and the colon [26]. Khacha-ananda et al. 2016 [19] found that ethanolic extracts of propolis (EEP) obtained from Chiang Mai, Thailand, exhibited higher antioxidant activity than EEP from other sources. In 2005, Hu et al. [23] showed that both the ethanol and the water extracts of propolis had anti-inflammatory activities in mice and rats [21]. Significant anti-HIV activities [EC(50) < 0.1 µg/mL, TI > 186] resulted from moronic acid (triterpenoids) isolated from a Brazilian propolis [25]. Additionally, because of its antiviral, antibacterial, and antifungal activities, propolis has been used in human healthcare to treat colds, wounds, ulcers, and rheumatism [27,28]. Propolis was found to exhibit antagonistic effects against a number of Gram-positive cocci and rods [29]. A recent study by Shimizu et al. 2011 [30], showed that the ethanol extract of propolis from Brazil had antiviral activities. When administered orally or cutaneously to herpes simplex virus type 1 (HSV-1)-infected mice, the ethanol extract of propolis significantly reduced the herpetic skin lesions and enhanced delayed-type hypersensitivity [30]. Silici et al. 2006 [31] reported that propolis had antifungal activities against 15 strains belonging to four species of yeasts isolated from patients with superficial mycoses.

Traditionally, studies on the medicinal benefits of propolis have attributed its effects to its complex composition and to the synergistic effects among its complex chemical constituents [32,33]. Another emerging theme is that the chemical composition of propolis is highly dependent on the geographical location, botanical origin [34], and bee species [35]. In different ecosystems, there are different plant species, and these plants can vary in their secretion and exudates, and therefore provide diverse food sources to bees [16]. Thus, the variability in chemical composition among propolis from different sources can be large. For example, propolis produced in the Pacific region contains geranyl flavanones which are also a typical component for the African propolis [17]. The green propolis of Brazil has prenylated phenylpropanoids (e.g., artepillin C) and diterpenes as major components [17], while the propolis of temperate regions consists of flavonoids lacking the B-ring substituents, namely, chrysin, galangin, pinocembrin, pinobanksin, caffeic acid phenethyl ester [36]. These unique mixtures of constituents from different sources likely contribute to the observed multiple effects including not only the broad biological effects described above, but also the inhibition of nuclear factor κ-B, cell proliferation, cell arrest, and apoptosis [17,36].

In this study, we tested the effectiveness of the commercially available propolis purchased from Natural Factors in Coquitlam, British Columbia, Canada on the WNS agent *Pd*. We investigated the in vitro antagonistic properties of propolis against *Pd*. We also tested the inhibition of germule development when incubated with propolis. This study is the first investigation of the anti-*Pd* activities of propolis.

2. Results

2.1. Kirby–Bauer Diffusion Assay

Propolis exhibited anti-Pd activities at all the concentrations (1–25%) we tested (in quadruplets), as revealed by a clear 'zone of inhibition' around each of the impregnated paper discs, in comparison to discs treated with water or anhydrous ethanol (Figure 1(Ai,ii,xii,xiii)). ANOVA tests showed that the different concentrations of propolis differed significantly in their inhibitory effects (Figure 1(Aiii–xi,xiv–xxii)). Propolis significantly inhibited the growth of Pd at 8 °C (one-way ANOVA; F = 8.309; df = 8; $p = 0.100^{-4}$) as well as at 15 °C (one-way ANOVA; F = 8.704; df = 8; $p = 0.839^{-5}$). Along the concentration gradient, at 8 °C, the diameter of the inhibitory zones initially increased with the increase in propolis concentration, reaching the highest value at the propolis concentration of 10%, and showed some decline at higher propolis concentrations. At 15 °C, though there were some variations, the inhibition also increased with increasing propolis concentrations, reaching the highest level at the concentration of 25% of propolis. The pairwise post-hoc T-test results are shown in Supplementary Tables S1 and S2.

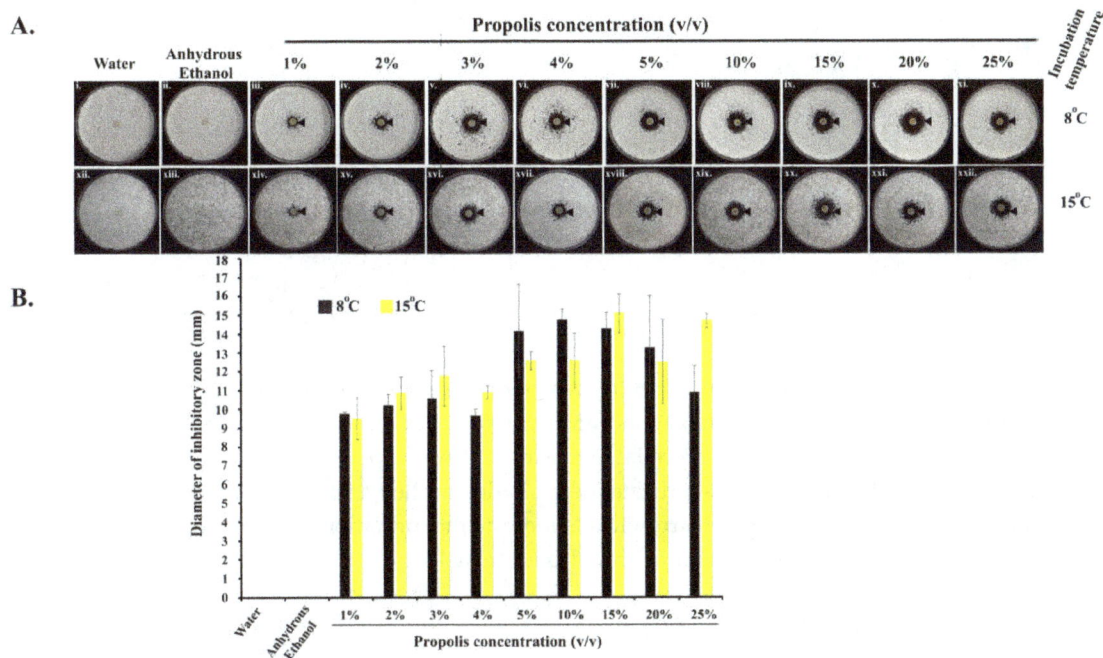

Figure 1. Anti-Pd activity of propolis. (**A**) Images (i–xi) and (xii–xxii) indicate the activity of propolis at 8 °C and 15 °C, respectively. The black arrowheads indicate the zone of inhibition of Pd when treated with different concentrations of propolis in comparison to water and anhydrous ethanol treatments; (**B**) diameter of the zones of inhibition at 8 °C and 15 °C. The error bars are standard deviations of the diameters.

2.2. Suppression of Germination of Pd Spores

As revealed by the macroscopic and microscopic assay images (Figure 2A,B), there was a complete inhibition of Pd sporulation with all propolis concentrations throughout the entire incubation period (16 days) at both incubation temperatures tested. On the seventh day of incubation at 8 °C, more mycelial extensions ($4\times$ microscopic images, Figure 2(Axxiii,xxiv)) were observed in the samples treated with water or anhydrous ethanol. The mycelial growth became more confluent amongst the Pd spores treated with water and ethanol by the 16th day of incubation (Figure 2(Axxxiv,xxxv)). At 15 °C, the Pd spores treated with water and ethanol exhibited a confluent growth from the seventh day of incubation (Figure 2(Bi,ii,xxiii,xxiv)).

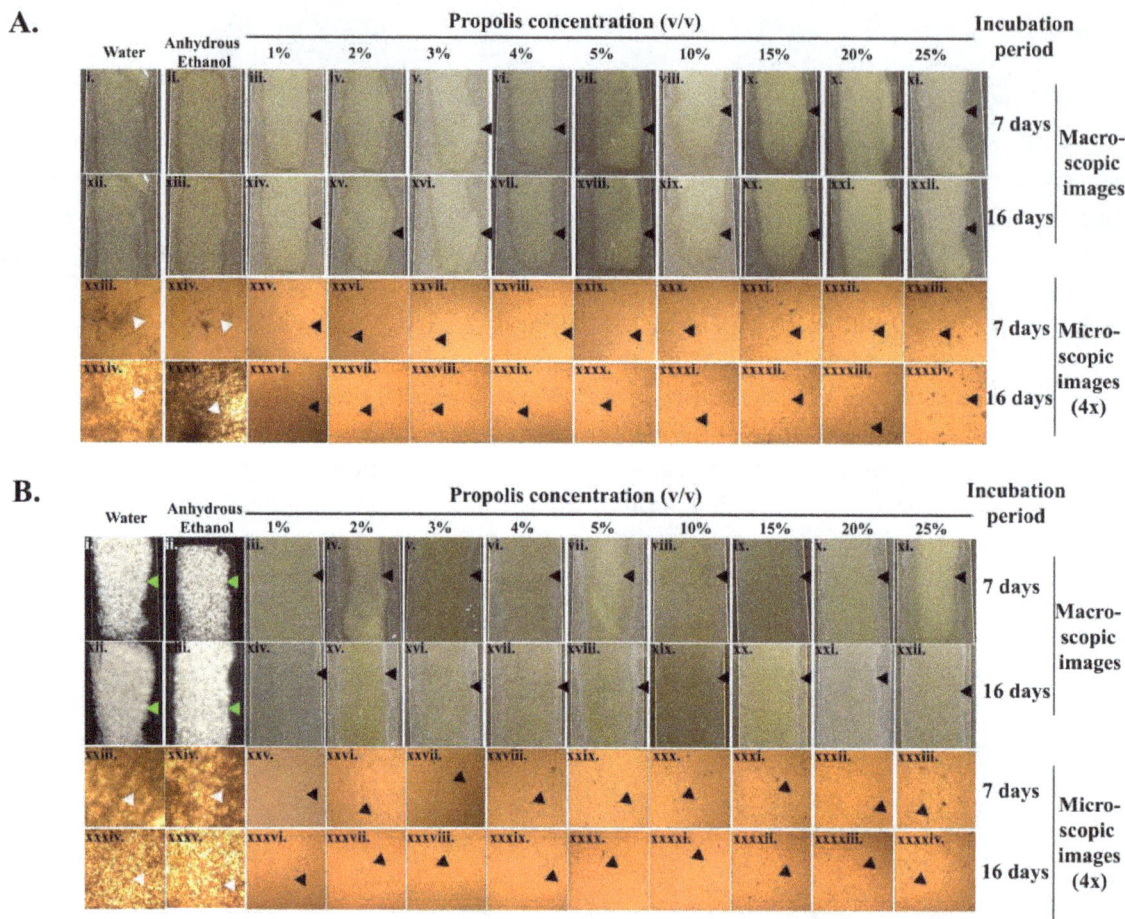

Figure 2. Germule suppression assay. (**A,B**) represent the *Pd* germination assay for treatments with water, anhydrous ethanol, and various concentrations of propolis at 8 °C and 15 °C, respectively. The white arrowheads indicate the mycelial extension of the *Pd* spores at two different incubation temperatures. The black arrowheads indicate the inhibition of the *Pd* spores on exposure to propolis at different concentrations. The green arrowheads indicate the formation of white *Pd* lawns resulting from the treatment of spores with water or anhydrous ethanol.

2.3. Microscopic Examination of the Treated Pd Spores

Pd spores treated with 1% propolis revealed a complete deformation (Microscopic images at 10× and 40×, Figure 3(iii,iv)) in vitro when compared to the untreated spores that exhibited elliptical shapes, typical of *Pd* spores. (Figure 3(i,ii)).

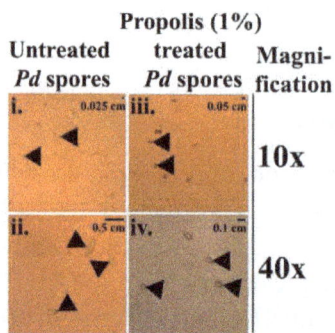

Figure 3. Micrographs of *Pd* spores displayed at 10× and 40× magnification: (**i–ii**) elliptical shape of untreated *Pd* spores; (**iii–iv**) deformed *Pd* spores treated with 1% propolis.

2.4. Chemical Composition of Propolis

MALDI spectra (Figure 4) revealed that the major constituents of the propolis used in this study were aromatic acids, i.e., cinnamic acid and p-coumaric acid; dihydrochalcones, i.e., 2,4,6-trihydroxydihydrochalcone; fatty acids, i.e., stearic acid, palmitic acid; esters, i.e., benzyl methoxybenzoate.

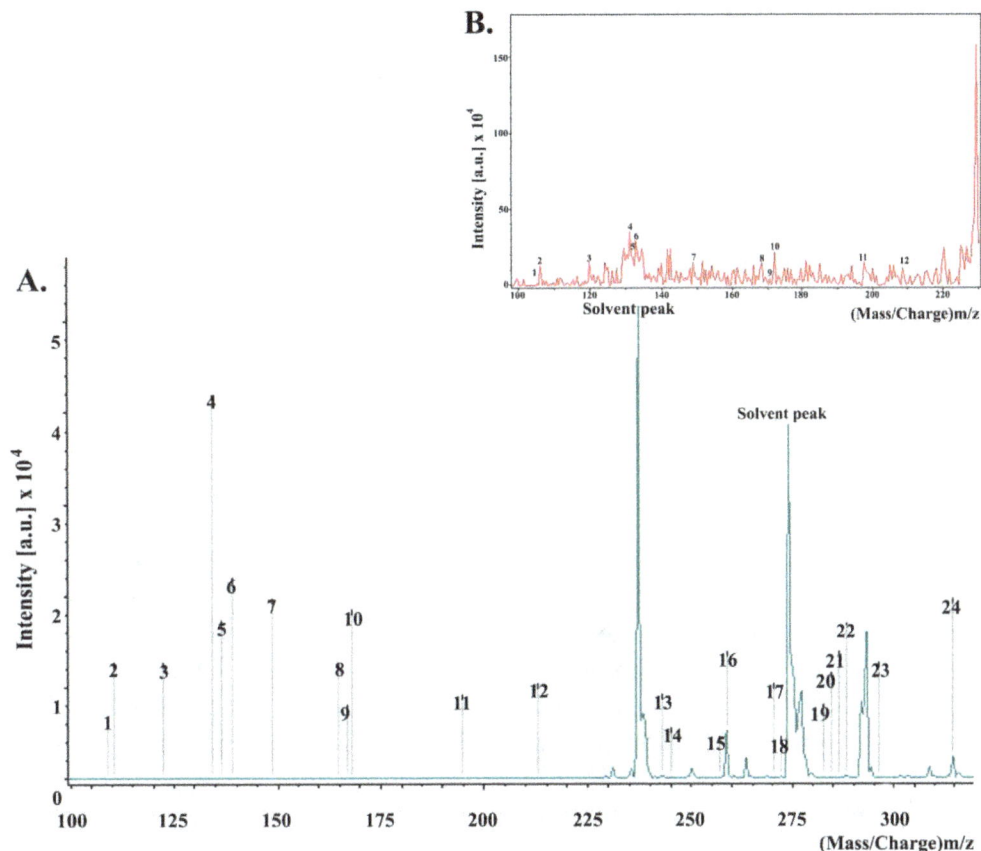

Figure 4. (**A**) MALDI-TOF-MS of a propolis sample at a mass range of 100–400 Da. Each of the peaks on the mass spectrum represents a distinctive compound in our propolis sample. The numbers above the peaks correspond to the compounds listed in Table 1; (**B**) magnified version of the mass spectrum at a mass range of the 100–225 Da.

Table 1. Composition of propolis as determined by MALDI-TOF-MS (the peaks corresponding to these values can be seen in the mass spectrum in Figure 4).

Peak	Constituents Identified	Mass/Charge (*m/z*)	Intensity
1	Benzyl alcohol	108.14	0.77
2	Hydroquinone	110.11	5.00
3	Benzoic acid	122.12	5.93
4	Cinnamyl alcohol	134.17	23.81
5	Hydroxyacetophenone	136.15	7.82
6	4-Hydroxybenzoic acid	138.12	10.98
7	Cinnamic acid	148.16	14.81
8	p-coumaric acid	164.16	4.91
9	3-Phenyl-3-hydroxypropanoic acid	166.18	5.91
10	Sesquiterpenes	168.31	13.90
11	Ferulic acid	194.18	3.91
12	Benzyl benzoate	212.25	6.85
13	Benzyl methoxybenzoate	242.27	211.88
14	Benzyl dihydroxybenzoate	244.24	105.16
15	Palmitic acid	256.43	64.16

Table 1. *Cont.*

Peak	Constituents Identified	Mass/Charge (*m/z*)	Intensity
16	2,4,6-Trihydroxydihydrochalcone	258.27	5184.70
17	Pinostrobin chalcone	270.28	47.98
18	2,6-Dihydroxy-4-methoxydihydrochalcone	272.25	132.69
19	Oleic acid	282.47	28.64
20	Stearic acid	284.31	50.69
21	Sakuranetin	286.27	44.71
22	2,4,6-Trihydroxy-4-methoxydihydrochalcone	288.30	247.59
23	Cinnamyl caffeate	296.32	44.87
24	Pinobanksin 3-O-acetate	314.29	2331.83

3. Discussion

The populations of hibernating bats in North America are declining at unprecedented rates because of WNS [1,37]. Because insectivorous bats usually eat insects, they play important roles in the ecosystem and provide valuable pest control services to the agricultural and forestry sectors of the North American economy [11]. Our research has identified a new potential tool for combatting WNS that is threatening many bats across the continent. We have discovered that bee propolis may be used as an effective antifungal agent against *Pd*, the causative agent of WNS.

Our study has revealed that even low concentration (1%) of commercially available propolis (65% tincture) can completely inhibit *Pd* spore germination at both 8 °C and 15 °C. Unfortunately, *Pd* grows optimally between 8–16 °C [3], and the hibernating environment creates an ideal condition for Pd growth on hibernating bats. The incubation temperatures used in our testing were thus representative of the effective hibernation and fungal infection range that are also found in cave environments [38]. Additionally, the bioassay plates were kept until the 60th day after the 22nd day of observation, and we never found any encroachment of growth of *Pd* spores in the observed ZOI. This may indicate that propolis can completely inhibit *Pd* spore germination for up to 60 days when tested in the lab setting.

Propolis has previously been shown to exhibit antifungal, antibacterial, and antiviral properties and therefore has been widely used in human healthcare for treating ulcers, wounds, and rheumatisms [27,28]. We employed the Kirby–Bauer diffusion assay to identify fungicidal activities of propolis, while the germule suppression assay was performed in order to understand the possible inhibitory mechanism of the propolis against *Pd* spores germination. Similar studies by Cornelison el al. 2014 [13,39] have shown that bacteria-derived volatile compounds that include decanal, 2-ethyl-hexanol, nonanal, benzothiole, and N, N-dimethyloctylamine, completely inhibited the growth of conidia and radial mycelial extensions. Moreover, our findings show a deformation of the *Pd* spores exposed to propolis, a result consistent with a possible fungicidal mechanism of action. The deformation of the fungal conidia by propolis has never been reported before.

Though the propolis used in this study was purchased from a western Canadian company, Natural Factors, the company obtained the raw propolis materials from a variety of sources and geographic regions. Further examinations of our purchased propolis traced its origin to Mongolia. Unfortunately, no further information could be obtained, including the specific region within Mongolia, or the plants that bees were feeding on (personal communication). However, consistent with previous findings [40–42], our MALDI-TOF analysis of the tested propolis identified a range of constituents. These included benzyl benzoate, benzyl methoxybenzoate, benzyl dihydroxybenzoate, hydroxyacetophenone, 2,4,6-trihydroxydihydrochalcone, pinostrobin chalcone, 2,6-dihydroxy-4-methoxydihydrochalcone, 2,4,6-trihydroxy-4-methoxydihydrochalcone, cinnamic acid, and p-coumaric acid as major constituents. A previous study of Canadian propolis from two regions showed that the propolis from Victoria contained mainly p-hydroxyacetophenone, benzyl hydroxybenzoate, cinnamic acid, and dihydrochalcones, while that from Richmond had large amounts of cinnamic acid and p-coumaric acid [40]. However, both propolis samples showed significant antioxidant properties with a high level of radical scavenging activity. The other remaining compounds identified in our propolis also showed some geographic specificity in previous studies. For example, 3,3-dimethylallyl caffeate was reported from European poplar-type propolis [41,42], while we identified cinnamyl caffeate in our propolis. Other compounds from diverse locations include hydroquinone (Burdock et al. 1998 [42]) and benzyl alcohol [43]. Benzyl alcohol has anti-inflammatory, antibacterial, antitumour, hepatoprotective, and antioxidant activities [41]. Benzoic acid and 4-hydroxybenoic acid found in our samples were previously found in an Iranian propolis, and have shown antibacterial properties [44]. Other constituents revealed in our propolis included ferulic acid, oleic acid, stearic acid, palmitic acid, and pinobanksin 3-O-acetate. An earlier analysis of Anatolian propolis also identified the above mentioned compounds and showed that they exhibited antibacterial activities against Gram-positive bacteria such as *Staphylococcus aureus* (6538-P), *Streptococcus sobrinus*, *Staphylococcus epidermidis*, *Streptococcus mutans*, *Enterococcus faecalis*, and *Micrococcus luteus* [45]. Certain Gram-negative bacteria, such as *Escherichia coli*, *Salmonella typhimurium*, *Pseudomonas aeruginosa*, and *Enterobacter aerogenes* and yeast such as *Candida albicans*, *C. tropicalis*, and *C. krusei* were reported to be susceptible to the Anatolian propolis [45]. Lastly, Sakuranetin, one of the flavonoids identified in our propolis, was reported to exhibit antimicrobial activities against oral pathogens [46].

We have confirmed the complete inhibition of *Pd* spore germination even at a low concentration of propolis (1%). Propolis, also called "bee glue" [21,47], is soluble in anhydrous ethanol, which eliminates the resinous and sticky properties of this substance making it suitable for application on roost substrates. Our study contributes to a growing portfolio of biological and chemical measures for controlling the growth of *Pd* [10,12,13,42]. Future applications on bats, and tests in wild hibernacula are required to test the effectiveness of propolis outside of a laboratory setting.

The US Fish and Wildlife Service (USFWS) has also recommended a number of decontaminants. The only appropriate methods for laboratory and field decontamination of equipment and clothing include ethanol ($\geq$60%), isopropanol ($\geq$60%), isopropyl alcohol wipes (70%), hydrogen peroxide wipes (3%), Accel®, Clorox® bleach, Clorox® wipes, Clorox® Clean-Up cleaner + bleach, Hibiclens®, and Lysol® IC quaternary disinfectant cleaner. Whether propolis would be useful as a decontamination substance is yet to be seen, in any case the substances listed in the current US national WNS decontamination protocol are more readily available. The toxicity of many of these listed decontamination substances is of minor concern for an equipment decontamination protocol, but it is of utmost concern when these substances are employed for the mitigation of a disease. Naturally sourced anti-*Pd* substances like propolis could provide treatment options that are generally considered safe for mammals. Previous studies reported that Greek and Roman physicians prescribed propolis as a mouth disinfectant and for the topical therapy of cutaneous and mucosal wounds in humans [16]. More recently, a study showed that propolis paste applied on dogs' cutaneous wounds resulted in better wound re-epithelization, contraction, and total wound healing than a placebo [48]. However, no study has examined the effects of propolis on bats.

Overall, our study has demonstrated the complete inhibition of *Pd* spore germination by propolis. However, significant research is still required, for example an investigation on whether a longer period of testing time in the laboratory would yield any additional results further indicating a real potential of propolis as one of the treatment options for WNS. The potential activities of the individual constituents of propolis and their combinations, as well as their synergistic interactions against *Pd* spore germination and mycelial growth also need to be identified. At present, the medicinal benefits of propolis have been attributed to its complex composition and to the potential synergistic effects of its chemical constituents. In addition, the chemical composition of propolis is highly dependent on its geographical origin, on bee species, and on the botanical food sources of the bees. Further investigations are needed in order to determine whether propolis, or its individual ingredients or combinations thereof may be an option for the treatment of *Pd*-infected cave or bats.

4. Materials and Methods

4.1. Cultivation of Pd Spores

The *P. destructans* M3906-2 strain was used in this study. This *Pd* strain was previously described by Khankhet et al. (2014) [49]. The cultivation and isolation of the *Pd* spores were performed as previously described [37]. *Pd* cultures were maintained on Sabouraud dextrose agar (SDA) plates at 15 °C. *Pd* spores were isolated from cultures by submerging the conidial lawn in Conidia Harvesting Solution (CHS) (0.05% Tween 80, 0.9% NaCl) for 5 min followed by mechanical scrapping and filtration through glass wool as previously described [13,14]. The concentration of the *Pd* spores was quantified by a haemocytometer and the spores were stored in phosphate buffer saline (PBS) at 4 °C until further use.

4.2. Kirby–Bauer Diffusion Assay

One hundred microliter of isolated *Pd* spores (1×10^7 spores/mL) were mixed with 250 mL of Sabouraud dextrose agar (SDA) media supplemented with chloramphenicol (34 mg/L) at 50 °C (Fisher Scientific, Fairlawn, NJ, USA) to avoid bacterial contamination. Approximately 20–22 mL of the mixture was poured into each of the 85 mm petri plates. Plates were air-dried in a laminar airflow hood. Eight millimeter (diameter) paper discs (Toyo Roshi Kaisha Ltd., Tokyo, Japan) were soaked in different concentrations (1%, 2%, 3%, 4%, 5%, 10%, 15%, 20%, and 25%) of commercially available propolis (65% extract) (Natural Factors, Coquitlam, BC, Canada), air-dried, and placed in the center of each seeded SDA medium plate along with sterile water and anhydrous ethanol (<0.005% water) (Sigma Aldrich, St. Louis, MO, USA); the latter two conditions were used as controls. Anhydrous ethanol was tested since it was used as a solvent to dissolve propolis in all dilutions (as per the manufacturer's instructions). All plates with different propolis concentrations were incubated at 8 °C or 15 °C, including control plates, in duplicate. Anti-*Pd* activities were identified as zones of inhibition around the impregnated paper discs, and the diameters were measured in millimeters with an electronic Vernier caliper (Guilin, Guangxi, China). Notably, the measurement of the diameters for the zones of inhibition were recorded on the 22nd and 15th day of incubation at 8 °C and 15 °C, respectively, since *Pd* spores germinated slower at 8 °C than at 15 °C. Each treatment was repeated four times. The bioassay plates were kept until the 60th day after the observation performed at the 22nd day.

To determine whether the concentrations of propolis differed in their inhibitory effects, we used a single-factor ANOVA to analyze the quantitative-zone-of-inhibition data. If an overall difference was found, all pairwise comparisons were made using the two-tailed t-test. Since there were 36 pairwise comparisons [9 concentrations × (9 − 1)/2 = 36] at each of the two temperatures, a Bonferroni correction was applied to the typical p value of < 0.05 considered statistically significant. The corrected *p* value was 0.05/36 = 0.0013888.

4.3. Germule Suppression Assay

Sterile microscopic slides (24.5 × 76.2 mm) were layered with 600 µL of molten SDA (10%) at a temperature of 50 °C and premixed with 5 µL of *Pd* spores (1×10^7 spores/mL) and 5 µL of each of the indicated concentrations of propolis. Quadruplet slides were prepared for each of the propolis concentrations and were incubated in duplicate at 8 °C and 15 °C. The germination of the *Pd* spores was measured macroscopically by visualizing the white growth confluence of the *Pd* lawn, and microscopically by the *Pd* hyphal extension. Both macroscopic and microscopic images were acquired from slides on the 7th and 16th day of incubation. The microscopic images were taken using a DCM 130E digital camera for microscope (1.3 M pixels, CMOS chip) (AmScope, Irvine, CA, USA). The microscopic images were imported with the Scope Photo Software (AmScope, Irvine, CA, USA).

4.4. Analysis of Chemical Constituents

The chemical composition of propolis was determined using matrix-assisted laser desorption ionization time-of-flight mass spectrometry (MALDI-TOF-MS). The propolis sample consisted of 50% diluted propolis in methanol covered with 0.1020 M of α-cyano-4-hydroxy cinnamic acid (HCCA) in 1:4 (v/v) H_2O/acetonitrile. A 1.0 μL diluted aliquot of the sample was first spotted on the plate and covered with 2.0 μL of matrix. The mass spectra were obtained using a bench-top Microflex MALDI-TOF MS from Bruker Daltonics® (Bremen, Germany) equipped with a pulsed nitrogen laser at 355 nm wavelength. The spectra were recorded from 40 to 2000 Da (positive mode), and from 100 to 400 Da (positive mode) using FlexControl 3.3 software (ion source 1: 19 kV; ion source 2: 15.5 kV; lens voltage: 9.45 kV; laser frequency: 60 Hz; pulsed ion extraction (PIE) delay: 120 ns). Other parameters are shown in Table 2. Mass gates of 400 m/z (positive mode) were set for all experiments. Individual mass spectra from each spot were acquired by averaging 350 laser shots. Data acquisition was set to automate, and the "random walk" movement was activated at 10 shots per raster during the sequence. The peak lists and intensities were calculated using the peak-picking centroid algorithm in FlexAnalysis 3.3 software.

Table 2. Parameters of MALDI-TOF-MS.

Parameters	Values
Laser	Pulsed nitrogen
Laser power	20–80%
Peak selection (mass range)	40–2000 Da
Sample rate	0.05 GS/s
Mass range	Low range
Electronic gain	Enhanced 100 mV
Realtime smooth	Off
Spectrum size	2069 pts
Spectrum delay	307 pts
Laser frequency	60.0 Hz
Laser attenuator offset	17%
Laser attenuator range	30%
Target	MSP 96 target polished steel
Matrix	α-cyano-4-hydroxy-cinnamic acid, HCCA
Sample	50% diluted propolis in MeOH covered with 0.1020 M of HCCA in 1:4 (v/v) H_2O/acetonitrile

Acknowledgments: We are thankful to the United States Fish and Wildlife Service (Cheeptham and Lausen's Grant #F15AS00188) for funding. Our sincere appreciation also goes to Cori Lausen of the Wildlife Conservation Society Canada and Mark Rakobowchuk of TRU for their time and assistance in editing this manuscript.

Author Contributions: N.C. conceived the idea to use propolis. S.G. and R.M.A. designed all the experiments under the close guidance and supervision of N.C. S.G. drafted the manuscript. R.M.A. conducted the experiments. N.C. secured funding. K.D. designed the experiments used to determine the chemical composition of propolis. Z.C.G. and R.M.K. conducted the experiments under the supervision of K.D. K.D. drafted the chemistry section of the manuscript. J.P.X. provided the *P. destructans* M3906-2 strain and contributed to the statistical analyses. N.C., S.G., J.P.X. and K.D. read and edited the manuscript.

References

1. United States Fish and Wildlife Service (USFWS). North American bat death toll exceeds 5.5 million from white-nose syndrome. In *USFWS News Release*; United States Fish and Wildlife Service (USFWS): Washington, DC, USA, 2012; pp. 1–2.

2. United States Fish and Wildlife Service (USFWS). *White Nose Sydromes: Where Is It Now? In USFWS News Release*; United States Fish and Wildlife Service (USFWS): Washington, DC, USA, 2017.

3. Verant, M.L.; Boyles, J.G.; Waldrep, W., Jr.; Wibbelt, G.; Blehert, D.S. Temperature-dependent growth of *Geomyces destructans*, the fungus that causes bat white-nose syndrome. *PLoS ONE* **2012**, *7*, e46280. [CrossRef] [PubMed]

4. O'Donoghue, A.J.; Knudsen, G.M.; Beekman, C.; Perry, J.A.; Johnson, A.D.; DeRisi, J.L.; Craik, C.S.; Bennett, R.J. Destructin-1 is a collagen-degrading endopeptidase secreted by *pseudogymnoascus destructans*, the causative agent of white-nose syndrome. *Proc. Natl. Acad. Sci. USA* **2015**, *112*, 7478–7483. [CrossRef] [PubMed]

5. Webb, P.I.; Speakman, J.R.; Racey, P.A. How hot is a hibernaculum? A review of the temperatures at which bats hibernate. *Can. J. Zool.* **1996**, *74*, 761–765.

6. Davies, W.H. Hibernation: Ecology and physiological ecology. In *Biology of Bats*; Wimsatt, W.A., Ed.; Acedemic Press: New York, NY, USA; London, UK, 1970; Volume 1, pp. 265–300.

7. Humphries, M.M.; Thomas, D.W.; Speakman, J.R. Climate-mediated energetic constraints on the distribution of hibernating mammals. *Nature* **2002**, *418*, 313–316. [CrossRef] [PubMed]

8. Speakman, J.R.; Thomas, D.W. Physiological ecology and enegetics of bats. In *Bat Ecology*; Kunz, T.H., Fenton, M.B., Eds.; The University of Chicago Press: Chicago, IL, USA; London, UK, 2003; pp. 431–434.

9. Warnecke, L.; Turner, J.M.; Bollinger, T.K.; Misra, V.; Cryan, P.M.; Blehert, D.S.; Wibbelt, G.; Willis, C.K. Pathophysiology of white-nose syndrome in bats: A mechanistic model linking wing damage to mortality. *Biol. Lett.* **2013**, *9*, 20130177. [CrossRef] [PubMed]

10. Cryan, P.M.; Meteyer, C.U.; Boyles, J.G.; Blehert, D.S. Wing pathology of white-nose syndrome in bats suggests life-threatening disruption of physiology. *BMC Biol.* **2010**, *8*, 135. [CrossRef] [PubMed]

11. Boyles, J.G.; Cryan, P.M.; McCracken, G.F.; Kunz, T.H. Conservation. Economic importance of bats in agriculture. *Science* **2011**, *332*, 41–42. [CrossRef] [PubMed]

12. Kunz, T.H.; Braun de Torrez, E.; Bauer, D.; Lobova, T.; Fleming, T.H. Ecosystem services provided by bats. *Ann. N. Y. Acad. Sci.* **2011**, *1223*, 1–38. [CrossRef] [PubMed]

13. Cornelison, C.T.; Keel, M.K.; Gabriel, K.T.; Barlament, C.K.; Tucker, T.A.; Pierce, G.E.; Crow, S.A. A preliminary report on the contact-independent antagonism of *Pseudogymnoascus destructans* by *Rhodococcus rhodochrous* strain DAP96253. *BMC Microbiol.* **2014**, *14*, 246. [CrossRef] [PubMed]

14. Hoyt, J.R.; Cheng, T.L.; Langwig, K.E.; Hee, M.M.; Frick, W.F.; Kilpatrick, A.M. Bacteria isolated from bats inhibit the growth of *Pseudogymnoascus destructans*, the causative agent of white-nose syndrome. *PLoS ONE* **2015**, *10*, e0121329. [CrossRef] [PubMed]

15. Boire, N.; Zhang, S.; Khuvis, J.; Lee, R.; Rivers, J.; Crandall, P.; Keel, M.K.; Parrish, N. Potent inhibition of *Pseudogymnoascus destructans*, the causative agent of white-nose syndrome in bats, by cold-pressed, terpeneless, valencia orange oil. *PLoS ONE* **2016**, *11*, e0148473. [CrossRef] [PubMed]

16. Bankova, V.S.; de Castro, S.L.; Marcucci, M.C. Propolis: Recent advances in chemistry and plant origin. *Apidologie* **2000**, *31*, 3–15. [CrossRef]

17. Huang, S.; Zhang, C.P.; Wang, K.; Li, G.Q.; Hu, F.L. Recent advances in the chemical composition of propolis. *Molecules* **2014**, *19*, 19610–19632. [CrossRef] [PubMed]

18. Choudhari, M.K.; Punekar, S.A.; Ranade, R.V.; Paknikar, K.M. Antimicrobial activity of stingless bee (*Trigona* sp.) propolis used in the folk medicine of western Maharashtra, India. *J. Ethnopharmacol.* **2012**, *141*, 363–367. [CrossRef] [PubMed]

19. Khacha-ananda, S.; Tragoolpua, K.; Chantawannakul, P.; Tragoolpua, Y. Propolis extracts from the northern region of Thailand suppress cancer cell growth through induction of apoptosis pathways. *Investig. New Drugs* **2016**, *34*, 707–722. [CrossRef] [PubMed]

20. Wagh, V.D. Propolis: A wonder bees product and its pharmacological potentials. *Adv. Pharmacol. Sci.* **2013**, *2013*, 308249. [CrossRef] [PubMed]

21. Hu, F.; Hepburn, H.R.; Li, Y.; Chen, M.; Radloff, S.E.; Daya, S. Effects of ethanol and water extracts of propolis (bee glue) on acute inflammatory animal models. *J. Ethnopharmacol.* **2005**, *100*, 276–283. [CrossRef] [PubMed]

22. Wang, K.; Ping, S.; Huang, S.; Hu, L.; Xuan, H.Z.; Zhang, C.P.; Hu, F.L. Molecular mechanisms underlying the in vitro anti-inflammatory effects of a Ffavonoid-rich ethanol extract from Chinese propolis (poplar type). *Evid. Based Complement. Altern. Med.* **2013**, *2013*, 127672.

23. Xuan, H.; Zhao, J.; Miao, J.; Li, Y.; Chu, Y.; Hu, F. Effect of Brazilian propolis on human umbilical vein endothelial cell apoptosis. *Food Chem. Toxicol.* **2011**, *49*, 78–85. [CrossRef] [PubMed]

24. Xuan, H.; Zhu, R.; Li, Y.; Hu, F. Inhibitory effect of chinese propolis on phosphatidylcholine-specific phospholipase C activity in vascular endothelial cells. *Evid. Based Complement. Altern. Med.* **2011**, *2011*, 985278. [CrossRef] [PubMed]

25. Ito, J.; Chang, F.R.; Wang, H.K.; Park, Y.K.; Ikegaki, M.; Kilgore, N.; Lee, K.H. Anti-AIDS agents. 48.(1) ANTI-HIV activity of moronic acid derivatives and the new melliferone-related triterpenoid isolated from Brazilian propolis. *J. Nat. Prod.* **2001**, *64*, 1278–1281. [CrossRef] [PubMed]

26. Teerasripreecha, D.; Phuwapraisirisan, P.; Puthong, S.; Kimura, K.; Okuyama, M.; Mori, H.; Kimura, A.; Chanchao, C. In vitro antiproliferative/cytotoxic activity on cancer cell lines of a cardanol and a cardol enriched from Thai *Apis mellifera* propolis. *BMC Complement. Altern. Med.* **2012**, *12*, 27. [CrossRef] [PubMed]

27. Silici, S.; Kutluca, S. Chemical composition and antibacterial activity of propolis collected by three different races of honeybees in the same region. *J. Ethnopharmacol.* **2005**, *99*, 69–73. [CrossRef] [PubMed]

28. Kujumgiev, A.; Tsvetkova, I.; Serkedjieva, Y.; Bankova, V.; Christov, R.; Popov, S. Antibacterial, antifungal and antiviral activity of propolis of different geographic origin. *J. Ethnopharmacol.* **1999**, *64*, 235–240. [CrossRef]

29. Grange, J.M.; Davey, R.W. Antibacterial properties of propolis (bee glue). *J. R. Soc. Med.* **1990**, *83*, 159–160. [PubMed]

30. Shimizu, T.; Takeshita, Y.; Takamori, Y.; Kai, H.; Sawamura, R.; Yoshida, H.; Watanabe, W.; Tsutsumi, A.; Park, Y.K.; Yasukawa, K.; et al. Efficacy of Brazilian propolis against herpes simplex virus type 1 infection in mice and their modes of antiherpetic efficacies. *Evid. Based Complement. Altern. Med.* **2011**, *2011*, 976196. [CrossRef] [PubMed]

31. Silici, S.; Koc, A.N. Comparative study of in vitro methods to analyse the antifungal activity of propolis against yeasts isolated from patients with superficial mycoses. *Lett. Appl. Microbiol.* **2006**, *43*, 318–324. [CrossRef] [PubMed]

32. Amoros, M.; Simoes, C.M.; Girre, L.; Sauvager, F.; Cormier, M. Synergistic effect of flavones and flavonols against herpes simplex virus type 1 in cell culture. Comparison with the antiviral activity of propolis. *J. Nat. Prod.* **1992**, *55*, 1732–1740. [CrossRef] [PubMed]

33. Bueno-Silva, B.; Alencar, S.M.; Koo, H.; Ikegaki, M.; Silva, G.V.; Napimoga, M.H.; Rosalen, P.L. Anti-inflammatory and antimicrobial evaluation of neovestitol and vestitol isolated from Brazilian red propolis. *J. Agric. Food Chem.* **2013**, *61*, 4546–4550. [CrossRef] [PubMed]

34. Salatino, A.; Fernandes-Silva, C.C.; Righi, A.A.; Salatino, M.L. Propolis research and the chemistry of plant products. *Nat. Prod. Rep.* **2011**, *28*, 925–936. [CrossRef] [PubMed]

35. Simon, C.; Buckley, T.R.; Frati, F.; Stewart, J.B.; Beckenbach, A.T. Incorporating molecular evolution into phylogenetic analysis, and a new compilation of conserved polymerase chain reaction primers for animal mitochondrial DNA. *Annu. Rev. Ecol. Evol. Syst.* **2006**, *37*, 545–579. [CrossRef]

36. Fernandes-Silva, C.C.; Freitas, J.C.; Salatino, A.; Salatino, M.L. Cytotoxic activity of six samples of Brazilian propolis on sea urchin (*Lytechinus variegatus*) eggs. *Evid. Based Complement. Altern. Med.* **2013**, *2013*, 619361. [CrossRef] [PubMed]

37. McArthur, R.L.; Ghosh, S.; Cheeptham, N. Improvement of protocols for the screening of biological control agents against white-nose syndrome. *JEMI+* **2017**, *2*, 1–7.

38. Langwig, K.E.; Frick, W.F.; Hoyt, J.R.; Parise, K.L.; Drees, K.P.; Kunz, T.H.; Foster, J.T.; Kilpatrick, A.M. Drivers of variation in species impacts for a multi-host fungal disease of bats. *Philos. Trans. R. Soc. Lond. B Biol. Sci.* **2016**, *371*. [CrossRef] [PubMed]

39. Cornelison, C.T.; Gabriel, K.T.; Barlament, C.; Crow, S.A., Jr. Inhibition of *Pseudogymnoascus destructans* growth from conidia and mycelial extension by bacterially produced volatile organic compounds. *Mycopathologia* **2014**, *177*, 1–10. [CrossRef] [PubMed]

40. Christov, R.; Trusheva, B.; Popova, M.; Bankova, V.; Bertrand, M. Chemical composition of propolis from Canada, its antiradical activity and plant origin. *Nat. Prod. Res.* **2006**, *20*, 531–536. [CrossRef] [PubMed]

41. Bankova, V. Recent trends and important developments in propolis research. *Evid. Based Complement. Altern. Med.* **2005**, *2*, 29–32. [CrossRef] [PubMed]

42. Burdock, G.A. Review of the biological properties and toxicity of bee propolis (propolis). *Food Chem. Toxicol.* **1998**, *36*, 347–363. [CrossRef]

43. Bankova, V.; Popova, M.; Trusheva, B. Propolis volatile compounds: Chemical diversity and biological activity: A review. *Chem. Cent. J.* **2014**, *8*, 28. [CrossRef] [PubMed]

44. Trusheva, B.; Todorov, I.; Ninova, M.; Najdenski, H.; Daneshmand, A.; Bankova, V. Antibacterial mono- and sesquiterpene esters of benzoic acids from iranian propolis. *Chem. Cent. J.* **2010**, *4*, 8. [CrossRef] [PubMed]

45. Uzel, A.; Sorkun, K.; Oncag, O.; Cogulu, D.; Gencay, O.; Salih, B. Chemical compositions and antimicrobial activities of four different Anatolian propolis samples. *Microbiol. Res.* **2005**, *160*, 189–195. [CrossRef] [PubMed]

46. Koo, H.; Gomes, B.P.; Rosalen, P.L.; Ambrosano, G.M.; Park, Y.K.; Cury, J.A. In vitro antimicrobial activity of propolis and Arnica montana against oral pathogens. *Arch. Oral Biol.* **2000**, *45*, 141–148. [CrossRef]

47. Santos, F.A.; Bastos, E.M.; Rodrigues, P.H.; de Uzeda, M.; de Carvalho, M.A.; Farias Lde, M.; Moreira, E.S. Susceptibility of Prevotella intermedia/Prevotella nigrescens (and Porphyromonas gingivalis) to propolis (bee glue) and other antimicrobial agents. *Anaerobe* **2002**, *8*, 9–15. [CrossRef] [PubMed]

48. Abu-Seida, A.M. Effect of propolis on experimental cutaneous wound healing in dogs. *Vet. Med. Int.* **2015**, *2015*, 1–4. [CrossRef] [PubMed]

49. Khankhet, J.; Vanderwolf, K.J.; McAlpine, D.F.; McBurney, S.; Overy, D.P.; Slavic, D.; Xu, J. Clonal expansion of the *Pseudogymnoascus destructans* genotype in North America is accompanied by significant variation in phenotypic expression. *PLoS ONE* **2014**, *9*, e104684. [CrossRef] [PubMed]

11

Biotin Protein Ligase Is a Target for New Antibacterials

Jiage Feng [1], Ashleigh S. Paparella [2], Grant W. Booker [2], Steven W. Polyak [2,*] and Andrew D. Abell [2,3,*]

[1]   Department of Chemistry, University of Adelaide, North Tce, Adelaide, SA 5005, Australia; dovekey_feng@hotmail.com
[2]   School of Biological Sciences, University of Adelaide, North Tce, Adelaide, SA 5005, Australia; ashleigh.paparella@adelaide.edu.au (A.S.P.); grant.booker@adelaide.edu.au (G.W.B.)
[3]   Centre for Nanoscale BioPhotonics (CNBP), University of Adelaide, Adelaide, SA 5005, Australia
*   Correspondence: steven.polyak@adelaide.edu.au (S.W.P.); andrew.abell@adelaide.edu.au (A.D.A.)

Academic Editor: Naresh Kumar

Abstract: There is a desperate need for novel antibiotic classes to combat the rise of drug resistant pathogenic bacteria, such as *Staphylococcus aureus*. Inhibitors of the essential metabolic enzyme biotin protein ligase (BPL) represent a promising drug target for new antibacterials. Structural and biochemical studies on the BPL from *S. aureus* have paved the way for the design and development of new antibacterial chemotherapeutics. BPL employs an ordered ligand binding mechanism for the synthesis of the reaction intermediate biotinyl-5′-AMP from substrates biotin and ATP. Here we review the structure and catalytic mechanism of the target enzyme, along with an overview of chemical analogues of biotin and biotinyl-5′-AMP as BPL inhibitors reported to date. Of particular promise are studies to replace the labile phosphoroanhydride linker present in biotinyl-5′-AMP with alternative bioisosteres. A novel in situ click approach using a mutant of *S. aureus* BPL as a template for the synthesis of triazole-based inhibitors is also presented. These approaches can be widely applied to BPLs from other bacteria, as well as other closely related metabolic enzymes and antibacterial drug targets.

Keywords: antibiotic; biotin; biotin protein ligase; *Staphylococcus aureus*; inhibitor design; X-ray crystallography; in situ click chemistry

1. Introduction

Infectious diseases caused by pathogenic bacteria, such as *Staphylococcus aureus*, are a major threat to human health. The spread of antibiotic resistant strains, such as methicillin resistant *S. aureus* (MRSA), is particularly problematic with resistance having been developed to most penicillin-based antibiotics [1,2]. Antibiotic resistance arises in two major subsets of MRSA, hospital acquired MRSA and community acquired MRSA. Both have been described over the past decade in the USA [3], UK [4] and Australia amongst other countries [5]. The impact of MRSA is overwhelming, as these infections are more difficult to treat with increased associated healthcare costs. In the USA alone, the cost to treat hospital acquired-MRSA stands at $USD 9.7 billion annually [6], and community acquired-MRSA accounts for 18% of all MRSA incidents [3]. Overall, these factors have contributed to an increase in the mortality rate due to MRSA infections worldwide [7]. One critical strategy to combat drug resistant *S. aureus* is to develop new classes of antibacterials that are not subject to pre-existing resistance mechanisms [8]. This review presents biotin protein ligase (BPL) as a novel drug target, and discusses the design of small molecule inhibitors for antibacterial discovery.

2. Biotin Protein Ligase as a Novel Antibacterial Target

BPL, a vital enzyme present in all organisms, is responsible for the post-translational attachment of biotin 1 onto a specific lysine residue present in the active site of biotin-dependent enzymes, as shown in Scheme 1 [9,10]. *S. aureus* expresses two such enzymes, namely acetyl CoA carboxylase (ACC) [11] and pyruvate carboxylase (PC) [12], which are known to catalyze key reactions in important metabolic pathways. ACC is a critical enzyme for the carboxylation of acetyl-CoA to malonyl-CoA in fatty acid biosynthesis that is essential for cell membrane biogenesis and maintenance [13]. Biotin-activated PC is involved in the conversion of pyruvate to oxaloacetate required in the citric acid cycle that is central to a number of key metabolic pathways, such as gluconeogenesis and amino acid biosynthesis [14]. These metabolic pathways are essential for the survival and virulence of *S. aureus*, and, as such, BPL presents as an attractive drug target for new antibacterial drugs. Moreover, genetic knockout studies on various bacteria, including *S. aureus* [15,16], abolished cell growth in the absence of the *bpl* gene, highlighting that an alternative pathway for protein biotinylation does not exist in bacteria.

BPL acts as a transcriptional repressor [17–19] in addition to its pivotal role in the activation of ACC and PC. In the absence of non-biotinylated biotin-dependent enzymes, *S. aureus* BPL (*Sa*BPL) can form a dimer that is responsive to DNA binding. The *Sa*BPL dimer is a transcriptional repressor that controls the uptake and biosynthesis of biotin by binding specific DNA sequences in the promoters of the genes encoding these proteins. Therefore, BPL not only utilizes biotin, but it is also the key regulator that co-ordinates the import and synthesis of biotin in response to cellular demand. This bifunctionality makes BPL an attractive drug target as *S. aureus* is unlikely to readily develop target based resistance through mutation due to the intimate role played by BPL in multiple metabolic pathways [19].

Step 1

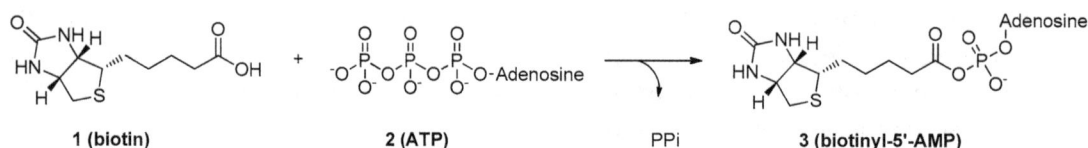

Step 2

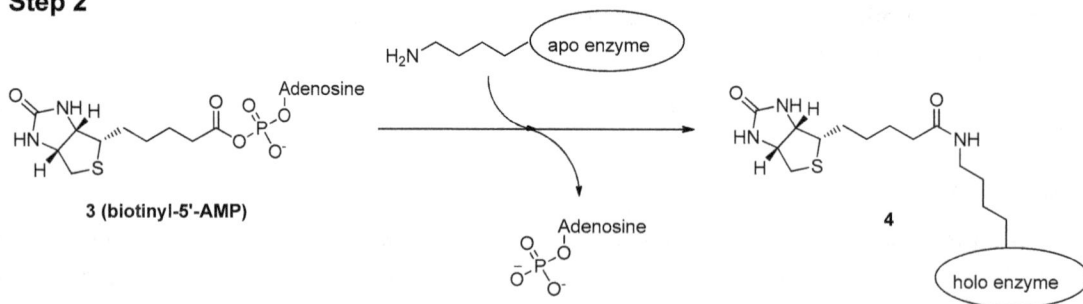

Scheme 1. The catalytic mechanism of protein biotinylation catalyzed by biotin protein ligase (BPL).

3. Mechanism of Protein Biotinylation

BPL catalyzes protein biotinylation through a two-step reaction mechanism, as shown in Scheme 1 [10,20]. In the first step, BPL catalyzes a condensation reaction between biotin 1 and ATP 2 to form the reaction intermediate biotinyl-5'-AMP 3, with the release of pyrophosphate (PPi). During this first step, biotin 1 binds to the biotin-binding pocket in BPL, which induces ordering of a biotin-binding loop within the enzyme (Figure 1). This disordered-to-ordered conformational change positions a key tryptophan residue (Trp127) in the active site, thereby creating the nucleotide binding pocket that facilitates binding of ATP 2. Reaction of biotin with the α-phosphate of ATP then produces the intermediate biotinyl-5′-AMP 3 to complete the first partial reaction. The complex of BPL with biotinyl-5′-AMP 3 then forms a protein: protein interaction with the unliganded biotin-dependent enzyme (i.e., the apo enzyme in Figure 1) to allow biotinyl transfer in the second partial reaction. During this final step, biotin is attached to the ε-amino group of the target lysine residue present in apo protein substrate to afford biotinylated ACC or PC (4, i.e., the holo enzyme in Figure 1), with the release of AMP. This reaction mechanism is conserved in all species, suggesting a high degree of homology amongst different BPL enzymes [21–23].

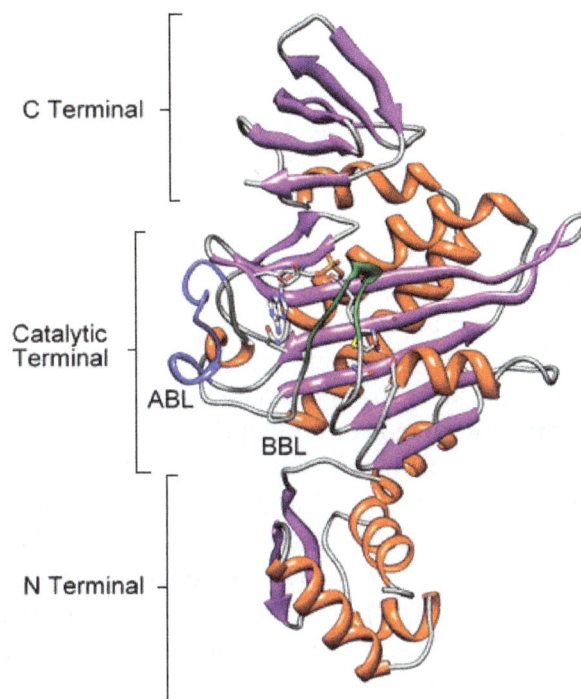

Figure 1. 3D depiction of *Sa*BPL with biotinyl-5′-AMP 3 bound (PDB: 3V8L). The β sheets are shown in purple, α helices in orange, biotin-binding loop in green and ATP-binding loop in blue.

4. BPL Structure

BPL can be divided into three distinct structural classes, as depicted in Figure 2. Classes I and II include BPLs from Archaea, prokaryotes and plants. Class III contains BPLs from yeast, insects and mammals. All three classes of BPLs contain a conserved catalytic domain and a C-terminal cap domain that are essential for protein biotinylation [21]. Class I BPLs consists solely of the conserved catalytic and C-terminal domains. Class II BPLs contain an additional N-terminal domain that facilitates binding to DNA in the regulation of cellular uptake of biotin and biosynthesis of biotin, as described above. Class III BPLs have a larger N-terminal extension that is distinct from the DNA-binding domain of class II enzymes [24–27]. X-ray crystal structures of class I BPLs from *Mycobacteria tuberculosis* [28], *Aquifex aeolicus* [29] and *Pyrococcus horikoshii* [10], and class II BPL from *S. aureus* [30] and *Escherichia coli* [20] have been reported. An examination of these structural data reveals that all BPLs adopt a highly conserved protein fold within the catalytic domain. Of particular note are the biotin-binding loop (highlighted in green in Figure 1) and an ATP-binding loop (highlighted by blue ribbons in Figure 1) that are responsible for the ordered binding mechanism described above. A closer examination of these structural features is detailed below, with a view to designing inhibitors that can occupy the BPL active site.

Class I

Eg *M. tuberculosis*

Class II

Bifunctional proteins
Eg *E. coli, S. aureus*

DNA binding

Class III

Eg *Homo sapiens*

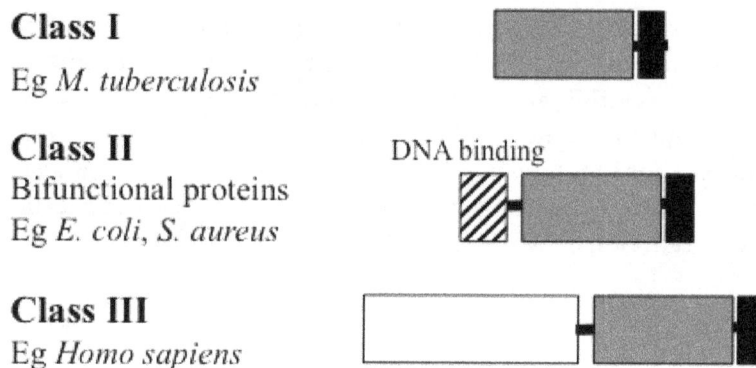

Figure 2. Schematic diagram of the three classes of BPL. The conserved catalytic (grey) and C-terminal domains (black) are highlighted. The relative sizes of the N-terminal extensions on class II and class III BPLs are represented.

Catalytic Domain

As mentioned above, the catalytic domain of BPL contains two major ligand-binding pockets, one for biotin and the other ATP. The biotin-binding site consists of two distinct regions, a hydrophobic wall to accommodate the valeric acid chain on biotin and a glycine rich hydrophilic pocket to accommodate the heterocycle of biotin. Multiple hydrogen bonds are formed between the ureido ring of biotin and amino acid residues in the hydrophilic region of *Sa*BPL [31], namely Ser92, Thr93, Gln115 and Arg119, as depicted in Figure 3. These residues are highly conserved in BPLs from all species [32]. Biotin forms additional hydrophobic interactions with Trp127 and Gly209. The carbon chain on the valeric acid tail of biotin is orientated to a hydrophobic tunnel consisting of Gly118, Gly209, Gly188, Leu191 and Ile208 by induced fit binding of biotin in the first catalytic step of BPL [21,22]. The biotin-binding loop is believed to enclose the active site, thereby preventing the dissociation of ligand from the active site. Structural analysis with all the available crystal structures reveals a high degree of conservation in the biotin-binding pocket, as highlighted in Figure 3.

A highly conserved phosphate-binding domain is located between the biotin and ATP binding pockets of *Sa*BPL. A number of hydrogen bonds are observed between the phosphoroanhydride linker of biotinyl-5′-AMP 3 and the side chains of Lys187 and Arg125, as well as the backbone of Arg122 (Figure 4) [31]. The conserved "Gly-Arg-Gly-Arg[122]-X" motif present in the biotin-binding loop is critical in stabilizing binding of biotinyl-5′-AMP 3 by shielding it from solvent [20]. Of particular note is Arg122, which is central to a complex network of water-mediated hydrogen bonds with the side chain of Asp180 (Figure 4) [31,32]. This observation is also supported by studies with *E. coli* BPL where a point mutation of the equivalent residue (Arg118) results in dissociation rates enhanced by 100-fold for biotin 1 and 400-fold for biotinyl-5′-AMP 3 [32]. Mutation of Arg122 to glycine results in a "leaky phenotype" that has been exploited using in situ click chemistry to develop BPL inhibitors (described later) [33].

The previously mentioned, induced-fit binding of the biotin-binding loop (highlighted in green as in Figure 4) orientates the side chain of Trp127 of *Sa*BPL such that it creates a binding pocket for nucleotide binding. This binding is stabilized by a displaced parallel π interaction between the adenine ring of ATP and the indole ring of Trp127 [32,34]. It is noteworthy that this key binding interaction does not occur in the absence of biotin [10]. A number of hydrogen bonds are also observed between the adenine ring of ATP and Asn212 and Ser128 at the base of the ATP-binding pocket (Figure 5). Following ATP binding, the previously discussed condensation reaction between biotin and ATP occurs to give biotinyl-5′-AMP 3 [31]. The reaction intermediate adopts a distinctive "U-shaped" geometry so the biotinyl and adenyl moieties can bind in their respective binding pockets. The ATP-binding loop (highlighted in blue in Figure 5) helps to stabilize the reaction intermediate (3) via a disordered-to-ordered conformational change. Here, the ATP-binding loop folds over the adenosine moiety of 3 with associated hydrophobic interactions with 3 through Ile224, Ala228 and Phe220. This structural data provides a molecular explanation for the ordered ligand binding mechanism that is critical for the design of inhibitors.

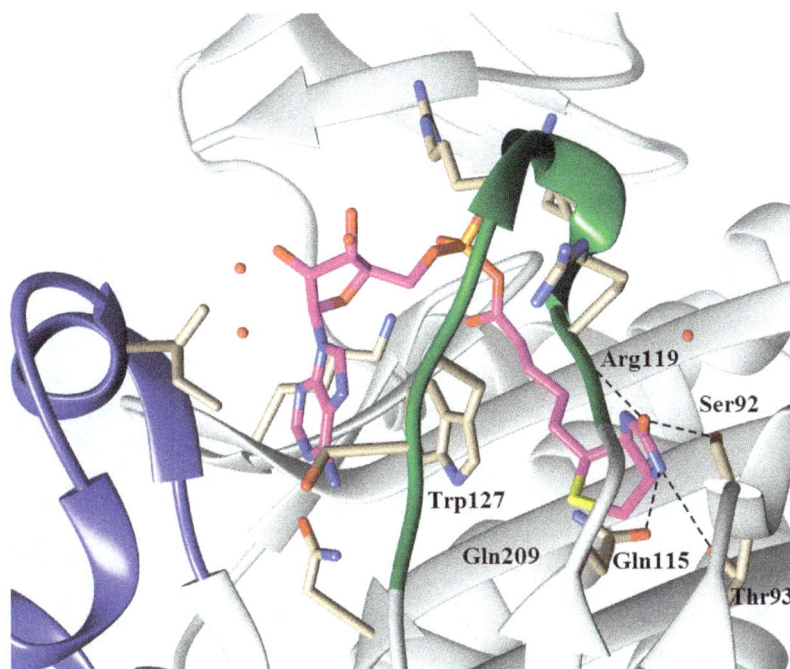

Figure 3. 3D depiction of reaction intermediate biotinyl-5′-AMP 3 (highlighted in magenta) bound to *Sa*BPL (PDB: 3V8L) with a close examination of the biotin-binding pocket. Green ribbon highlights the biotin-binding loop and black dashes indicating hydrogen-bonding interactions between the ureido ring of biotin and *Sa*BPL.

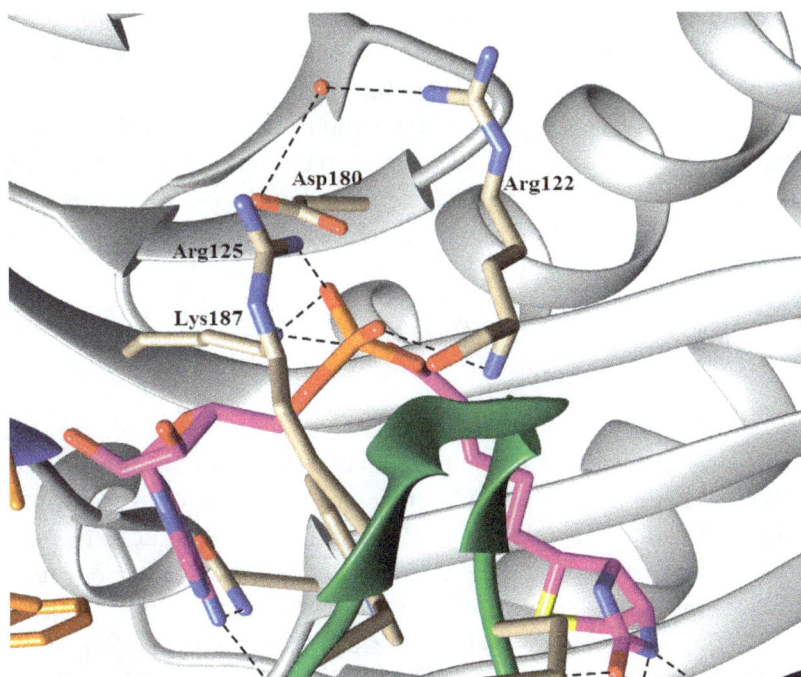

Figure 4. 3D depiction of reaction intermediate biotinyl-5′-AMP 3 (highlighted in magenta) bound to *Sa*BPL (PDB: 3V8L) with a close examination of the phosphate-binding pocket. The biotin-binding loop is shown in green.

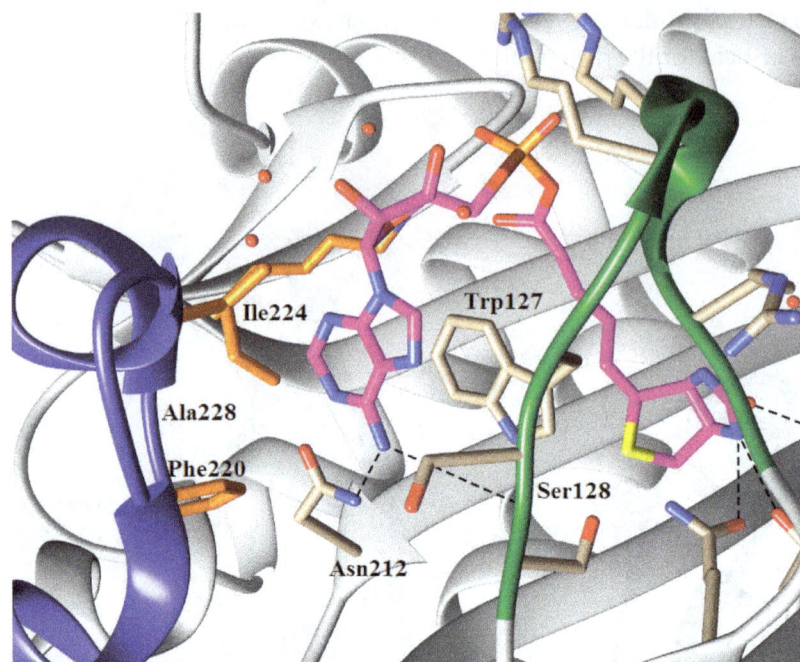

Figure 5. 3D depiction of reaction intermediate biotinyl-5'-AMP 3 (highlighted in magenta) bound to *Sa*BPL (PDB: 3V8L) with a close examination of the ATP-binding pocket. Green ribbon highlighting the biotin-binding loop and blue ribbon highlighting the ATP-binding loop [31].

5. BPL Inhibitors as New Antibacterials

*Sa*BPL is an attractive novel target for antibacterial development for three main reasons. Firstly, *Sa*BPL is the sole enzyme responsible for the biotinylation, and subsequent activation, of ACC and PC of *S. aureus* [35]. As these biotin-dependent enzymes play key roles in metabolic pathways critical for survival and virulence, BPL is an essential enzyme. Secondly, *Sa*BPL is the only enzyme in *S. aureus* responsible for regulation of biotin biosynthesis and import on cellular demand. Thus, targeting *Sa*BPL targets both the source of biotin and its utilization [17,18]. Thirdly, *Sa*BPL is not the target of any antibacterial currently in clinical use, thereby providing a novel mechanism of action. Recent structure-guided approaches to the design of small molecule inhibitors against *Sa*BPL have led to the discovery of BPL inhibitors that bind selectively to bacterial BPL over the human homolog. These studies are described further below.

5.1. Biotin Analogues as Antibacterial Agents

An effective approach to disrupt protein biotinylation is to design small molecule inhibitors that bind tightly and specifically to the active site of bacterial BPL, thereby blocking all protein biotinylation. For example, modification to the ureido and thiophene ring of biotin gave rise to analogues 5 and 6 as shown in Figure 6 [31]. The study revealed that BPLs were highly specific to the natural structure of biotin 1 and did not utilize other biotin analogues as substrates [31]. In addition, amino acid sequence alignments highlight that the biotin-binding pocket is highly conserved amongst BPLs from all species, including human [30,31,36]. This presents a challenge for the design of selective inhibitors that target bacterial BPLs over the human equivalent. Moreover, analysis of available X-ray structures reveals a relatively small biotin-binding pocket for *Sa*BPL, thereby restricting opportunities to chemically modify the heterocycles of biotin 1.

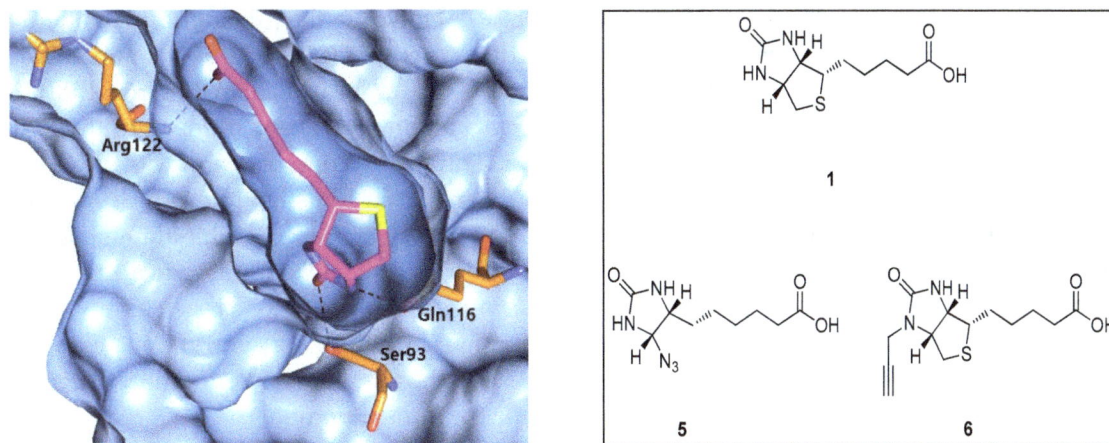

Figure 6. 3D depiction of biotin 1 (highlighted in magenta) bound to *Sa*BPL (PDB: 3V8K) with a side view of biotin binding pocket (**left**); Chemical structures of biotin 1 and its analogues 5 and 6 (**right**).

Specific chemical modification of the carboxyl group of biotin 1 gave rise to a series of BPL inhibitors 7–13 as shown in Table 1 [31]. These compounds contain a hydroxyl, alkane and alkyne in place of the carboxyl group of biotin 1. The alcohol derivative 7 was found to be equally active against *Sa*BPL and *E. coli* BPLs with a K_i between 3 and 4 μM. However, 7 displayed limited selectivity with only a 2.6-fold difference in K_i for *H. sapiens* BPL (*Hs*BPL) versus *Sa*BPL ($K_i \approx 9.0$ μM) [31]. The more hydrophobic analogues 9–13 were more selective, e.g., 10 displayed approximately 12-fold selectivity for *Sa*BPL compared to *Hs*BPL [31]. An X-ray structure of *Sa*BPL in complex with biotin alkene 12 revealed a key hydrophobic interaction between the terminal carbon on the ligand and the side-chain of Trp127. Interestingly, increasing the length of the alkyl chain by a single carbon as in 13, resulted in reduced potency, presumably due to the disruption of this key bonding interaction [31]. Overall, this study suggests that biotin derivatives with chemical modifications at the biotin heterocycles and the valeric acid moiety are not ideal for achieving optimal potency and selectivity towards *Sa*BPL. However, derivatives 11 and 12 do provide an important starting point for further inhibitor development as discussed in section 5.3 below.

Table 1. Biotin analogue series [30].

	n	R	*Sa*BPL K_i (μM)	*Ec*BPL K_i (μM)	*Hs*BPL K_i (μM)
7	2	OH	3.4	4.0	9.0
8	3	OH	>20	>20	>20
9	1	CH$_3$	0.05	1.1	0.1
10	2	CH$_3$	0.5	7.3	6.4
11	1	C≡C	0.08	0.9	0.2
12	2	C≡C	0.3	7.3	3.5
13	3	C≡C	2.4	20	12

5.2. BPL Reaction Intermediate Analogues as Antibacterial Agents

As discussed earlier, the first step of the BPL reaction yields biotinyl-5′-AMP 3. The acyl phosphate group of 3 can be replaced with the non-hydrolysable and enzymatically stable phosphodiester bioisostere as in biotinol-5′-AMP 14 (Figure 7, below) [37]. Biotinol-5′-AMP 14 proved to be a potent inhibitor of *Sa*BPL (K_i = 0.03 μM) while critically also possessing anti-*S. aureus* activity with a minimal inhibitory concentration of 1–8 μg/mL [38]. However, progressing biotinol-5′-AMP 14 as drug candidate is limited by its activity against *Hs*BPL with K_i = 0.42 μM and also difficulty of synthesis. Two other phosphonate-based isosteres, as in 15 and 16, respectively, were initially developed by Sittiwong et al. for investigation of *Hs*BPL [39]. However, the β-ketophosphonate 15 and β-hydroxyphosphonate 16 analogues both showed reduced activity (IC_{50} of 39.7 μM and 203.7 μM, respectively) against *Hs*BPL compared to biotinol-5′-AMP 14 (IC_{50} = 7 μM against human BPL) [39].

Brown and co workers [37,40] described a sulfamoyl analogue 17 as a mimetic of the natural reaction intermediate 3 (Figure 7). However, this analogue rapidly decomposes and was thus difficult to assay [28,37]. A recent study identified sulfonamide analogue 18 as having improved stability compared to the sulfamoyl analogue 17 [28]. Significantly, 18 is a competitive inhibitor against biotin when assayed against *M. tuberculosis* BPL with an IC_{50} of 135 nM [28]. This analogue also displayed anti-mycobacterial activity against the virulent *M. tuberculosis* strain H37Rv as well as a number of multi-drug resistant *M. tuberculosis* strains, with a minimal inhibitory concentration ranging from 0.625 to 0.16 μM [28]. However, cytotoxicity was observed in the mammalian Vero cell line suggesting potential issue with selectivity for the bacterial BPL over the human homolog.

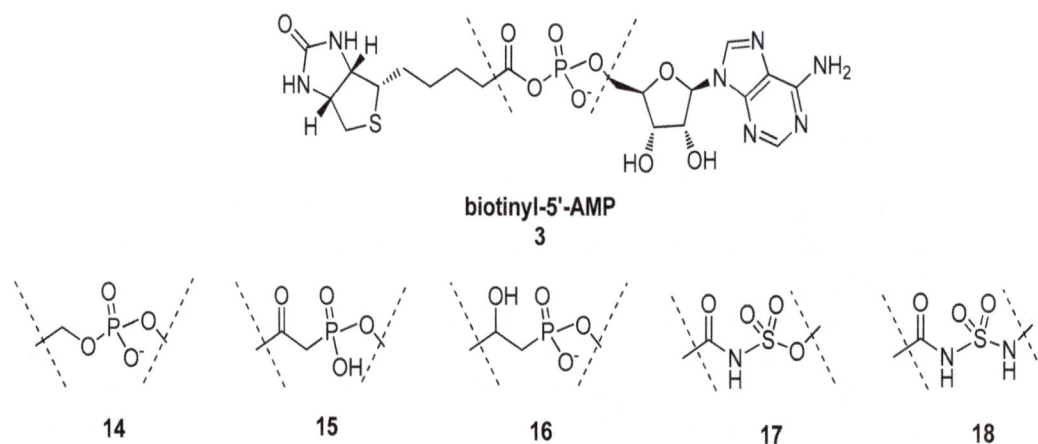

biotinyl-5'-AMP
3

14   **15**   **16**   **17**   **18**

Figure 7. Reaction intermediate biotinyl-5′-AMP 3 and its mimics, biotinol-5′-AMP 14, β-ketophosphonate 15, β-hydroxyphosphonate 16, acylsulfamate 17, and acylsulfonamide 18.

5.3. 1,2,3-Triazole Based Analogues

Soares da Costa et al. identified a 1,2,3-triazole as a new and effective bioisostere for the labile phosphoroanhydride linker of biotinyl-5′-AMP 3 [41]. A triazole offers a number of advantages over the natural phosphate linker of 3. It is stable to acid/base hydrolysis, reductive and oxidative conditions, as well as typical physiological conditions. This makes it resistant to metabolic degradation [42]. In addition, the 1,2,3-triazole motif has potential sites for hydrogen bonding (Figure 8), an ability to participate in π-π stacking interactions and it is easy to prepare.

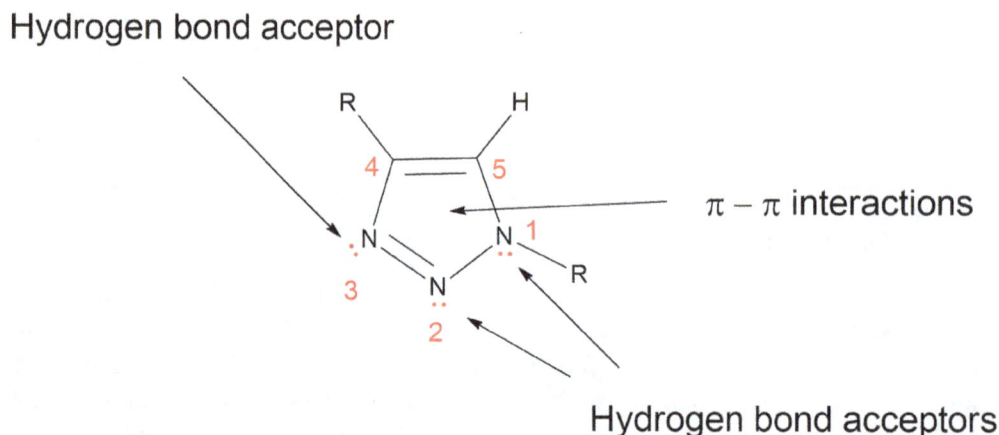

Figure 8. The assignment of 1,2,3-triazole with the potential intermolecular interaction sites.

A series of 1,2,3-triazole based analogues of 20–23 (see Scheme 2 and Figure 9) was synthesized by alkyne azide cycloaddition (CuAAC) and these were tested for inhibitory activity against *S. aureus* and human BPLs [41]. In particular, reaction of biotin acetylene 12 and adenosine azide 19 gave the 1,4 disubstituted triazole 20 which displayed modest activity against *Sa*BPL ($K_i = 1.8$ µM) but was effectively inactive against *Hs*BPL ($K_i > 33$ µM) in vitro [41]. This was an important finding as it represented the first example of a BPL inhibitor with high selectivity for *S. aureus* BPL over the human equivalent. In addition, the 1,4-triazole 20 was not toxic against mammalian HepG2 cells in culture. Importantly, the 1,5-triazole regioisomer 21 (Scheme 2) prepared via ruthenium alkyne azide cycloaddition (RuAAC) proved to be inactive against *Sa*BPL [41]. An X-ray crystallographic structure of *Sa*BPL in complex with 20 revealed that the 1,4-triazole provides the desired U-shape geometry on binding to *Sa*BPL, as observed for biotinyl-5′-AMP 3.

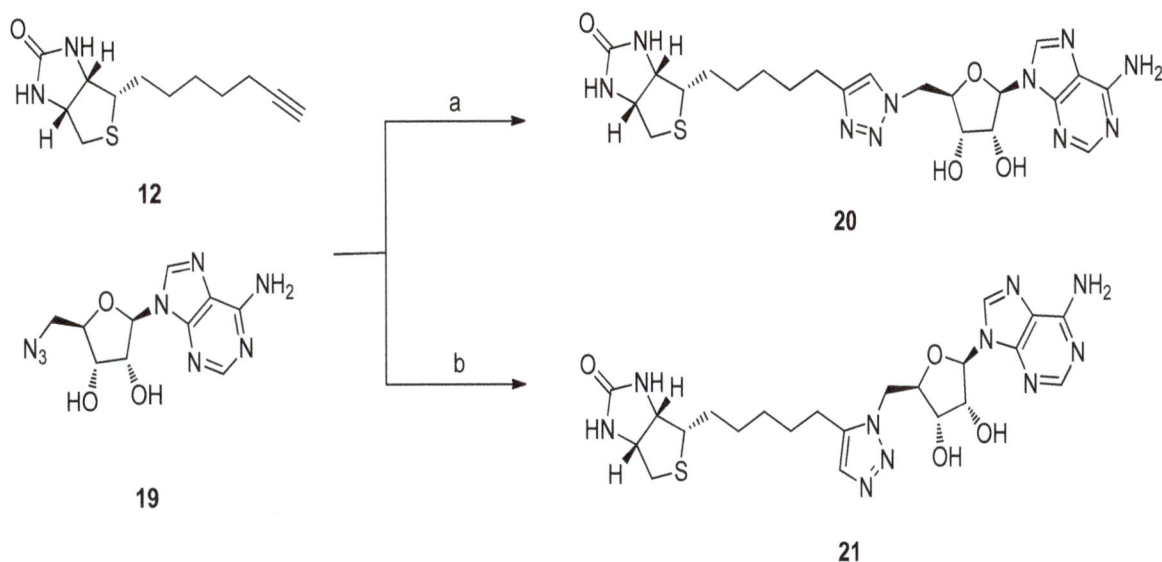

Scheme 2. Synthesis of 1,4-triazole 20 and 1,5-triazole 21 from biotin acetylene 12 and azide 19. Conditions and reagents. (**a**) (i) copper nano powder, 2:1 AcCN/H₂O, 4 h, sonication, 35 °C; (**b**) (i) Cp*RuCl(PPh₃)₂, 1:1 THF/DMF, 4 h, 70 °C.

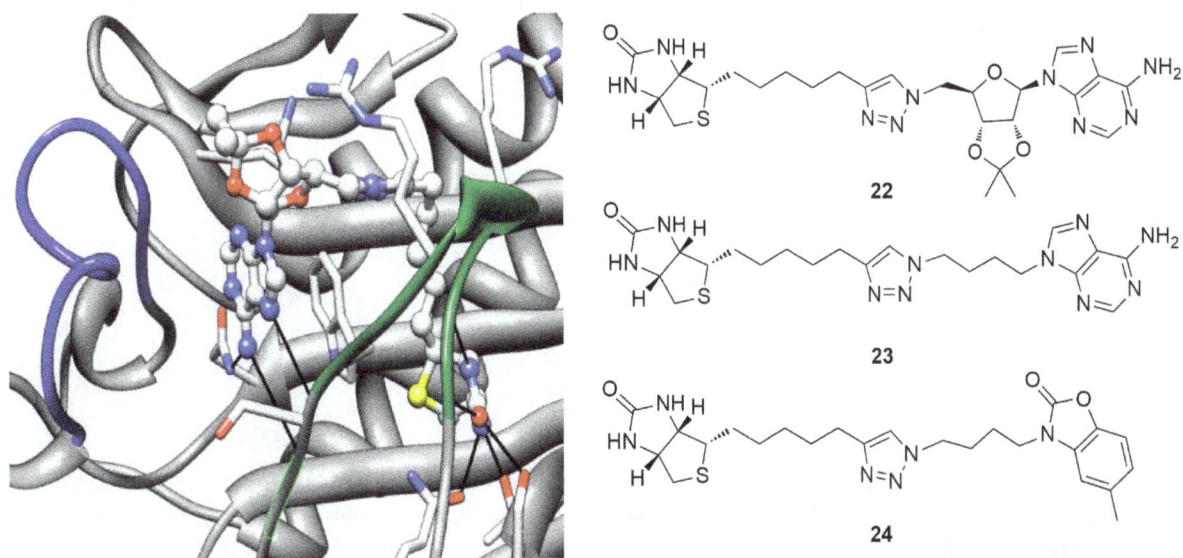

Figure 9. 3D depiction of 1,4-triazole 22 bound to *Sa*BPL (PDB: 3V7C) (**left**); Chemical structures of 1,2,3-triazole analogues: 1,4-triazole 22 and 1,4-triazole 23 (**right**).

Based on the above assessment, a new generation of *Sa*BPL inhibitors was designed to target the ATP-binding site. A detailed analysis of the crystal structure of 20 bound to *Sa*BPL revealed an absence of hydrogen bonding between the ribose moiety of 20 and *Sa*BPL (Figure 9) [33,41]. Gratifyingly, the 1,4-triazole analogue 23, which lacks the ribose group, proved to be more potent than 20 against *Sa*BPL with K_i of 0.7 µM [33] while retaining selectivity for the bacterial enzyme over the human homologue. Furthermore, the study also identified a biotin 1,4-triazole analogue containing a 2-benzoxalone group as a mimic of the adenine of 23 to target the ATP-binding pocket [41]. The 2-benzoxazolone containing 1,4-triazole 24 proved to be the most potent *Sa*BPL inhibitor with a $K_i = 0.09$ µM [41]. Significantly, 24 exhibited >1100 fold selectivity for *Sa*BPL compared to human BPL. Thus, 24 represents the most potent and selective inhibitor of *Sa*BPL reported to date. Bacteriostatic activity was observed for 1,4-triazole 24 against *S. aureus* ATCC strain 49775, with the compound effectively reducing *S. aureus* cell growth by 80% at 8 µg/mL [41]. Both 1,4-triazoles 23 and 24 were not toxic in a cell culture model using HepG2 cells, highlighting these biotin triazoles as exciting hits for further antibiotic development [33,41].

6. In Situ Click Chemistry

In situ click chemistry has recently been reported as an alternative and more facile approach to optimize the biotin triazole series as inhibitors of *Sa*BPL [33,43–45]. Here, the target enzyme is used as a template to identify and bind optimum azide and acetylene fragments from a library of such structures. Once each azide and acetylene bind to their respective pockets, a cycloaddition reaction occurs in the absence of external catalysts (i.e., copper or ruthenium) to assemble the triazole. Moreover, as the biological target is actively involved in selecting its most potent inhibitor from a library of precursors, in situ click chemistry is able to circumvent the need to individually synthesize and screen all possible triazole combinations [46–48]. The BPL is only one of a select few examples of enzymes shown to catalyse the alkene azide cycloaddition reaction, as exemplified with biotin acetylene 12 and adenosine azide 19 in Scheme 3 [33]. This is possible because *Sa*BPL contains two well defined binding pockets, one capable of binding a biotin analogue and the other an adenine analogue, as revealed in the before mentioned X-ray structures.

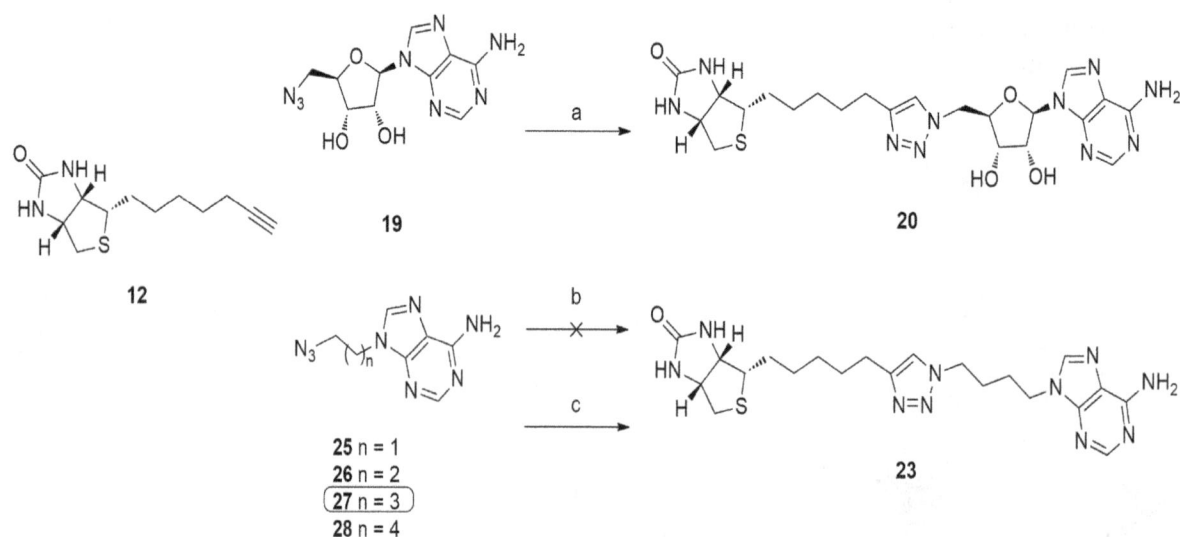

Scheme 3. (**a**) In situ click reactions of acetylene 12 with azides 19 in the presence of wild type *Sa*BPL, 1,4-triazole 20 was confirmed by HPLC; (**b**) In situ click reactions of acetylene 12 with azides 25–28 in the presence of wild type *Sa*BPL, no triazole products were observed by HPLC; (**c**) In situ click reactions of acetylene 12 with azides 25–28 in the presence of *Sa*BPL Arg122-Gly, 1,4-triazole 23 was confirmed by HPLC.

An initial in situ click reaction was performed between biotin acetylene 12 (K_i = 0.3 µM) and adenosine azide 19 using wild type SaBPL as a template in an attempt to form 20 (Scheme 3). Analysis of the reaction mixture by HPLC and mass spectrometry revealed 1.07 ± 0.1 mol of triazole 20 was formed per mol of SaBPL [33]. The triazole formed by SaBPL is presumed to be the 1,4-triazole 20 (K_i = 1.18 µM), given that the 1,5-triazole 21 (see Scheme 2) had earlier been shown to be inactive against SaBPL [41]. An in situ experiment was then performed between biotin acetylene 12 and a small library of azides (25–28), as shown in Scheme 3. The azide 19 was used as a reference, while 25–28 were designed to probe the importance of the furanose ring and also the length of the azide spacer with regards to potency. However, in this case triazole products were not detected by HPLC. This likely reflects a low turnover rate for the native BPL.

Attention was then focused upon improving the catalytic efficiency of the target enzyme, SaBPL. The structural biology demonstrated that the before mentioned biotin-binding loop closes over the active site to prevent diffusion of the synthesized triazole from the active site and thereby preventing efficient turnover [33]. Of particular significance is Arg122, which is known to stabilize the "closed" conformation through a complex network of interactions with amino acid residues in the SaBPL dimer interface and the C-terminal domain, as well as a water-mediated hydrogen bond with Asp180 [23,41]. It was proposed that an engineered variant of SaBPL, with Arg122 substituted by glycine, would improve production of triazole 20 by increasing the enzyme's turnover rate. This proposal is supported by studies with Escherichia coli BPL that have demonstrated that mutation of the equivalent residue (Arg118) results in enhanced dissociation rates for both biotin and biotinyl-5′-AMP [33].

A subsequent in situ click reaction of biotin alkyne 12 and azide 19 with SaBPL-Arg122Gly gave vastly improved formation of triazole 20 (11.9 ± 0.7 moles per mol of enzyme) [33]. This clearly demonstrated that the mutant enzyme provides a template for cycloaddition, with an increased turnover rate compared to the wild-type enzyme. The "leaky mutant" thus provided much improved efficiency of reaction and sensitivity of detection. The library experiment using biotin alkyne 12 and azides 25–28 was repeated using the "leaky mutant". Analysis of the product mixture by HPLC and LC/MS revealed efficient formation of 1,4-triazole 23 with a smaller quantity of a second 1,4-triazole 20 detected by MS but not HPLC. This observation was consistent with other multi-component in situ experiments where the higher affinity triazoles are formed to a greater extent. In our case, there is an overwhelming bias towards the formation of the more potent triazole 23 (K_i = 0.66 ± 0.1 µM) over triazole 20 (K_i = 1.83 ± 0.3 µM) [33,41]. None of the other possible triazole products were detected. This methodology provides a powerful tool for the identification of new inhibitors that target the BPL active site from libraries of precursor fragments. In addition, the study represents an important advance in in situ inhibitor optimization, where it was shown for the first time that a target enzyme can be engineered to improve efficiency and hence utility in such studies.

7. Future Directions

The emergence of bacteria resistant to chemotherapy is rendering our current arsenal of antibiotics less effective and in certain cases totally ineffectual. An important approach to address drug resistance is to develop new antibiotic classes that work through novel modes of action and that are not subject to existing resistance mechanisms. BPL inhibitors presents one such promising example as it is not the target of any chemotherapeutic currently in clinical use, thereby providing a novel mechanism of action. Importantly, we have identified a novel class of 1,2,3-triazole based BPL inhibitor (23 and 24) that (1) with a unique mode of antibacterial action; (2) unique selectivity for the bacterial BPL target over the human isozyme; (3) have antimicrobial activity against S. aureus; and (4) does not show toxicity either against a cultured human cell line or preliminary studies in rodent models. New analogues with improved solubility and/or new formulations are required to continue the development of lead compounds 23 and 24 towards pre-clinical antibacterial candidates.

The biotin triazole pharmacophore provides a valuable starting point for the chemical optimization of improved BPL inhibitors. X-ray analysis of lead compounds 23 and 24 bound to

*Sa*BPL reveal that the adenosine and benzoxalone moieties bind into the nucleotide-binding pocket of the drug target. However, these approaches yield compounds with molecular masses greater than the 500 limit proposed as being optimum by Lipinski for drug-like candidates. One current strategy is to identify smaller structures that specifically bind into the ribose-binding pocket of *Sa*BPL. This latter approach with simplified structures is being pursued with the goal of optimizing simplified structures with greater drug-like properties and improved solubility. Moreover, we are extending our "smart" in situ click chemistry as an alternative approach to inhibitor optimization using our leaky mutant of the target enzyme (BPL) and new chemically diverse libraries of acetylene and azide coupling partners. These approaches provide valuable tools to aid in the development of new inhibitors against the BPLs of other clinically important bacteria and fungi. Furthermore, other enzymes that are targets for other diseases beyond antibacterial discovery can adopt the in situ guided approaches for inhibitor discovery we describe here for BPL. Particularly amendable to these methods are other ligases that synthesize an adenylated reaction intermediate from an organic acid and ATP, analogous to the BPL reaction mechanism. Of importance are ligases such as amino-acyl tRNA synthethases [49–51], bi-functional salicyl-AMP ligase [52,53], indole-3-acetic acid-amido synthetase [54] and pantothenate synthetase [55,56].

Acknowledgments: This work was supported by the National Health and Medical Research Council of Australia (application APP1068885), the Centre for Molecular Pathology, University of Adelaide, and Adelaide Research and Innovation's Commercial Accelerator Scheme. We are grateful to the Wallace and Carthew families for their financial support of this work.

Author Contributions: Jiage Feng, Andrew D. Abell and Steven W. Polyak wrote the paper. Critical proof reading and development of the project was provided by all authors.

Abbreviations

The following abbreviations are used in this manuscript:

ACC	Acetyl CoA carboxylase
AMP	Adenosine-5′-monophosphate
ATP	Adenosine-5′-triphosphate
BPL	Biotin protein ligase
CuAAC	Copper mediated alkyne azide cycloaddition
HPLC	High-performance liquid chromatography
*Hs*BPL	*Homo sapiens* biotin protein ligase
K_i	Inhibition constant
MRSA	Methicillin resistant *S. aureus*
PC	Pyruvate carboxylase
RuAAC	Ruthenium mediated Alkyne Azide cycloaddition
*Sa*BPL	*Staphylococcus aureus* biotin protein ligase

References

1. Boucher, H.W.; Talbot, G.H.; Bradley, J.S.; Edwards, J.E.; Gilbert, D.; Rice, L.B.; Scheld, M.; Spellberg, B.; Bartlett, J. Bad bugs, no drugs: No eskape! An update from the Infectious Diseases Society of America. *Clin. Infect. Dis.* **2009**, *48*, 1–12. [CrossRef] [PubMed]

2. Lewis, K. Antibiotics: Recover the lost art of drug discovery. *Nature* **2012**, *485*, 439–440. [CrossRef] [PubMed]

3. Kallen, A.J.; Mu, Y.; Bulens, S.; Reingold, A.; Petit, S.; Gershman, K.; Ray, S.M.; Harrison, L.H.; Lynfield, R.; Dumyati, G.; et al. Health care-associated invasive MRSA infections, 2005–2008. *J. Am. Med. Assoc.* **2010**, *304*, 641–647. [CrossRef] [PubMed]

4. Pearson, A.; Chronias, A.; Murray, M. Voluntary and mandatory surveillance for methicillin-resistant *Staphylococcus aureus* (MRSA) and methicillin-susceptible *S. aureus* (MSSA) bacteraemia in England. *J. Antimicrob. Chemother.* **2009**, *64*, i11–i17. [CrossRef] [PubMed]

5. Ferguson, J. Healthcare-associated methicillin-resistant Staph aureus (MRSA) control in Australia and New Zealand—2007 Australasian Society for Infectious Diseases (ASID) conference forum convened by healthcare infection control special interest group (HICSIG). *Healthc. Infect.* **2007**, *12*, 60–66. [CrossRef]

6. Klein, E.; Smith, D.; Laxminarayan, R. Hospitalizations and deaths caused by methicillin-resistant *Staphylococcus aureus*, United States. *Emerg. Infect. Dis. J.* **2007**, *13*, 1840–1846. [CrossRef] [PubMed]

7. Holmes, N.E.; Turnidge, J.D.; Munckhof, W.J.; Robinson, J.O.; Korman, T.M.; O'Sullivan, M.V.; Anderson, T.L.; Roberts, S.A.; Gao, W.; Christiansen, K.J. Antibiotic choice may not explain poorer outcomes in patients with *Staphylococcus aureus* bacteremia and high vancomycin minimum inhibitory concentrations. *J. Infect. Dis.* **2011**, *204*, 340–347. [CrossRef] [PubMed]

8. Fischbach, M.A.; Walsh, C.T. Antibiotics for emerging pathogens. *Science* **2009**, *325*, 1089–1093. [CrossRef] [PubMed]

9. Pendini, N.R.; Bailey, L.M.; Booker, G.W.; Wilce, M.; Wallace, J.C.; Polyak, S.W. Microbial biotin protein ligases aid in understanding holocarboxylase synthetase deficiency. *Biochim. Biophys. Acta Prot. Proteom.* **2008**, *784*, 973–982. [CrossRef] [PubMed]

10. Bagautdinov, B.; Kuroishi, C.; Sugahara, M.; Kunishima, N. Crystal structures of biotin protein ligase from *Pyrococcus horikoshii* OT3 and its complexes: Structural basis of biotin activation. *J. Mol. Biol.* **2005**, *353*, 322–333. [CrossRef] [PubMed]

11. Polyak, S.W.; Abell, A.D.; Wilce, M.C.J.; Zhang, L.; Booker, G.W. Structure, function and selective inhibition of bacterial acetyl CoA carboxylase. *Appl. Microbiol. Biotechnol.* **2012**, *93*, 983–992. [CrossRef] [PubMed]

12. Arpornsuwan, T.; Carey, K.J.; Stojkoski, C.; Booker, G.W.; Polyak, S.W.; Wallace, J.C. Localization of inhibitory antibodies to the biotin domain of human pyruvate carboxylase. *Hybridoma* **2012**, *31*, 305–313. [CrossRef] [PubMed]

13. Salaemae, W.; Azhar, A.; Booker, G.W.; Polyak, S.W. Biotin biosynthesis in *Mycobacterium tuberculosis*: Physiology, biochemistry and molecular intervention. *Protein Cell* **2011**, *2*, 691–695. [CrossRef] [PubMed]

14. Wallace, J.C.; Jitrapakdee, S.; Chapman-Smith, A. Pyruvate carboxylase. *Int. J. Biochem. Cell Biol.* **1998**, *30*, 1–5. [CrossRef]

15. Payne, D.J.; Gwynn, M.N.; Holmes, D.J.; Pompliano, D.L. Drugs for bad bugs: Confronting the challenges of antibacterial discovery. *Nat. Rev. Drug Discov.* **2007**, *6*, 29–40. [CrossRef] [PubMed]

16. Forsyth, R.; Haselbeck, R.J.; Ohlsen, K.L.; Yamamoto, R.T.; Xu, H.; Trawick, J.D.; Wall, D.; Wang, L.; Brown-Driver, V.; Froelich, J.M. A genome-wide strategy for the identification of essential genes in *Staphylococcus aureus*. *Mol. Microbiol.* **2002**, *43*, 1387–1400. [CrossRef] [PubMed]

17. Abbott, J.; Beckett, D. Cooperative binding of the *Escherichia coli* repressor of biotin biosynthesis to the biotin operator sequence. *Biochemistry* **1993**, *32*, 9649–9656. [CrossRef] [PubMed]

18. Rodionov, D.A.; Mironov, A.A.; Gelfand, M.S. Conservation of the biotin regulon and the BirA regulatory signal in eubacteria and archaea. *Genome Res.* **2002**, *12*, 1507–1516. [CrossRef] [PubMed]

19. Beckett, D. Biotin sensing at the molecular level. *J. Nutr.* **2009**, *139*, 167–170. [CrossRef] [PubMed]

20. Wood, Z.A.; Weaver, L.H.; Brown, P.H.; Beckett, D.; Matthews, B.W. Co-repressor induced order and biotin repressor dimerization: A case for divergent followed by convergent evolution. *J. Mol. Biol.* **2006**, *357*, 509–523. [CrossRef] [PubMed]

21. Chapman-Smith, A.; Cronan, J.E., Jr. In vivo enzymatic protein biotinylation. *Biomol. Eng.* **1999**, *16*, 119–125. [CrossRef]

22. Bagautdinov, B.; Matsuura, Y.; Bagautdinova, S.; Kunishima, N. Protein biotinylation visualized by a complex structure of biotin protein ligase with a substrate. *J. Biol. Chem.* **2008**, *283*, 14739–14750. [CrossRef] [PubMed]

23. Paparella, A.S.; Soares da Costa, T.P.; Yap, M.Y.; Tieu, W.; Wilce, M.C.; Booker, G.W.; Abell, A.D.; Polyak, S.W. Structure guided design of biotin protein ligase inhibitors for antibiotic discovery. *Curr. Top. Med. Chem.* **2014**, *14*, 4–20. [CrossRef] [PubMed]

24. Mayende, L.; Swift, R.D.; Bailey, L.M.; da Costa, T.P.S.; Wallace, J.C.; Booker, G.W.; Polyak, S.W. A novel molecular mechanism to explain biotin-unresponsive holocarboxylase synthetase deficiency. *J. Mol. Med.* **2012**, *90*, 81–88. [CrossRef] [PubMed]

25. Polyak, S.W.; Chapman-Smith, A.; Brautigan, P.J.; Wallace, J.C. Biotin protein ligase from *Saccharomyces cerevisiae*: The N-terminal domain is required for complete activity. *J. Biol. Chem.* **1999**, *274*, 32847–32854. [CrossRef] [PubMed]

26. Pendini, N.R.; Bailey, L.M.; Booker, G.W.; Wilce, M.C.; Wallace, J.C.; Polyak, S.W. Biotin protein ligase from Candida albicans: Expression, purification and development of a novel assay. *Arch. Biochem. Biophys.* **2008**, *479*, 163–169. [CrossRef] [PubMed]

27. Campeau, E.; Gravel, R.A. Expression in *Escherichia coli* of N- and C-terminally deleted human holocarboxylase synthetase influence of the N-terminus on biotinylation and identification of a minimum functional protein. *J. Biol. Chem.* **2001**, *276*, 12310–12316. [CrossRef] [PubMed]

28. Duckworth, B.P.; Geders, T.W.; Tiwari, D.; Boshoff, H.I.; Sibbald, P.A.; Barry, C.E., 3rd; Schnappinger, D.; Finzel, B.C.; Aldrich, C.C. Bisubstrate adenylation inhibitors of biotin protein ligase from *Mycobacterium tuberculosis*. *Chem. Biol.* **2011**, *18*, 1432–1441. [CrossRef] [PubMed]

29. Tron, C.M.; McNae, I.W.; Nutley, M.; Clarke, D.J.; Cooper, A.; Walkinshaw, M.D.; Baxter, R.L.; Campopiano, D.J. Structural and functional studies of the biotin protein ligase from *Aquifex aeolicus* reveal a critical role for a conserved residue in target specificity. *J. Mol. Biol.* **2009**, *387*, 129–146. [CrossRef] [PubMed]

30. Pendini, N.R.; Yap, M.Y.; Polyak, S.W.; Cowieson, N.P.; Abell, A.; Booker, G.W.; Wallace, J.C.; Wilce, J.A.; Wilce, M.C. Structural characterization of *Staphylococcus aureus* biotin protein ligase and interaction partners: An antibiotic target. *Protein Sci.* **2013**, *22*, 762–773. [CrossRef] [PubMed]

31. Soares da Costa, T.P.; Tieu, W.; Yap, M.Y.; Zvarec, O.; Bell, J.M.; Turnidge, J.D.; Wallace, J.C.; Booker, G.W.; Wilce, M.C.; Abell, A.D. Biotin analogues with antibacterial activity are potent inhibitors of biotin protein ligase. *ACS Med. Chem. Lett.* **2012**, *3*, 509–514. [CrossRef] [PubMed]

32. Kwon, K.; Beckett, D. Function of a conserved sequence motif in biotin holoenzyme synthetases. *Protein Sci.* **2000**, *9*, 1530–1539. [CrossRef] [PubMed]

33. Tieu, W.; Soares da Costa, T.P.; Yap, M.Y.; Keeling, K.L.; Wilce, M.C.; Wallace, J.C.; Booker, G.W.; Polyak, S.W.; Abell, A.D. Optimising in situ click chemistry: The screening and identification of biotin protein ligase inhibitors. *Chem. Sci.* **2013**, *4*, 3533–3537. [CrossRef]

34. Naganathan, S.; Beckett, D. Nucleation of an allosteric response via ligand-induced loop folding. *J. Mol. Biol.* **2007**, *373*, 96–111. [CrossRef] [PubMed]

35. Rozwarski, D.A.; Vilchèze, C.; Sugantino, M.; Bittman, R.; Sacchettini, J.C. Crystal structure of the *Mycobacterium tuberculosis* enoyl-ACP reductase, InhA, in complex with NAD$^+$ and a C16 fatty acyl substrate. *J. Biol. Chem.* **1999**, *274*, 15582–15589. [CrossRef] [PubMed]

36. Chapman-Smith, A.; Cronan, J.E. The enzymatic biotinylation of proteins: A post-translational modification of exceptional specificity. *Trends Biochem. Sci.* **1999**, *24*, 359–363. [CrossRef]

37. Brown, P.H.; Cronan, J.E.; Grøtli, M.; Beckett, D. The biotin repressor: Modulation of allostery by corepressor analogs. *J. Mol. Biol.* **2004**, *337*, 857–869. [CrossRef] [PubMed]

38. Tieu, W.; Polyak, S.W.; Paparella, A.S.; Yap, M.Y.; Soares da Costa, T.P.; Ng, B.; Wang, G.; Lumb, R.; Bell, J.M.; Turnidge, J.D. Improved synthesis of biotinol-5'-AMP: Implications for antibacterial discovery. *ACS Med. Chem. Lett.* **2014**, *6*, 216–220. [CrossRef] [PubMed]

39. Sittiwong, W.; Cordonier, E.L.; Zempleni, J.; Dussault, P.H. B-keto and β-hydroxyphosphonate analogs of biotin-5'-AMP are inhibitors of holocarboxylase synthetase. *Bioorg. Med. Chem. Lett.* **2014**, *24*, 5568–5571. [CrossRef] [PubMed]

40. Brown, P.H.; Beckett, D. Use of binding enthalpy to drive an allosteric transition. *Biochemistry* **2005**, *44*, 3112–3121. [CrossRef] [PubMed]

41. Soares da Costa, T.P.; Tieu, W.; Yap, M.Y.; Pendini, N.R.; Polyak, S.W.; Sejer Pedersen, D.; Morona, R.; Turnidge, J.D.; Wallace, J.C.; Wilce, M.C.; et al. Selective inhibition of biotin protein ligase from *Staphylococcus aureus*. *J. Biol. Chem.* **2012**, *287*, 17823–17832. [CrossRef] [PubMed]

42. Rostovtsev, V.V.; Green, L.G.; Fokin, V.V.; Sharpless, K.B. A stepwise huisgen cycloaddition process: Copper (I)-catalyzed regioselective "ligation" of azides and terminal alkynes. *Angew. Chem.* **2002**, *114*, 2708–2711. [CrossRef]

43. Mamidyala, S.K.; Finn, M.G. In situ click chemistry: Probing the binding landscapes of biological molecules. *Chem. Soc. Rev.* **2010**, *39*, 1252–1261. [CrossRef] [PubMed]

44. Sharpless, K.B.; Manetsch, R. In situ click chemistry: A powerful means for lead discovery. *Expert Opin. Drug Discov.* **2006**, *1*, 525–538. [CrossRef] [PubMed]

45. Thirumurugan, P.; Matosiuk, D.; Jozwiak, K. Click chemistry for drug development and diverse chemical-biology applications. *Chem. Rev.* **2013**, *113*, 4905–4979. [CrossRef] [PubMed]

46. Krasiński, A.; Radić, Z.; Manetsch, R.; Raushel, J.; Taylor, P.; Sharpless, K.B.; Kolb, H.C. In situ selection of lead compounds by click chemistry: Target-guided optimization of acetylcholinesterase inhibitors. *J. Am. Chem. Soc.* **2005**, *127*, 6686–6692. [CrossRef] [PubMed]

47. Mocharla, V.P.; Colasson, B.; Lee, L.V.; Röper, S.; Sharpless, K.B.; Wong, C.-H.; Kolb, H.C. In situ click chemistry: Enzyme-generated inhibitors of carbonic anhydrase II. *Angew. Chem. Int. Ed.* **2005**, *44*, 116–120. [CrossRef] [PubMed]

48. Hirose, T.; Sunazuka, T.; Sugawara, A.; Endo, A.; Iguchi, K.; Yamamoto, T.; Ui, H.; Shiomi, K.; Watanabe, T.; Sharpless, K.B.; et al. Chitinase inhibitors: Extraction of the active framework from natural argifin and use of in situ click chemistry. *J. Antibiot.* **2009**, *62*, 277–282. [CrossRef] [PubMed]

49. Hurdle, J.G.; O'Neill, A.J.; Chopra, I. Prospects for aminoacyl-tRNA synthetase inhibitors as new antimicrobial agents. *Antimicrob. Agents Chemother.* **2005**, *49*, 4821–4833. [CrossRef] [PubMed]

50. Brown, M.J.B.; Mensah, L.M.; Doyle, M.L.; Broom, N.J.P.; Osbourne, N.; Forrest, A.K.; Richardson, C.M.; O'Hanlon, P.J.; Pope, A.J. Rational design of femtomolar inhibitors of isoleucyl tRNA synthetase from a binding model for pseudomonic acid-A. *Biochemistry* **2000**, *39*, 6003–6011. [CrossRef] [PubMed]

51. Brown, P.; Richardson, C.M.; Mensah, L.M.; O'Hanlon, P.J.; Osborne, N.F.; Pope, A.J.; Walker, G. Molecular recognition of tyrosinyl adenylate analogues by prokaryotic tyrosyl tRNA synthetases. *Bioorg. Med. Chem.* **1999**, *7*, 2473–2485. [CrossRef]

52. Somu, R.V.; Boshoff, H.; Qiao, C.; Bennett, E.M.; Barry, C.E.; Aldrich, C.C. Rationally designed nucleoside antibiotics that inhibit siderophore biosynthesis of *Mycobacterium tuberculosis. J. Med. Chem.* **2005**, *49*, 31–34. [CrossRef] [PubMed]

53. Ferreras, J.A.; Ryu, J.-S.; di Lello, F.; Tan, D.S.; Quadri, L.E.N. Small-molecule inhibition of siderophore biosynthesis in *Mycobacterium tuberculosis* and *Yersinia pestis. Nat. Chem. Biol.* **2005**, *1*, 29–32. [CrossRef] [PubMed]

54. Tuck, K.L.; Saldanha, S.A.; Birch, L.M.; Smith, A.G.; Abell, C. The design and synthesis of inhibitors of pantothenate synthetase. *Org. Biomol. Chem.* **2006**, *4*, 3598–3610. [CrossRef] [PubMed]

55. Ciulli, A.; Scott, D.E.; Ando, M.; Reyes, F.; Saldanha, S.A.; Tuck, K.L.; Chirgadze, D.Y.; Blundell, T.L.; Abell, C. Inhibition of *Mycobacterium tuberculosis* pantothenate synthetase by analogues of the reaction intermediate. *Chem. Bio. Chem.* **2008**, *9*, 2606–2611. [CrossRef] [PubMed]

56. Böttcher, C.; Dennis, E.G.; Booker, G.W.; Polyak, S.W.; Boss, P.K.; Davies, C. A novel tool for studying auxin-metabolism: The inhibition of grapevine indole-3-acetic acid-amido synthetases by a reaction intermediate analogue. *PLoS ONE* **2012**, *7*, e37632. [CrossRef] [PubMed]

12

First Description of Colistin and Tigecycline-Resistant *Acinetobacter baumannii* Producing KPC-3 Carbapenemase

Cátia Caneiras [1,2,*] ⓘ, **Filipa Calisto** [1,3] ⓘ, **Gabriela Jorge da Silva** [4], **Luis Lito** [5], **José Melo-Cristino** [5,6] **and Aida Duarte** [1] ⓘ

1. Microbiology and Immunology Department, Interdisciplinary Research Centre Egas Moniz (CiiEM), Faculty of Pharmacy, Universidade de Lisboa, 1649-003 Lisboa, Portugal; fcalisto@itqb.unl.pt (F.C.); aduarte@ff.ulisboa.pt (A.D.)
2. Institute of Environmental Health (ISAMB), Faculty of Medicine, Universidade de Lisboa, 1649-028 Lisboa, Portugal
3. Instituto de Tecnologia Química e Biológica António Xavier, Universidade Nova de Lisboa, 2780-157 Oeiras, Portugal
4. Faculty of Pharmacy, Universidade de Coimbra, Polo das Ciências da Saúde, Azinhaga de Santa Comba, 3000-548 Coimbra, Portugal; gjsilva@ci.uc.pt
5. Laboratory of Microbiology, Centro Hospitalar Lisboa Norte, 1649-035 Lisboa, Portugal; lmlito@chln.min-saude.pt (L.L.); melo_cristino@medicina.ulisboa.pt (J.M.-C.)
6. Institute of Microbiology, Institute of Molecular Medicine, Faculty of Medicine, Universidade de Lisboa, 1649-028 Lisboa, Portugal
* Correspondence: ccaneiras@gmail.com

Abstract: Herein, we describe a case report of carbapenem-resistant *Acinetobacter baumannii* and *Klebsiella pneumoniae* isolates that were identified from the same patient at a Tertiary University Hospital Centre in Portugal. Antimicrobial susceptibility and the molecular characterization of resistance and virulence determinants were performed. PCR screening identified the presence of the resistance genes bla_{KPC-3}, bla_{TEM-1} and bla_{SHV-1} in both isolates. The KPC-3 *K. pneumoniae* isolate belonged to the ST-14 high risk clone and accumulated an uncommon resistance and virulence profile additional to a horizontal dissemination capacity. In conclusion, the molecular screening led to the first identification of the *A. baumannii* KPC-3 producer in Portugal with a full antimicrobial resistance profile including tigecycline and colistin.

Keywords: antimicrobial resistance; Gram-negative bacteria; *K. pneumoniae*; *A. baumannii*; KPC-3 carbapenemase; colistin; tigecycline

---

1. Introduction

The acquisition and emergence of carbapenem resistance among Gram-negative bacteria (GNB) is a major cause of concern since carbapenems currently represent the treatment of choice for severe infections caused by multidrug-resistant (MDR) strains producing extended-spectrum β-lactamases (ESBL) which is a major global challenge in the treatment of these pathogens [1]. The carbapenemases frequently detected in *Enterobacteriaceae* are: (i) class A β-lactamases (e.g., *K. pneumoniae* carbapenemase; KPC); (ii) class B β-lactamases/metallo-β-lactamases (e.g., New Delhi metallo-β-lactamase-1; NDM-1) and (iii) class D β-lactamases (e.g., oxacillinase-48; OXA-48-like carbapenemases) [2,3]. Several reports have identified these plasmid-encoded carbapenemases worldwide but their prevalence varies geographically [2]. In 2017, the World Health Organization published a global priority pathogen list of antibiotic-resistant bacteria to help in prioritizing the research and development of new and effective antibiotic treatments. In this list, carbapenem-resistant *Enterobacteriaceae* and *Acinetobacter baumannii* are identified as two of the top three critical threats [4]. Antimicrobial resistance and bacterial virulence have developed on different timescales but they share some common characteristics and studies regarding the interplay between these factors are needed. Additionally, the development of new strategies involving new antimicrobial compounds, novel diagnostic methods that focus on high-risk clones and rapid tests to detect virulence markers may help to resolve the increasing problem of the association between virulence and resistance, which is becoming more beneficial for pathogenic bacteria with consequent therapeutic inefficacy [5]. Although great efforts have been made to enhance epidemiological surveillance in Europe, the detection of virulence traits and the molecular characterization of carbapenem-resistant isolates from some countries remain scarce.

This article aims to describe a case report of carbapenem-resistant *A. baumannii* and *K. pneumoniae* isolates that were identified from the same patient at a Tertiary University Hospital Centre in Portugal, leading, to the best of our knowledge, to the first description of the *A. baumannii* KPC-3 producer in Portugal.

2. Results

A 35-year-old Portuguese Caucasian female patient with a medical history of renal insufficiency was admitted to a Tertiary University Hospital Centre in Lisboa, Portugal at the beginning of January. At the end of the same month, the patient underwent gastro-enterotomy surgery. A carbapenem-resistant *K. pneumoniae* bacterial pathogen was identified in an infected wound at the beginning of February. One month later, a new surgery was done at the same general surgical ward. At the end of March, carbapenem-resistant *A. baumannii* was isolated from the same patient, also from an infected wound and in the same surgical department. Previous failed treatments with meropenem, linezolid and ciprofloxacin were documented. Considering the clinical instability of the patient, a prolonged hospitalization (from January to May) in the general surgery ward occurred. Despite all the efforts, the clinical condition worsened, an immunosuppression clinical state occurred and the patient died. Both clinical pathogens were preserved and sent to the Laboratory of Microbiology and Immunology in the Faculty of Pharmacy for specific and additional microbiological studies.

Carbapenem-resistant *K. pneumoniae* and *A. baumannii* were both recovered from the wound sample. After identification, the antimicrobial susceptibility profiling analysis indicated that the *K. pneumoniae* strain was resistant to all antibiotics tested, except tigecycline and colistin, while *A. baumanni* showed resistance to all antibiotics studied (Table 1). Screening for carbapenemase yielded positive results when using the Modified Hodge test.

PCR screening for β-lactamase genes followed by DNA sequencing identified the presence of the resistance genes bla_{KPC-3}, bla_{TEM-1} and bla_{SHV-1} in both isolates. The *OmpK35* and *OmpK36* porin genes were positive in the *K. pneumoniae* strain and no mutational changes were found by DNA sequencing. Multilocus sequence typing (MLST), based on the analysis of internal fragments of seven housekeeping genes (*gapA*, *infB*, *mdh*, *pgi*, *phoE*, *rpoB* and *tonB*) revealed that the *K. pneumoniae* clinical isolate belonged to sequence type 14 (ST-14). Additionally, *K. pneumoniae* virulence factors were assessed by PCR with specific primers for the K2 serotype, fimbrial adhesins type 1 and type 3, haemolysin, aerobactin, mucoid regulator and the hypermucoviscosity phenotype. All except the mucoid and hypermucoviscosity phenotype virulence factors were identified (Table 2).

Table 1. Phenotypic characterization of the *K. pneumoniae* an-d *A. baumannii* isolates.

Classes of Antibiotics	List of Antibiotics [1] (*n* = 15 Agents)	*K. pneumoniae* 69633	*A. baumannii* [4] 86982
Penicillins	Ampicillin	R	R
β-lactam/β-lactamase inhibitor combinations	Amoxicillin-clavulanic acid	R	R
	Piperacillin-tazobactam	R	R
Cephalosporins	Cefoxitin-C2G [2]	R	R
	Cefotaxime-C3G [3]	R	R
	Ceftazidime-C3G [3]	R	R
Monobactams	Aztreonam	R	R
Carbapenems	Imipenem	R	R
	Meropenem	R	R
	Ertapenem	R	R
Aminoglycosides	Gentamicin	R	R
Fluoroquinolones	Ciprofloxacin	R	R
	Levofloxacin	R	R
Polymyxins	Colistin	S	R
Tetracyclines	Tigecycline	S	R

[1] β-lactam antibiotics classes are shaded grey. Red/R indicates resistance and green/S indicates susceptible, standard dosing regimen. Strains were recovered from the same patient. [2] C2G: second generation cephalosporin; [3] C3G: third generation cephalosporin [4] *A. baumannii* is considered to be intrinsically resistant to ampicillin, cefotaxime, aztreonam and ertapenem.

Table 2. Resistance and virulence molecular characteristics of *K. pneumoniae* carbapenemase (KPC)-3 producer isolates.

Strain	β-Lactamases Identified	PBRT [1]	MLST	Virulence Profile
K. pneumoniae 69633	KPC-3 + SHV-1 + TEM-1	IncFrepB	ST-14	K2 + fimH + mrkDV1 + mrkDV2-4 + khe + iucC
A. baumannii 86982	KPC-3 + SHV-1 + TEM-1	IncFrepB	-	-

[1] Legend: PBRT: PCR-based replicon typing; MLST: multilocus sequence typing.

In order to study the transferability of the resistance profile, biparental mating between the *K. pneumoniae* isolate and the *E. coli* strain J53AziR was conducted and a transconjugant strain was selected. Replicon typing classified this plasmid within the incompatibility group IncFrepB. The transconjungant strain showed a susceptibility profile similar to the donor strain, with resistance to amoxicillin/clavulanic acid, cefotaxime and ceftazidime, whereas the carbapenems and cefoxitin showed decreased susceptibility, since they were not under the influence of porins. The genetic environment of the bla_{KPC-3} gene was characterized, namely, we searched for the genes associated with Tn*4401*, a Tn3-based transposon involved in bla_{KPC} gene mobilization transposon, in the *K. pneumoniae* and *A. baumannii* isolates. The Tn*4401b* transposon was identified in both isolates. The plasmid incompatibility group IncFrepB was also identified in the *A. baumannii* isolate.

3. Discussion

K. pneumoniae is the causative agent of several different healthcare-associated infections, such as wound infections, bloodstream infections, meningitis and pneumonia [6]. The extensive use of antimicrobials has led to a high incidence of resistance [7]. In our study, the firstly identified *K. pneumoniae* isolate showed a multidrug resistance profile to all β-lactams (including carbapenems) but also to aminoglycosides and fluoroquinolones. Tigecycline, colistin and carbapenem were the most commonly used drugs in combination antibiotic treatment in carbapenem-resistant infections [7]. However, carbapenemase-producing *A. baumannii*, which was identified three months later, was resistant to all antibiotics studied, limiting treatment options. In Portugal, the carbapenem resistance rates in *K. pneumoniae* increased from 0.9% (2009) to 5.2% (2016) and a worryingly resistance rate of 51.9% (2016) was reported for *A. baumannii* isolates, [8] despite the reduction trends in carbapenem antimicrobial consumption (ESAC-Net) [9].

Regardless of the efforts, our patient died. Pang et al. studied the prevalence and treatment for carbapenem-resistant *Enterobacteriaceae* infections in three tertiary care hospitals and showed poor mortality outcomes (23% at 28 days) but an effective treatment with the quinolone antibiotic [10]. Worryingly, infection with carbapenem-resistant *A. baumannii* is associated with a risk of mortality that is twice that of infection with its carbapenem-susceptible counterparts [11] as the high patient mortality rate (44% at 28 days) found in the AIDA trial demonstrated [12]. So, it is critical to effectively treat the primary infection in order to avoid co-infections or secondary infections with more resistant pathogens with consequent therapeutic failure. The role of old antibiotics in the era of antibiotic resistance should be promoted, such as the case of fosfomycin, which may be indicated for infections of the central nervous system, soft tissues, bone, lungs and abscesses due to its extensive tissue penetration [13,14].

The outer membrane of Gram-negative bacteria is a unique architecture that acts as a potent permeability barrier against toxic molecules, such as antibiotics [15]. It has been reported that a loss of porins OmpK35 and OmpK36 led to an increase in carbapenem and ciprofloxacin resistance [16]. DNA sequence analyses and protein homology searches were conducted and no changes were found when compared with *K. pneumoniae* isolates (GenBank accession number AJ303057 and GU461279), which is in accordance with studies described by other authors, namely in wound specimens [6] and KPC-3 producers [17], with the results being indicative that carbapenemase production is the main carbapenem resistance mechanism.

The genetic characterization confirmed the phenotypic features described since it identified the gene coding of the carbapenemase KPC-3 in co-expression with broad-spectrum β-lactamases (TEM-1 and SHV-1). Also, the *A. baumannii* showed the same resistance profile. The most common carbapenemase described worldwide is KPC-2 [18–22] but KPC-3 has already been identified in the United States [23], Israel [22], Italy [24] and Spain [25]. In Portugal, the first carbapenem-resistant *K. pneumoniae* was identified in 2009 [26] and since then, dissemination to other *Enterobacteriaceae* [27] and the increasing frequency of hospital outbreaks [28] has led to the creation of the Epidemiological Surveillance of Antimicrobial Resistance Guidelines, which contains mandatory notification of these pathogens [29].

The genetic environment of the *K. pneumoniae* strain was determined in order to understand if there had been a horizontal spread of the *KPC-3* gene between the *K. pneumoniae* and *A. baumannii* isolates. Our study describes a horizontal dissemination ability of the bla_{KPC-3} gene found in the *K. pneumoniae* isolate by an identical mobile genetic element, the Tn*4401b* isoform which is associated with a high resistance to carbapenems [17,30], propagated by a single type of plasmid, IncFrepB. The *K. pneumoniae* and *A. baummanii* isolates found in the same patient shared the same IncFrepB replicon origin which is indicative of a potential horizontal dissemination between these distinct species [31,32]. Additional studies should clearly demonstrate the interspecies transfer of bla_{KPC-3} by whole-plasmid sequencing.

Type 1 fimbriae is the most common adhesin in *Enterobacteriaceae* and can lead to persistent urinary tract infections [33]. Type 3 fimbrial adhesins mediate the binding of *K. pneumoniae* to endothelial and epithelial cells of the urinary and respiratory tracts. Many *K. pneumoniae* clinical isolates express both type 1 and type 3 fimbrial adhesins [33,34] but interestingly, in the current study, we found the coding genes to both of these adhesive structures but also to the K2 capsular serotype, which is predominantly associated with virulent strains [35], the iron siderophore aerobactin and hemolysin virulence factors.

Wasfi et al. demonstrated that only 7% of MDR *K. pneumoniae* isolates have the K2 capsular genotype [6]. The hemolysin virulence factor was detected in enterohemorrhagic *Escherichia coli* [36] and recently, also in uropathogenic bacteria, where has been described as causing programmed cell necrosis by altering mitochondrial dynamics [37]. The aerobactin mediates the acquisition of iron to help virulent bacteria to overcome iron starvation while bacteria invade and proliferate in the human system [38]. Russo et al. showed that aerobactin accounts for increased siderophore production, resulting in a 100% mortality rate and demonstrating the virulence of the isolates and their ability to cause infection at a low dose [39]. The virulence gene *aerobactin* has been previously detected in *Enterobacteriaceae* [40] including carbapenem-resistant *K. pneumoniae* isolates [6].

The carbapenemase producers are usually associated with highly resistant but low virulent strains [40–42]. In Brazil, De Cassia Andrade et al. reported the accumulation of virulence genes of KPC-2 *K. pneumoniae* isolates, along with the multi-resistance profile [43]. Also, in the United States, Krapp et al. described one *K. pneumoniae* KPC-3, SHV-28 and OXA-9 producer with the following virulence genes: enterobactin (*entABCDEF*), aerobactin receptor (*iutA*), type 1 and 3 fimbrial adhesion genes and the salmochelin receptor (*iroN*) [44]. These studies align with our findings in Portugal and suggest that the carbapenem-resistant *K. pneumoniae* strains are increasing in virulence. However, considering that we only described one clinical situation with one *K. pneumoniae* isolate, additional studies should be promoted, specifically regarding the interplay between resistance and virulence in *K. pneumoniae*. However, of note, our preliminary results indicate that variability in virulence profiles can exist according to the geographic origin of the isolate.

The MLST International clone ST-258 has been recognized as the prevalent ST of carbapenem-resistant *K. pneumoniae* isolates worldwide [45–48]. Herein, we described an isolate that belongs to sequence type ST-14 which has been associated with pan resistant isolates and the production of OXA-48 and NDM carbapenemases with a higher colistin rate of resistance when compared with isolates outside the cluster (37.1% vs. 27.1%) [49]. We should continuously highlight the importance of monitoring the emergence of highly virulent and resistant *K. pneumoniae*.

Future research regarding the colistin resistance molecular mechanisms in Gram-negative bacteria is needed. Furthermore, additional studies exploring the dangerous connections between resistance and virulence in Gram-negative infections and their impact on therapeutic efficacy should be incentivized.

4. Materials and Methods

4.1. Bacterial Isolates

The isolates were recovered using standard clinical operating procedures. Bacterial identification and antimicrobial susceptibility testing were performed at the microbiology laboratory by automated systems (Vitek2®, BioMérieux, Marcy, l'Etoile, France) and confirmed by the disk diffusion test in accordance with the methodology of the European Committee on Antimicrobial Susceptibility Testing (EUCAST), available at the European Society of Clinical Microbiology and Infectious Diseases (ESCMID) website (http://www.eucast.org/ast_of_bacteria/disk_diffusion_methodology/). Isolates with reduced susceptibility to carbapenems were selected and send to the Microbiology and Immunology Department in the Faculty of Pharmacy for specific and additional microbiological studies. The isolates were held in stock frozen in brain heart infusion (BHI) broth (VWR Prolabo®, Lisboa, Portugal) with 15% glycerol at −80 °C. For the analysis, the strains were grown in BHI broth for 18 h at 37 °C and seeded in Lysogeny broth (LB), more commonly known as Luria–Bertani agar (VWR Prolabo®, Lisboa, Portugal). Both isolates were recovered from wound infections.

4.2. Antimicrobial Susceptibility Testing

Bacterial antimicrobial susceptibility testing was performed in accordance with the EUCAST standardized disk diffusion method in Mueller–Hinton (MH) agar medium (VWR Prolabo®, Lisboa, Portugal). The detailed methodology and the preparation and storage of MH agar are described in the EUCAST Disk Diffusion Method for Antimicrobial Susceptibility Testing guidelines, which are available at (http://www.eucast.org/ast_of_bacteria/disk_diffusion_methodology/). Quality control was carried out in accordance with EUCAST (version 6.0, 2016) and the Clinical and Laboratory

Standards Institute (CLSI) guidelines (M100-S20), namely, *Escherichia coli* ATCC 25922 and *Escherichia coli* ATCC 35218 were used as controls for the inhibitor component of beta-lactam inhibitor-combination disks. Susceptibility was tested by a panel of antibiotics: amoxicillin/clavulanic acid (20/10 µg), cefoxitin (30 µg), cefotaxime (5 µg), ceftazidime (10 µg), imipenem (10 µg), gentamicin (10 µg), ciprofloxacin (5 µg) and tigecycline (15 µg). The inhibition zones were interpreted in accordance with EUCAST. The isolates were categorized as susceptible, standard dosing regimen (S); susceptible, increased exposure (I); and resistant (R) by applying the breakpoints in the phenotypic test results. Multidrug-resistant (MDR) bacteria were defined as those that acquired non-susceptibility to at least one agent in three or more antimicrobial categories, in accordance with the United States Center for Disease Control and Prevention (CDC) and the European Centre for Disease Prevention and Control (ECDC) consensual definition [50].

4.3. Resistance and Virulence Determinants

PCR-based screening for the most commonly found β-lactamase families was performed with specific primers that have already been described (*bla*$_{SHV}$ [51], *bla*$_{DHA}$ [52], *bla*$_{CMY}$ [53], *bla*$_{CTX-M}$ [54]) including carbapenemase genes (*bla*$_{KPC}$ [55], *bla*$_{IMP}$ [56], *bla*$_{VIM}$ [57] and *bla*$_{OXA}$ [58]). The virulence factors were assessed by PCR with specific primers for the K2 serotype (*K2A*), fimbrial adhesins type 1 (*fimH*) and type 3 (*mrkD*$_{v1}$ and *mrkD*$_{v2-4}$), haemolysin (*khe*), aerobactin (*iucC*), regulator of mucoid phenotype (*rmpA*) and the hypermucoviscosity phenotype (*magA*). The primers for *bla*$_{TEM}$, *bla*$_{NDM}$, *OmpK35* and *OmpK36* and for virulence genes were designed in our laboratory in accordance with the sequences'(5′–3′) available on Genbank (Table 3).

Table 3. List of primer designs in the current study and expected amplicon size.

Gene	DNA Sequence (5′ to 3′)	Amplicon Size (bp)	EMBL Accession Number (Genbank)
bla$_{NDM}$	F: TATCGCCGTCTAGTTCTGCTG R: ACTGCCCGTTGACGCCCAAT	871	AB604954
K2A	F: CAACCATGGTGGTCGATTAG R: TGGTAGCCATATCCCTTTGG	531	EF221827
fimH	F: TGTTCACCACCCTGCTGCTG R: CACCACGTCGTTCTTGGCGT	512	NC_012731.1
mrkD$_{V1}$	F: CGGTGATGCTGGACATGGT R: CCTCTAGCGAATAGTTGGTG	300	EU682505.2
mrkD$_{V2-4}$	F: CTTAATGGCGMTGGGCACCA R: TCATATGCGACTCCACCTCG	950	AY225463.1 AY225464.1 AY225465.1
khe	F: TGATTGCATTCGCCACTGG R: GGTCAACCCAACGATCCTGG	428	NC_012731.1
iucC	F: GTGCTGTCGATGAGCGATGC R: GTGAGCCAGGTTTCAGCGTC	944	NC_005249.1
rmpA	F: ACTGGGCTACCTCTGCTTCA R: CTTGCATGAGCCATCTTTCA	516	NC_012731.1
magA	F: TCTGTCATGGCTTAGACCGAT R: GCAATCGAAGTGAAGAGTGC	1137	NC_012731.1
ompK35	F: ATATTCTGGCAGTGGTGATCC R:GCTTTGGTGTAATCGTTGTC	1012	AJ303057
ompK36	F: TAGCAGGCGCAGCAAATGC R: TGCAACCACGTCGTCGGTA	1031	GU461279

Legend: F—forward primer; R—reverse primer.

4.4. Molecular Methods

Polymerase chain reactions (PCRs) were performed using the commercial kit puReTaq Ready-To-Go PCR Beads (GE Healthcare®, Lisboa, Portugal) in accordance with the manufacturer's instructions. Subsequently, the PCR products were resolved in 1% agarose gel in 1× concentrated Tris-Borate-EDTA (TBE) buffer (Sigma-Aldrich®, Lisboa, Portugal) (89 mM Tris-borate and 2 mM EDTA) and stained with GelRed (Biotium®, Lisboa, Portugal). Positive and negative controls were included in all PCR assays. The positive controls used were positive strains from the Laboratory of Microbiology collection that had been sequenced previously and the negative controls were provided by the PCR commercial kit puReTaq Ready-To-Go PCR Beads. The resulting PCR products were submitted to purification using the JETquick Spin Column Technique PCR Purification Kit (Genomed®, Lisboa, Portugal), in accordance with the producer's instructions and were sequenced at Macrogen Korea and STABVida Portugal. Searches for nucleotide sequences were performed with the BLAST program, which is available at the National Center for Biotechnology Information website (http://www.ncbi.nim.nih.gov/). Multiple-sequence alignments were performed with the ClustalX program, which is available at the European Bioinformatics Institute website (http://www.ebi.ac.uk/Tools/msa/clustalw2).

4.5. Transfer of blaKPC-3 and Plasmid Characterization

The identification of the incompatibility groups of plasmids was performed by the Replicon Typing technique [59]. This technique allowed us to identify the origins of replication of plasmids belonging to different incompatibility groups (*IncHI1, IncHI2, IncI1-I, IncX, IncL/M, IncN, IncFIA, IncFIB, IncW, IncY, IncP, IncFIC, IncA/C, IncT, IncFIIAs, IncK, IncB/O, IncF*). Subsequently, the transfer of the bla_{KPC-3} gene to the *E. coli* J53 resistant azide (AziR) receptor was performed by conjugation [60]. The transconjugants were selected in Müller–Hinton agar (VWR Prolabo®) supplemented with sodium azide (100 µg/mL) and cefotaxime (1 µg/mL).

4.6. Multilocus Sequence Typing (MLST)

MLST was performed on the *K. pneumoniae* isolate as previously described [61]. The sequence was performed at Macrogen Korea and submitted to the MLST database for allele attribution. The *K. pneumoniae* database is available at the Pasteur MLST.

4.7. Ethical Approval

Isolates were obtained as part of routine diagnostic testing and were analysed anonymously. All data were collected in accordance with the European Parliament and Council Decision on the Epidemiological Surveillance and Control of Communicable Disease in the European Community. Clinical and epidemiological data were collected from clinical records. The study proposal was also approved by the Research Ethics Committee of the Faculty of Medicine, University of Lisboa, Portugal.

5. Conclusions

In conclusion, we identified the first KPC-3 carbapenemase-producing *A. baumannii* isolate in Portugal associated with a fateful opportunistic infection preceded by a highly resistant and virulent *K. pneumoniae* KPC-3 producer belonging to the ST-14 high-risk clone. This illustrates a previously undescribed situation in our country with significant impact regarding the therapeutic antibiotics available for severe infections. The knowledge of specific genotyping patterns, resistance and virulence determinants of pathogens is crucial for the development of new antibacterial agents and adjuvants against antimicrobial resistant Gram-negative bacteria.

Author Contributions: Conceptualization, C.C. and A.D.; Methodology, C.C. and F.C.; Investigation, C.C.; Formal Analysis, C.C., F.C., G.J.d.S., A.D.; Resources, L.L, A.D. and J.M.-C.; Data Curation, C.C., A.D., L.L. and J.M.-C.; Writing—Original Draft Preparation, C.C.; Writing—Review & Editing, A.D.; Supervision, A.D.

Funding: This research was funded by the Research Institute for Medicines (iMed.ULisboa), Faculty of Pharmacy, University of Lisbon.

Acknowledgments: The authors would like to thank to all the members of the Microbiology Laboratory of the Hospital for the collaboration in the isolation and identification of bacteria.

References

1. Butler, C.C. Antibiotics: Responding to a Global Challenge. *Antibiotics* **2012**, *1*, 14–16. [CrossRef] [PubMed]

2. European Centre for Disease Prevention and Control. *Antimicrobial Resistance Surveillance in Europe 2014*; European Centre for Disease Prevention and Control: Stockholm, Sweden, 2015.

3. Perez, F.; Bonomo, R.A. Evidence to improve the treatment of infections caused by carbapenem-resistant Gram-negative bacteria. *Lancet Infect. Dis.* **2018**, *18*, 358–360. [CrossRef]

4. Tacconelli, E.; Magrini, N. *Global Priority List of Antibiotic-Resistant Bacteria to Guide Research, Discovery, and Development of New Antibiotics*; World Health Organization: Geneva, Switzerland, 2017.

5. Beceiro, A.; Tomas, M.; Bou, G. Antimicrobial resistance and virulence: A successful or deleterious association in the bacterial world? *Clin. Microbiol. Rev.* **2013**, *26*, 185–230. [CrossRef] [PubMed]

6. Wasfi, R.; Elkhatib, W.F.; Ashour, H.M. Molecular typing and virulence analysis of multidrug resistant *Klebsiella pneumoniae* clinical isolates recovered from Egyptian hospitals. *Sci Rep.* **2016**, *6*, 38929. [CrossRef] [PubMed]

7. Falagas, M.E.; Lourida, P.; Poulikakos, P.; Rafailidis, P.I.; Tansarli, G.S. Antibiotic treatment of infections due to carbapenem-resistant Enterobacteriaceae: Systematic evaluation of the available evidence. *Antimicrob. Agents Chemother.* **2014**, *58*, 654–663. [CrossRef] [PubMed]

8. Data from the ECDC Surveillance Atlas—Antimicrobial Resistance. Available online: https://ecdc.europa.eu/en/antimicrobial-resistance/surveillance-and-disease-data/data-ecdc (accessed on 7 September 2018).

9. Antimicrobial Consumption Database (ESAC-Net). Available online: https://ecdc.europa.eu/en/antimicrobial-consumption/database/country-overview (accessed on 7 September 2018).

10. Pang, F.; Jia, X.Q.; Zhao, Q.G.; Zhang, Y. Factors associated to prevalence and treatment of carbapenem-resistant Enterobacteriaceae infections: A seven years retrospective study in three tertiary care hospitals. *Ann. Clin. Microbiol. Antimicrob.* **2018**, *17*, 13. [CrossRef] [PubMed]

11. Lemos, E.V.; de la Hoz, F.P.; Einarson, T.R.; McGhan, W.F.; Quevedo, E.; Castaneda, C.; Kawai, K. Carbapenem resistance and mortality in patients with Acinetobacter baumannii infection: Systematic review and meta-analysis. *Clin. Microbiol. Infect.* **2014**, *20*, 416–423. [CrossRef] [PubMed]

12. Paul, M.; Daikos, G.L.; Durante-Mangoni, E.; Yahav, D.; Carmeli, Y.; Benattar, Y.D.; Skiada, A.; Andini, R.; Eliakim-Raz, N.; Nutman, A.; et al. Colistin alone versus colistin plus meropenem for treatment of severe infections caused by carbapenem-resistant Gram-negative bacteria: An open-label, randomised controlled trial. *Lancet Infect. Dis.* **2018**, *18*, 391–400. [CrossRef]

13. Castaneda-Garcia, A.; Blazquez, J.; Rodriguez-Rojas, A. Molecular Mechanisms and Clinical Impact of Acquired and Intrinsic Fosfomycin Resistance. *Antibiotics* **2013**, *2*, 217–236. [CrossRef] [PubMed]

14. Dijkmans, A.C.; Zacarias, N.V.O.; Burggraaf, J.; Mouton, J.W.; Wilms, E.B.; van Nieuwkoop, C.; Touw, D.J.; Stevens, J.; Kamerling, I.M.C. Fosfomycin: Pharmacological, Clinical and Future Perspectives. *Antibiotics* **2017**, *6*, 24. [CrossRef] [PubMed]

15. Choi, U.; Lee, C.R. Antimicrobial agents that inhibit the outer membrane assembly machines of Gram negative bacteria. *J. Microbiol. Biotechnol.* **2018**. [CrossRef]

16. Hamzaoui, Z.; Ocampo-Sosa, A.; Martinez, M.F.; Landolsi, S.; Ferjani, S.; Maamar, E.; Saidani, M.; Slim, A.; Martinez-Martinez, L.; Boubaker, I.B. Role of association of OmpK35 and OmpK36 alteration and blaESBL and/or blaAmpC in conferring carbapenem resistance among non-producing carbapenemase-*Klebsiella pneumoniae*. *Int. J. Antimicrob. Agents* **2018**. [CrossRef] [PubMed]

17. Leavitt, A.; Chmelnitsky, I.; Ofek, I.; Carmeli, Y.; Navon-Venezia, S. Plasmid pKpQIL encoding KPC-3 and TEM-1 confers carbapenem resistance in an extremely drug-resistant epidemic *Klebsiella pneumoniae* strain. *J. Antimicrob. Chemother.* **2010**, *65*, 243–248. [CrossRef] [PubMed]

18. Perilli, M.; Bottoni, C.; Grimaldi, A.; Segatore, B.; Celenza, G.; Mariani, M.; Bellio, P.; Frascaria, P.; Amicosante, G. Carbapenem-resistant *Klebsiella pneumoniae* harbouring blaKPC-3 and blaVIM-2 from central Italy. *Diagn. Microbiol. Infect. Dis.* **2013**, *75*, 218–221. [CrossRef] [PubMed]

19. Chan, W.W.; Peirano, G.; Smyth, D.J.; Pitout, J.D. The characteristics of *Klebsiella pneumoniae* that produce KPC-2 imported from Greece. *Diagn. Microbiol. Infect. Dis.* **2013**, *75*, 317–319. [CrossRef] [PubMed]

20. Yoo, J.S.; Kim, H.M.; Yoo, J.I.; Yang, J.W.; Kim, H.S.; Chung, G.T.; Lee, Y.S. Detection of clonal KPC-2-producing *Klebsiella pneumoniae* ST258 in Korea during nationwide surveillance in 2011. *J. Med. Microbiol.* **2013**, *62*, 1338–1342. [CrossRef] [PubMed]

21. Babouee, B.; Widmer, A.F.; Dubuis, O.; Ciardo, D.; Droz, S.; Betsch, B.Y.; Garzoni, C.; Fuhrer, U.; Battegay, M.; Frei, R.; et al. Emergence of four cases of KPC-2 and KPC-3-carrying *Klebsiella pneumoniae* introduced to Switzerland, 2009–10. *Euro Surveill.* **2011**, *16*, 19817. [CrossRef] [PubMed]

22. Leavitt, A.; Navon-Venezia, S.; Chmelnitsky, I.; Schwaber, M.J.; Carmeli, Y. Emergence of KPC-2 and KPC-3 in carbapenem-resistant *Klebsiella pneumoniae* strains in an Israeli hospital. *Antimicrob. Agents Chemother.* **2007**, *51*, 3026–3029. [CrossRef] [PubMed]

23. Le, J.; Castanheira, M.; Burgess, D.S.; McKee, B.; Iqbal, R.; Jones, R.N. Clonal dissemination of *Klebsiella pneumoniae* carbapenemase KPC-3 in Long Beach, California. *J. Clin. Microbiol.* **2010**, *48*, 623–625. [CrossRef] [PubMed]

24. Garcia-Fernandez, A.; Villa, L.; Carta, C.; Venditti, C.; Giordano, A.; Venditti, M.; Mancini, C.; Carattoli, A. *Klebsiella pneumoniae* ST258 producing KPC-3 identified in italy carries novel plasmids and OmpK36/OmpK35 porin variants. *Antimicrob. Agents Chemother.* **2012**, *56*, 2143–2145. [CrossRef] [PubMed]

25. Robustillo Rodela, A.; Diaz-Agero Perez, C.; Sanchez Sagrado, T.; Ruiz-Garbajosa, P.; Pita Lopez, M.J.; Monge, V. Emergence and outbreak of carbapenemase-producing KPC-3 *Klebsiella pneumoniae* in Spain, September 2009 to February 2010: Control measures. *Euro Surveill.* **2012**, *17*, 20086. [PubMed]

26. Machado, P.; Silva, A.; Lito, L.; Melo-Cristino, J.; Duarte, A. Emergence of *Klebsiella pneumoniae* ST-11 producing KPC-3 carbapenemase at a Lisbon hospital. *Clin. Microbiol. Infect.* **2010**, *16*, S28.

27. Caneiras, C.; Calisto, F.; Da Silva, G.; Lito, L.; Melo Cristino, J.; Duarte, A. Enterobacteriaceae isolates and KPC-3 carbapenemase in Portugal: Overview of 2010–2011. In Proceedings of the European Congress of Clinical Microbiology and Infectious Diseases, London, UK, 31 March–2 April 2012.

28. Pires, D.; Zagalo, A.; Santos, C.; Cota de Medeiros, F.; Duarte, A.; Lito, L.; Melo Cristino, J.; Caldeira, L. Evolving epidemiology of carbapenemase-producing Enterobacteriaceae in Portugal: 2012 retrospective cohort at a tertiary hospital in Lisbon. *J. Hosp. Infect.* **2016**, *92*, 82–85. [CrossRef] [PubMed]

29. Direção-Geral da Saúde. *Vigilância Epidemiológica das Resistências Aos Antimicrobianos*; Norma No. 004/2013 de 21/02/2013; Direção-Geral da Saúde: Lisboa, Portugal, 2013.

30. Chen, L.; Chavda, K.D.; Melano, R.G.; Jacobs, M.R.; Levi, M.H.; Bonomo, R.A.; Kreiswirth, B.N. Complete sequence of a bla(KPC-2)-harboring IncFII(K1) plasmid from a *Klebsiella pneumoniae* sequence type 258 strain. *Antimicrob. Agents Chemother.* **2013**, *57*, 1542–1545. [CrossRef] [PubMed]

31. Carattoli, A. Resistance plasmid families in Enterobacteriaceae. *Antimicrob. Agents Chemother.* **2009**, *53*, 2227–2238. [CrossRef] [PubMed]

32. Carattoli, A. Plasmids and the spread of resistance. *Int. J. Med. Microbiol.* **2013**, *303*, 298–304. [CrossRef] [PubMed]

33. Schroll, C.; Barken, K.B.; Krogfelt, K.A.; Struve, C. Role of type 1 and type 3 fimbriae in *Klebsiella pneumoniae* biofilm formation. *BMC Microbiol.* **2010**, *10*, 179. [CrossRef] [PubMed]

34. Murphy, C.N.; Mortensen, M.S.; Krogfelt, K.A.; Clegg, S. Role of *Klebsiella pneumoniae* type 1 and type 3 fimbriae in colonizing silicone tubes implanted into the bladders of mice as a model of catheter-associated urinary tract infections. *Infect. Immun.* **2013**, *81*, 3009–3017. [CrossRef] [PubMed]

35. Siu, L.K.; Huang, D.B.; Chiang, T. Plasmid transferability of KPC into a virulent K2 serotype *Klebsiella pneumoniae*. *BMC Infect. Dis.* **2014**, *14*, 176. [CrossRef] [PubMed]

36. Bielaszewska, M.; Aldick, T.; Bauwens, A.; Karch, H. Hemolysin of enterohemorrhagic Escherichia coli: Structure, transport, biological activity and putative role in virulence. *Int. J. Med. Microbiol.* **2014**, *304*, 521–529. [CrossRef] [PubMed]

37. Lu, Y.; Rafiq, A.; Zhang, Z.; Aslani, F.; Fijak, M.; Lei, T.; Wang, M.; Kumar, S.; Klug, J.; Bergmann, M.; et al. Uropathogenic Escherichia coli virulence factor hemolysin A causes programmed cell necrosis by altering mitochondrial dynamics. *FASEB J.* **2018**, *32*, 4107–4120. [CrossRef] [PubMed]

38. Ku, Y.H.; Chuang, Y.C.; Chen, C.C.; Lee, M.F.; Yang, Y.C.; Tang, H.J.; Yu, W.L. *Klebsiella pneumoniae* Isolates from Meningitis: Epidemiology, Virulence and Antibiotic Resistance. *Sci. Rep.* **2017**, *7*, 6634. [CrossRef] [PubMed]

39. Russo, T.A.; Olson, R.; Macdonald, U.; Metzger, D.; Maltese, L.M.; Drake, E.J.; Gulick, A.M. Aerobactin mediates virulence and accounts for increased siderophore production under iron-limiting conditions by hypervirulent (hypermucoviscous) *Klebsiella pneumoniae*. *Infect. Immun.* **2014**, *82*, 2356–2367. [CrossRef] [PubMed]

40. Hsieh, P.F.; Lin, T.L.; Lee, C.Z.; Tsai, S.F.; Wang, J.T. Serum-induced iron-acquisition systems and TonB contribute to virulence in *Klebsiella pneumoniae* causing primary pyogenic liver abscess. *J. Infect. Dis.* **2008**, *197*, 1717–1727. [CrossRef] [PubMed]

41. Yu, W.L.; Lee, L.M.; Tang, H.J.; Chang, M.C.; Chuang, Y.C. Low prevalence of rmpA and high tendency of rmpA mutation correspond to low virulence of extended spectrum β-lactamase-producing *Klebsiella pneumoniae* isolates. *Virulence* **2015**, *6*, 162–172. [CrossRef] [PubMed]

42. Tzouvelekis, L.S.; Miriagou, V.; Kotsakis, S.D.; Spyridopoulou, K.; Athanasiou, E.; Karagouni, E.; Tzelepi, E.; Daikos, G.L. KPC-producing, multidrug-resistant *Klebsiella pneumoniae* sequence type 258 as a typical opportunistic pathogen. *Antimicrob. Agents Chemother.* **2013**, *57*, 5144–5146. [CrossRef] [PubMed]

43. De Cassia Andrade Melo, R.; de Barros, E.M.; Loureiro, N.G.; de Melo, H.R.; Maciel, M.A.; Souza Lopes, A.C. Presence of fimH, mrkD, and irp2 Virulence Genes in KPC-2-Producing *Klebsiella pneumoniae* Isolates in Recife-PE, Brazil. *Curr. Microbiol.* **2014**. [CrossRef] [PubMed]

44. Krapp, F.; Morris, A.R.; Ozer, E.A.; Hauser, A.R. Virulence Characteristics of Carbapenem-Resistant *Klebsiella pneumoniae* Strains from Patients with Necrotizing Skin and Soft Tissue Infections. *Sci. Rep.* **2017**, *7*, 13533. [CrossRef] [PubMed]

45. Delfino, E.; Giacobbe, D.R.; Del Bono, V.; Coppo, E.; Marchese, A.; Manno, G.; Morelli, P.; Minicucci, L.; Viscoli, C. First report of chronic pulmonary infection by KPC-3-producing and colistin-resistant *Klebsiella pneumoniae* sequence type 258 (ST258) in an adult patient with cystic fibrosis. *J. Clin. Microbiol.* **2015**, *53*, 1442–1444. [CrossRef] [PubMed]

46. Gartzonika, K.; Rossen, J.W.A.; Sakkas, H.; Rosema, S.; Priavali, E.; Friedrich, A.W.; Levidiotou, S.; Bathoorn, E. Identification of a KPC-9-producing *Klebsiella pneumoniae* ST258 cluster among KPC-2-producing isolates of an ongoing outbreak in Northwestern Greece: A retrospective study. *Clin. Microbiol. Infect.* **2018**, *24*, 558–560. [CrossRef] [PubMed]

47. Jousset, A.B.; Bonnin, R.A.; Rosinski-Chupin, I.; Girlich, D.; Cuzon, G.; Cabanel, N.; Frech, H.; Farfour, E.; Dortet, L.; Glaser, P.; et al. 4.5 years within-patient evolution of a colistin resistant KPC-producing *Klebsiella pneumoniae* ST258. *Clin. Infect. Dis.* **2018**. [CrossRef] [PubMed]

48. Sorlozano-Puerto, A.; Esteva-Fernandez, D.; Oteo-Iglesias, J.; Navarro-Mari, J.M.; Gutierrez-Fernandez, J. A new case report of urinary tract infection due to KPC-3-producing klebsiella pneumoniae (ST258) in Spain. *Arch. Esp. Urol.* **2016**, *69*, 437–440. [PubMed]

49. Moubareck, C.A.; Mouftah, S.F.; Pal, T.; Ghazawi, A.; Halat, D.H.; Nabi, A.; AlSharhan, M.A.; AlDeesi, Z.O.; Peters, C.C.; Celiloglu, H.; et al. Clonal emergence of *Klebsiella pneumoniae* ST14 co-producing OXA-48-type and NDM carbapenemases with high rate of colistin resistance in Dubai, United Arab Emirates. *Int. J. Antimicrob. Agents* **2018**, *52*, 90–95. [CrossRef] [PubMed]

50. Magiorakos, A.P.; Srinivasan, A.; Carey, R.B.; Carmeli, Y.; Falagas, M.E.; Giske, C.G.; Harbarth, S.; Hindler, J.F.; Kahlmeter, G.; Olsson-Liljequist, B.; et al. Multidrug-resistant, extensively drug-resistant and pandrug-resistant bacteria: An international expert proposal for interim standard definitions for acquired resistance. *Clin. Microbiol. Infect.* **2012**, *18*, 268–281. [CrossRef] [PubMed]

51. Pitout, J.D.; Thomson, K.S.; Hanson, N.D.; Ehrhardt, A.F.; Moland, E.S.; Sanders, C.C. beta-Lactamases responsible for resistance to expanded-spectrum cephalosporins in *Klebsiella pneumoniae*, *Escherichia coli*, and Proteus mirabilis isolates recovered in South Africa. *Antimicrob. Agents Chemother.* **1998**, *42*, 1350–1354. [CrossRef] [PubMed]

52. Yan, J.J.; Ko, W.C.; Jung, Y.C.; Chuang, C.L.; Wu, J.J. Emergence of *Klebsiella pneumoniae* isolates producing inducible DHA-1 beta-lactamase in a university hospital in Taiwan. *J. Clin. Microbiol.* **2002**, *40*, 3121–3126. [CrossRef] [PubMed]

53. Navarro, F.; Perez-Trallero, E.; Marimon, J.M.; Aliaga, R.; Gomariz, M.; Mirelis, B. CMY-2-producing *Salmonella enterica*, *Klebsiella pneumoniae*, *Klebsiella oxytoca*, *Proteus mirabilis* and *Escherichia coli* strains isolated in Spain (October 1999–December 2000). *J. Antimicrob. Chemother.* **2001**, *48*, 383–389. [CrossRef] [PubMed]

54. Conceicao, T.; Brizio, A.; Duarte, A.; Lito, L.M.; Cristino, J.M.; Salgado, M.J. First description of CTX-M-15-producing *Klebsiella pneumoniae* in Portugal. *Antimicrob. Agents Chemother.* **2005**, *49*, 477–478. [CrossRef] [PubMed]

55. Yigit, H.; Queenan, A.M.; Anderson, G.J.; Domenech-Sanchez, A.; Biddle, J.W.; Steward, C.D.; Alberti, S.; Bush, K.; Tenover, F.C. Novel carbapenem-hydrolyzing beta-lactamase, KPC-1, from a carbapenem-resistant strain of *Klebsiella pneumoniae*. *Antimicrob. Agents Chemother.* **2001**, *45*, 1151–1161. [CrossRef] [PubMed]

56. Senda, K.; Arakawa, Y.; Ichiyama, S.; Nakashima, K.; Ito, H.; Ohsuka, S.; Shimokata, K.; Kato, N.; Ohta, M. PCR detection of metallo-beta-lactamase gene (blaIMP) in gram-negative rods resistant to broad-spectrum beta-lactams. *J. Clin. Microbiol.* **1996**, *34*, 2909–2913. [PubMed]

57. Lee, K.; Lim, J.B.; Yum, J.H.; Yong, D.; Chong, Y.; Kim, J.M.; Livermore, D.M. bla(VIM-2) cassette-containing novel integrons in metallo-beta-lactamase-producing Pseudomonas aeruginosa and Pseudomonas putida isolates disseminated in a Korean hospital. *Antimicrob. Agents Chemother.* **2002**, *46*, 1053–1058. [CrossRef] [PubMed]

58. Poirel, L.; Heritier, C.; Tolun, V.; Nordmann, P. Emergence of oxacillinase-mediated resistance to imipenem in *Klebsiella pneumoniae*. *Antimicrob. Agents Chemother.* **2004**, *48*, 15–22. [CrossRef] [PubMed]

59. Carattoli, A.; Bertini, A.; Villa, L.; Falbo, V.; Hopkins, K.L.; Threlfall, E.J. Identification of plasmids by PCR-based replicon typing. *J. Microbiol. Methods* **2005**, *63*, 219–228. [CrossRef] [PubMed]

60. Martinez-Martinez, L.; Pascual, A.; Jacoby, G.A. Quinolone resistance from a transferable plasmid. *Lancet* **1998**, *351*, 797–799. [CrossRef]

61. Diancourt, L.; Passet, V.; Verhoef, J.; Grimont, P.A.; Brisse, S. Multilocus sequence typing of *Klebsiella pneumoniae* nosocomial isolates. *J. Clin. Microbiol.* **2005**, *43*, 4178–4182. [CrossRef] [PubMed]

13

Establishing a System for Testing Replication Inhibition of the *Vibrio cholerae* Secondary Chromosome in *Escherichia coli*

Nadine Schallopp [1,†], Sarah Milbredt [1,†], Theodor Sperlea [1,†], Franziska S. Kemter [1,†], Matthias Bruhn [1], Daniel Schindler [1,2] and Torsten Waldminghaus [1,*]

1   LOEWE Center for Synthetic Microbiology-SYNMIKRO, Philipps-Universität Marburg, Marburg 35032, Germany; nadine@schallopp.de (N.S.); Sarah.Milbredt@ruhr-uni-bochum.de (S.M.); theodor.sperlea@staff.Uni-Marburg.DE (T.P.); Kemter@students.uni-marburg.de (F.S.K.); bruhnmatthias@aol.com (M.B.); daniel.schindler@manchester.ac.uk (D.S.)

2   School of Chemistry, Manchester Institute of Biotechnology, University of Manchester, Manchester M1 7DN, UK

*   Correspondence: torsten.waldminghaus@synmikro.uni-marburg.de

†   N.S., S.M., T.S. and F.S.K. contributed equally to this work.

Academic Editor: Anders Løbner-Olesen

Abstract: Regulators of DNA replication in bacteria are an attractive target for new antibiotics, as not only is replication essential for cell viability, but its underlying mechanisms also differ from those operating in eukaryotes. The genetic information of most bacteria is encoded on a single chromosome, but about 10% of species carry a split genome spanning multiple chromosomes. The best studied bacterium in this context is the human pathogen *Vibrio cholerae*, with a primary chromosome (Chr1) of 3 M bps, and a secondary one (Chr2) of about 1 M bps. Replication of Chr2 is under control of a unique mechanism, presenting a potential target in the development of *V. cholerae*-specific antibiotics. A common challenge in such endeavors is whether the effects of candidate chemicals can be focused on specific mechanisms, such as DNA replication. To test the specificity of antimicrobial substances independent of other features of the *V. cholerae* cell for the replication mechanism of the *V. cholerae* secondary chromosome, we establish the replication machinery in the heterologous *E. coli* system. We characterize an *E. coli* strain in which chromosomal replication is driven by the replication origin of *V. cholerae* Chr2. Surprisingly, the *E. coli ori2* strain was not inhibited by vibrepin, previously found to inhibit *ori2*-based replication.

Keywords: chromosome engineering; replication initiation; drug development

1. Introduction

While the genetic setup in eukaryotic cells comprises multiple linear chromosomes, the standard in prokaryotes is a single circular chromosome [1]. The number of replication start sites is also different, with eukaryotic chromosomes starting replication at multiple origins, while all known bacterial chromosomes are replicated from a single origin of replication. However, in bacteria, some interesting exceptions occur in alternative genetic setups, including linear chromosomes and separation of the genetic information onto multiple chromosomes [2,3]. When two chromosomes exist in one bacterial cell, new questions arise about, for example, the timing of initiation and coordination of segregation in comparison to single-chromosome bacteria. The best studied two-chromosome bacterium is *Vibrio cholerae*, the causative agent of the cholera disease [4,5]. Chr1 of *V. cholerae* strain El Tor N16961 has a size of about 3 M bps and Chr2 of about 1 M bps [6]. Each of the two chromosomes has its own initiator protein to start replication at each single replication origin [7]; for Chr1, the initiator is

DnaA, known to be the standard from studies in other model bacteria [8]. Meanwhile, the initiator for Chr2 is the protein RctB [8,9]. Although RctB is unique within the phylogenetic group of *Vibrionaceae*, it shows structural similarity to plasmid initiators [10,11]. This fits the common idea that Chr2 originates from a plasmid that was acquired by the cell early in evolution and then developed into a secondary chromosome [12]. One chromosome-like characteristic of Chr2 is its regulation in a cell-cycle dependent manner, attributed to the participation of SeqA and Dam methyltransferase in regulation of *ori2* [13–15]. Another feature of Chr2, further distinguishing it from plasmids, is that it encodes essential genes, although they are less frequent than when compared to the primary chromosome [16,17]. However, the plasmid ancestry of Chr2 is shown by the similarity of its replication initiation mechanism to plasmid systems; one such shared feature of both is the binding of the initiator protein to an array of specific binding sites, the so-called iterons [18]. In addition, handcuffing is involved in negative regulation of *ori2* as has also been shown for plasmid origins [12]. Although RctB alone is sufficient to melt the DNA double strand at *ori2*, this replication origin has been found to also depend on DnaA [8], the experimental evidence being the inability of the transfer of an *ori2*-based minichromosome to an *E. coli* strain lacking DnaA [5]. DnaA activity at *ori2* is probably linked to a conserved DnaA box some base pairs away from the iteron array [6,19]. Coordination of replication in the two-chromosome system of *V. cholerae* appears to work through the *crtS* site (=chromosome II replication triggering site), located on Chr1 and found to positively regulate initiation at *ori2* by binding RctB [20]. Regulation is thought to include physical contacts between *crtS* and *ori2*, as these two chromosome parts appeared to be coupled in chromatin conformation capture experiments [21]. Genetic changes of the *crtS* position on Chr1, either closer to *ori1* or further away, resulted in a corresponding shift of Chr2 initiation time as seen by a changed copy number [21], showing that the native position of the *crtS* sets the timing of Chr2 replication to finish in synchrony with Chr1 replication [21–23]. An important tool in studies on *V. cholerae* DNA replication was and is the use of *E. coli* as a heterologous host. First evidence of which sequences function as replication origins in *V. cholerae* came from testing their ability to replicate a corresponding minichromosome in *E. coli* [5]. Later, the native replication origin of *E. coli* was replaced by the very similar *ori1* of the primary *V. cholerae* chromosome [13,14], which was used to show that the Dam methyltransferase is not essential for *ori1* replication and can thus not be responsible for Dam being essential in *V. cholerae* (and not in *E. coli*). The conclusion was therefore that Dam-dependent methylation of *ori2* is crucial for initiation of replication; this assumption was confirmed by showing firstly that RctB binding sites need to be methylated in order to be bound by RctB, and secondly, that Dam loss selects for chromosome fusion in *V. cholerae*, omitting the need for a functional *ori2* since all genetic material can be replicated by *ori1* [13,24]. Attempts to construct an *E. coli* strain with *V. cholerae ori2* driving DNA replication instead of *oriC* as an important tool to study related questions had previously been unsuccessful [13]. Here, we study replication of such a strain with an insertion of *ori2* including the genes encoding *parAB* and *rctB* at position 4,422,941 of the *E. coli* chromosome and an *oriC* deletion that was constructed on the way toward developing an *E. coli* strain with two chromosomes [25]. We show that chromosomes over-replicate in *E. coli* with an *ori2* origin and that its replication is indeed dependent on Dam. Further experiments assess the relationship of *crtS* to *ori2* copy number, the role of DnaA in *ori2* initiation and make use of the genetic system to study a chemical compound that was described to act specifically on RctB. Finally, we show that *ori2* can replace *oriC* at its native location by constructing a corresponding strain.

2. Results

2.1. V. Cholerae ori2 Dependent Replication of the E. coli Chromosome

In order to establish a test system for replication inhibitors of *V. cholerae ori2* we analyzed an *E. coli* strain which has this origin including the flanking genes *rctB* and *parAB* inserted at an ectopic site and the native *oriC* being deleted (strain #16) [25]. Exponentially growing cultures were treated with rifampicin, which blocks replication initiation, and cephalexin, which inhibits cell division [26]. In wildtype *E. coli* (wt) cells, this treatment led to cells containing either 4 or 8 fully replicated chromosomes (Figure 1A). However, the flow cytometry histogram of a strain in which chromosomal replication is driven solely by *ori2* (strain #16) looks completely different (Figure 1A). Total DNA content in the strain driven by *ori2* is higher on average than when compared to the wt strain, and no distinct peaks are visible indicating unfinished replication rounds. Our analysis fits a chromosome replicated by *ori2* in this strain, as *ori2* was shown to be insensitive to rifampicin treatment in comparison to *oriC* in *E. coli* and *ori1* in *V. cholerae* [22,23]. Clearly, a different experimental approach is needed to assess if *ori2*-driven replication in *E. coli* has similar timing to *oriC*-based replication, or if initiation timing is different and/or potentially disturbed. To answer this question, we used quantitative fluorescence microscopy based on a recently constructed FROS array inserted into the *lacZ* locus [27] (Figure 1B,C). Since the FROS array marks one region of the chromosome, the number of respective foci should correlate with chromosome copy numbers. In exponentially growing cells of the *ori2*-strain (SM113), we could detect a clear increase in the number of foci compared to the control strain with *oriC* (SM112) (Figure 1B,C). This observation suggests that the *ori2*-based chromosome in *E. coli* over-initiates, in comparison to the native *oriC*-driven replication. To verify this finding, we performed microarray-based comparative genomic hybridization (CGH) to examine genome wide gene copy number patterns (Figure 1D). Over-initiation should lead to an increased origin to terminus copy number [28]; indeed, the strain with *ori2* had an origin copy number of 3.2, which is significantly more than the wt strain under similar growth conditions (Compare red and blue line in Figure 1D). These results indicate that replication of the primary *E. coli* chromosome by *ori2* increases the number of initiation events within one cell cycle in comparison to wt *E. coli*. The CGH experiments also confirmed *ori2* to be the only active replication origin in the analyzed strain because the copy number maximum appeared at the chromosomal position of *ori2* insertion (Figure 1D).

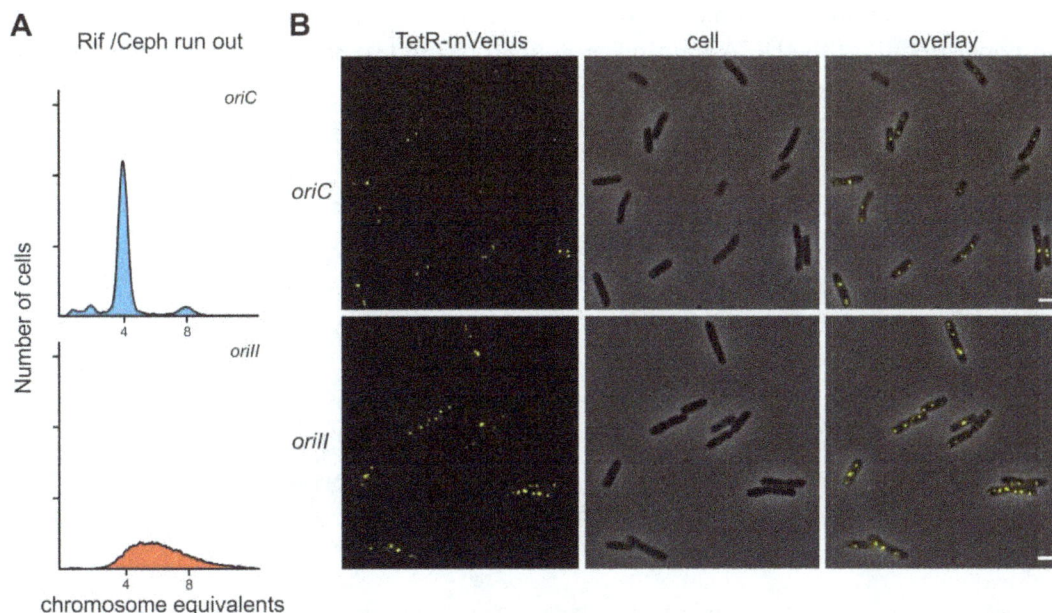

Figure 1. *Cont.*

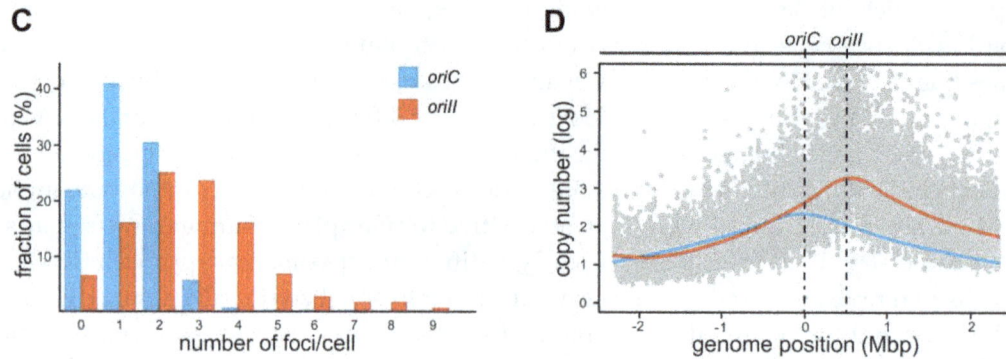

Figure 1. DNA replication in *E. coli* strains with *oriC* or *ori2* driven replication. (**A**) Flow cytometry analyses of DNA content in rifampicin/cephalexin treated *E. coli* cells with DNA replication starting at *oriC* (strain #1; top panel) or *V. cholerae ori2* (strain #16; bottom panel) [25]. (**B**) Fluorescence microscopy of *E. coli* cells harboring a plasmid encoding a TetR-mVenus fusion (pMA289), a FROS array insertion and either *oriC* (top panel; strain SM112) or *ori2* (bottom panel; strain SM113). The scale bar is 2 μm. (**C**) Quantification of fluorescence foci per cell for microscopy shown in B (n = 700). (**D**) Profile of genome-wide copy numbers based on comparative genomic hybridization (CGH). Grey dots represent values of single probes for the *ori2*-based strain (#16) with a Loess regression (red line, F = 0.2). For comparison, the Loess regression of the *oriC*-based strain #1 is shown based on published data [29] (blue line, F = 0.2). Positions of *oriC* and *ori2* are indicated and the genomic position as distance from *oriC*.

2.2. Initiation of Replication at ori2 in E. coli Depends on Dam Methylation

Dam methyltransferase was shown to be essential in *V. cholerae* [30]. An *E. coli* strain with *oriC* substituted by *V. cholerae ori1* was instrumental to show that this is due to effects of Dam on *ori2* and not *ori1*, as Dam was not essential in this strain [13,14]. Therefore, one conclusion would be that Dam should be essential in an *E. coli* strain with *ori2* driving chromosomal replication. To test this hypothesis, we analyzed the transfer of a Δ*dam* allele by P1 transduction to an *E. coli* strain in which replication is solely driven by *ori2* (#16). While the deletion could easily be introduced to *E. coli* wt cells, no transduction was found in strain #16 (Figure 2). In contrast, the positive control *hupA*, encoding one subunit of the DNA-binding protein HU, could be transduced into both strains with similar efficiencies (Figure 2). The same was observed for an antibiotic cassette insertion within the *seqA* locus. This result confirmed previous findings of SeqA not being essential for *ori2*-dependent initiation of DNA replication.

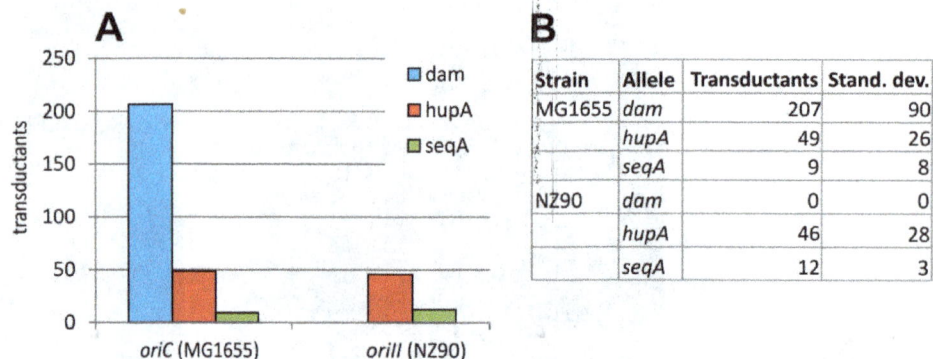

Strain	Allele	Transductants	Stand. dev.
MG1655	*dam*	207	90
	hupA	49	26
	seqA	9	8
NZ90	*dam*	0	0
	hupA	46	28
	seqA	12	3

Figure 2. Transduction efficiency of gene knockouts into *oriC* and *ori2 E. coli* strains. Colonies growing on plates supplemented with kanamycin were counted after P1 transduction of KanR-cassettes inserted in *dam*, *hapA* or *seqA* as indicated into *E. coli* strains, with chromosome replication based on *oriC* (MG1655 (#1)) or *ori2* (NZ90). Mean values of three replicates are shown in (**A**) with the actual numbers and standard deviation given in the table (**B**).

2.3. crtS-Dependent Regulation of ori2-Based Replication in E. coli

V. cholerae Chr1 was found to encode a short DNA sequence called *crtS* (*chromosome II replication triggering site*) that regulates initiation at *ori2* [20,21]. We hypothesized that the *ori2*-driven chromosome in strain #16 is dysregulated due to lacking a *crtS* site. The *crtS* site was found to increase the copy number of an *ori2*-minichromosome in *E. coli* [20]. However, in those experiments, *crtS* was supplied in multiple copies through a pBR322 plasmid, which is unlike the situation in *V. cholerae*. To analyze the effect of more physiological numbers of *crtS* on *ori2* replication, we inserted a *crtS* site on the *E. coli* wt chromosome driven by *oriC* between genes *fucR* and *rlmM* (genomic position ~2,940,120) about 1 M bps from *oriC*. The strain was transformed with an *ori2*-minichromosome and its copy number determined via quantification of the sensitivity towards elevated concentrations of antibiotics, the underlying logic being that higher replicon numbers lead to higher gene dosage of the encoded resistance gene and correspondingly to a higher tolerance towards respective antibiotics [31–33]. An increased copy number of the *ori2*-minichromosome was observed in a strain carrying the *crtS* insertion, compared to the wt lacking *crtS* (Figure 3A). Notably, this effect was *ori2* specific, since a replicon driven by the F-plasmid replication origin did not show differential copy numbers (Figure 3A). To verify these results, we measured *ori2*-minichromosome copy numbers relative to the primary *E. coli* chromosome by qPCR (Figure 3B). We found an increased copy number of the *ori2*-minichromosome from 0.31 ± 0.02 in wt to 0.82 ± 0.13 in the strain with a chromosomal insertion of *crtS*. Our data confirmed that *crtS* increases the *ori2*-minichromosome copy number and showed that a chromosomal *crtS* insertion is sufficient to this end.

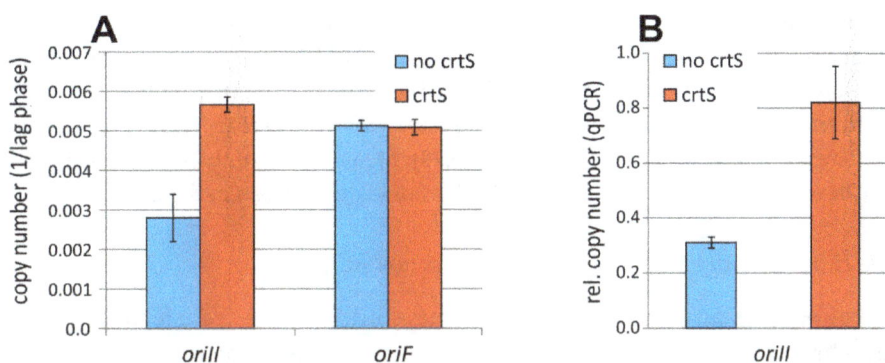

Figure 3. Copy numbers of secondary replicons in *E. coli* dependent on *crtS*. (**A**) Copy number of an *ori2*-based minichromosome in an *E. coli* strain without *crtS* (Strain NZ72) or with *crtS*-site insertion on the chromosome (Strain NZ140) was measured as inverse of the lag time for cells in medium with high concentrations of ampicillin (500 µg/ mL). Strains carrying an *oriF*-based replicon and the *crtS* (Strain NZ141) or no *crtS* on the chromosome (Strain NZ119) were used as control. Data are the mean of three biological replicates with the indicated standard deviations. (**B**) Copy number of an *ori2*-minichromosome (pMA568) analyzed by qPCR-based marker frequency analysis relative to *oriC*. Mean values of three biological replicates are shown with the respective standard deviations.

We speculated that a *crtS* site could lead to more regular replication timing of the primary chromosome in the *E. coli* strain #16 with *ori2*-driven chromosome replication. To make *crtS* replication dependent on the cell cycle, as is the case in *V. cholerae*, we constructed an *oriC*-minichromosome carrying a *crtS* site. However, transformation of strain #16 failed by this replicon failed. To study this phenomenon in detail we quantified the number of colonies as a result of conjugating the replicon from a donor strain to either an *E. coli* wt, or strain #16 with *ori2*-driven chromosomal replication. An *oriC*-minichromosome was efficiently transferred into a wt *E. coli* by conjugation, as was an *oriC*-minichromosome carrying a *crtS* site (Figure 4A). In contrast, neither of these two replicons could be transferred to strain #16 via conjugation. These results indicated that it is the *oriC* on the extra replicon which causes some problem in the *ori2 E. coli* strain. As an alternative to test the effect of *crtS* on chromosomal *ori2* replication, we constructed a replicon with the F-plasmid origin and a *crtS* site. Interestingly, this replicon could also not be transferred to strain #16 (Figure 4B). One explanation for lacking transconjugants could be that the *crtS* site leads to repression of the extra replicon for example by strong binding of RctB. An alternative explanation would be that the *crtS* site effects *ori2* replication on the primary chromosome in a way leading to cell death. To distinguish between these two possibilities we tested conjugation into a strain carrying *oriC* and *ori2* on the primary *E. coli* chromosome (Figure 4B). If replication problems would be due to events on the extra replicon it should not be possible to conjugate into this strain. However, transconjugants were observed, indicating that some interference of the *crtS* site with *ori2*-based replication on the *E. coli* chromosome hinders extra replicons carrying a *crtS* site to be transferred to strain #16.

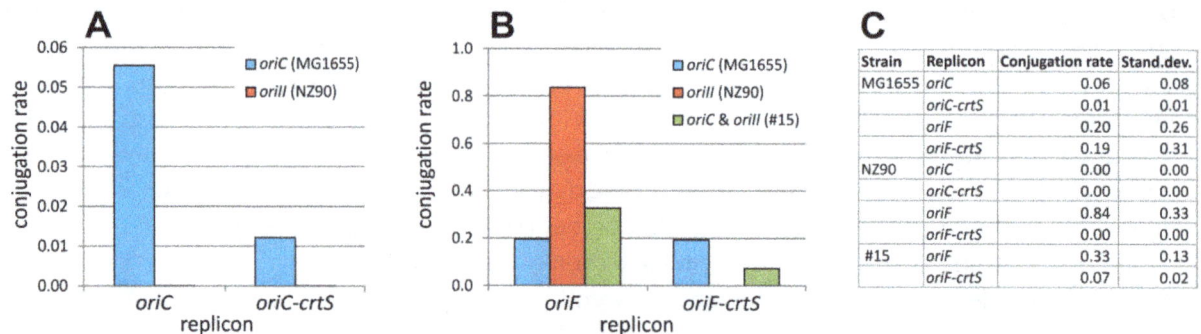

Figure 4. Conjugation rate of extra replicons to *oriC* and *ori2 E. coli* strains. (**A**) Transfer by conjugation was tested for *oriC*-minichromosomes carrying a *crtS* site (pMA200) or no *crtS* (pMA308) into *E. coli* with chromosome replication based on *oriC* (MG1655) or *ori2* (NZ90). (**B**) Conjugation of *oriF*-based replicons with *crtS* (pMA206) or without (pMA899) into *E. coli* with *oriC* (MG1655), *ori2* (NZ90) or *oriC* at the native site and *ori2* at an ectopic site (#15) [25,29]. Mean values of three biological replicates are shown in (**A,B**) with the actual numbers and standard deviations given in the table (**C**).

2.4. Assaying the DnaA-Box in ori2 for Its Role in Replication Initiation

Our observation that an *oriC*-minichromosome could not be transferred to an *E. coli* strain with *ori2*-based chromosome replication suggested a mechanism of interference. Such an effect has been observed in cases where the two origins differ in their efficiency to initiate replication [13,34]. However, such interference is usually due to the competition or interference of factors used by both replication origins. One factor that both *ori2* and *oriC* require for replication is DnaA. While the role of DnaA as initiator at *oriC* and *ori1* is well studied, much less is known about DnaA activity at *ori2*. It has been established that *ori2*-dependent replication requires DnaA and that *ori2* contains a DnaA box beside the RctB binding iterons, which appeared in a mutagenesis screen to be functionally important [5,19]. The role of the DnaA box was initially tested by the introduction of some mutations into a minichromosome carrying the minimal *ori2* sequence [19]. Here, we constructed and tested some of these mutations as well as additional ones in a minichromosome system including both the entire *ori2* and the flanking *rctB* and *parAB* genes. Functionality of minichromosomes was tested by measuring their transformation efficiency of a wt *E. coli*. This efficiency was measured relative to transformation of the same replicon into a strain encoding the λpir gene, which allowed replication based on the *oriR6K* of the *ori2*-minichromosomes. Deletion, inversion or scrambling of the DnaA-box rendered *ori2* nonfunctional, as seen by the inability of the respective replicons to transform a wt *E. coli* (Figure 5A). How well a DnaA box matches the consensus sequence determines the affinity of DnaA towards this site. Since the DnaA box within *ori2* has the sequence of a high-affinity binding site, we tested the effect of changing this sequence to a weak or medium-strength DnaA box (Figure 5B). Both alternative DnaA boxes allowed *ori2*-minichromosome replication; however, the transformation efficiency was reduced, indicating that a high affinity DnaA box is needed to allow optimal functioning of *ori2*. The distance between the DnaA box and the first of six RctB binding iterons is 22 bps, placing the two proteins on the same face of the DNA helix. We tested the insertion or deletion of 5 bps between these sites which should shift the binding sites half of a DNA turn along (Figure 5C). Insertion and deletion to the right of the DnaA box (between DnaA box and iteron) greatly reduced the transformation efficiency in comparison to wt or to an insertion to the left. This finding indicated that the distance between the DnaA box and the iterons is critical for its functionality. Interestingly, a deletion to the left of the DnaA box also reduced the transformation efficiency.

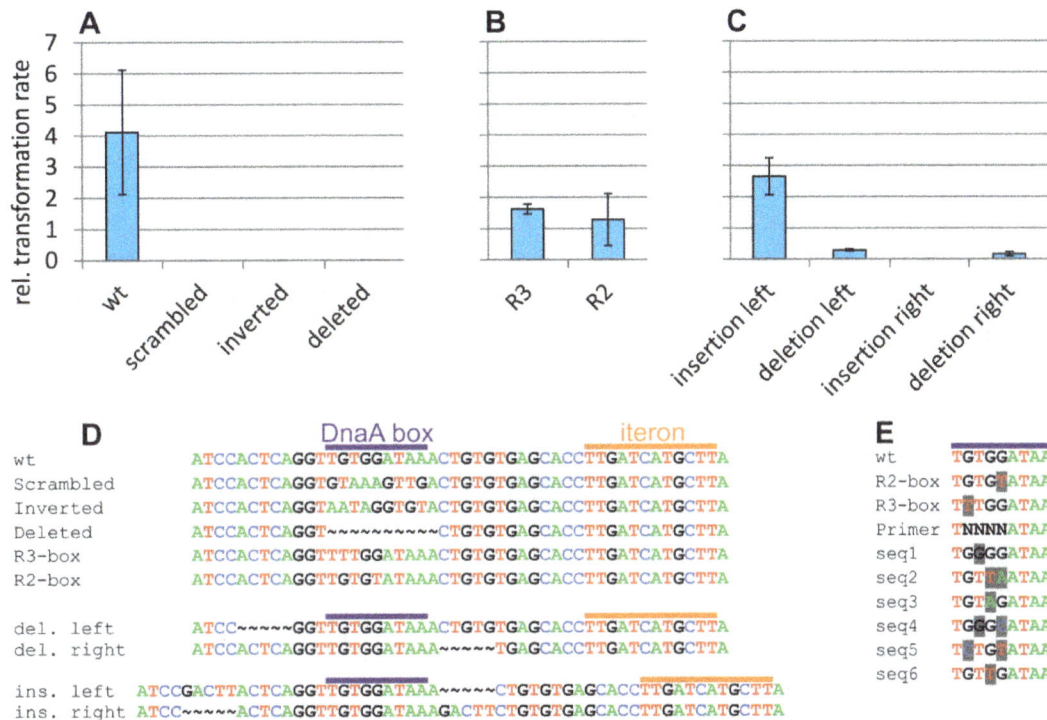

Figure 5. Mutation-based analysis of the DnaA box within *ori2*. (**A–C**) *Ori2*-based minichromosomes with different mutations at the DnaA box were tested for their ability to replicate by transformation into *E. coli* (XL1-Blue) or DH5α*λpir*. The latter was used as a control because all replicons carry an oriR6K which allows replication in strains encoding the initiator Pir. Values are ratios between respective colony numbers of three biological replicates with the indicated standard deviations. Relevant sequences are shown in (**D**) for DnaA boxes wt (pMA87), scrambled (pMA108), inverted (pMA109), deleted (pMA110), a weak DnaA box R3 (pMA111), a medium-strength DnaA box R2 (pMA112), a 5 bp insertion to the left of the DnaA box (pMA115) or the right (pMA114) or a 5 bp deletion to the left (pMA113) or right (pMA116) as indicated. (**E**) Sequences found by transformation of an assembled *ori2*-minichromosome with a mix of sequence combinations at positions 2–5 as indicated by "N" in the Primer sequence. DnaA-box sequences from *oriC* in *E. coli* are shown for comparison (wt, R2, R3). Six sequences found in the screen are shown with the nucleotides differing from the consensus DnaA box shaded in grey.

As an alternative approach to assess the importance of the DnaA box for *ori2* functionality, we cloned the *ori2* fragment into a plasmid based on a sequence library that substituted four nucleotides of the DnaA box with all possible 256 sequence combinations (Figure 5D). Transformation of the respective minichromosome mix into *E. coli* wt should then allow selection of functional replication origins. Sequencing of *ori2* sequences derived from such experiments revealed six different sequences that could function in place of the original DnaA box (Figure 5D). In all sequences found, two or three out of four nucleotides matched the DnaA box consensus, confirming the importance of the DnaA box on one hand and some potential for variation on the other, supporting the above results on introduction of weaker DnaA boxes.

2.5. Vibrepin Does Not Inhibit ori2-Dependent Replication

A screen for substances that lead to growth inhibition of an *E. coli* strain carrying an *ori2* minichromosome uncovered such activity of 3-(3,4-dichlorophenyl)cyclopropane-1,1,2,2-tetracarbonitrile, designated as "vibrepin" (for *Vibrio* replication inhibitor) [35]. It was found that vibrepin interferes with *ori2*-opening activity of RctB [35]. We reasoned that vibrepin should inhibit growth of *E. coli* strain #16 with chromosomal replication solely based on *ori2*, and as such the strain might be useful to identify additional *ori2*-specific inhibitors in the future in order to derive *V. cholerae*-selective antibiotics. Comparing the lag-phase duration of an *E. coli* wt with and without vibrepin revealed a slightly longer lag phase (13.5%) in medium supplemented with 16 µg/mL vibrepin (Figure 6A). Surprisingly, this difference was similar in the *ori2* strain (Figure 6A) indicating that vibrepin does not significantly inhibit *ori2* initiation in this context. As a second line of evidence, we compared the effect of vibrepin on *E. coli* cells carrying extra replicons based on either *ori2*, *oriC* or the F-plasmid origin (Figure 6B). The elongation of lag phases caused by vibrepin was similar for all three replicons, confirming the above results that vibrepin was not acting on *ori2* specifically (Figure 6B). To test vibrepin activity on *ori2* in *V. cholerae* directly, we compared its effect on growth of (i) strain N16961 carrying a secondary *ori2*-based chromosome [6], (ii) strain MCH1 with a fused chromosome driven by *ori1* and lacking *ori2* [36], and (iii) the recently characterized *V. cholerae* strain NSCVI with fused chromosomes and intact copies of *ori1* and *ori2* [37]. If vibrepin acts against *ori2* specifically, one would expect strain N16961 to be inhibited but not the two other strains. However, we found vibrepin to have an effect on the lag phase duration for all three strains, indicating that vibrepin inhibits *V. cholerae* growth, but not based on interference at *ori2* (Figure 6C).

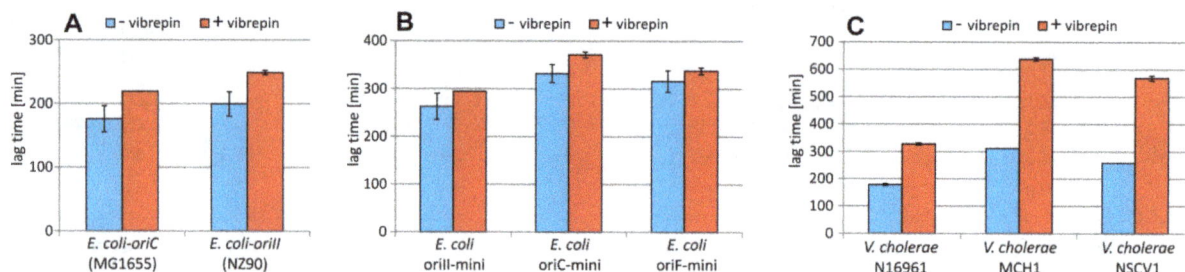

Figure 6. Effect of vibrepin on *ori2*-dependent replication. Lag time (time until OD = 0.1 was reached) is shown as the mean value of three replicates, with the respective standard deviations, in medium without vibrepin (blue) or with vibrepin (red). Vibrepin concentrations were 16 µg/mL for *E. coli* strains (**A–B**) and 1.6 µg/mL for *V. cholerae* strains (**C**). Analyzed *E. coli* strains replicated their chromosome based on *oriC* (MG1655) or *ori1* (NZ90) (**A**) or carried an extra minireplicon with *ori2* (pMA100), *oriC* (pMA106) or *oriF* (pMA129) [38] (**B**) as indicated. *V. cholerae* strains are the standard two-chromosome strain N16961 [6], an engineered derivative of N16961 with fused chromosomes (MCH1) [36] or a natural isolate with fused chromosomes (NSCV1) [37].

2.6. ori2 Can Replace oriC in E. coli

We have characterized here an *E. coli* strain with an ectopic *ori2* insertion about 500 kbps away from *oriC* combined with a deletion of *oriC* and used it to study biological features related to *ori2*-based replication. The value of such a system was appreciated before but attempts to replace *oriC* by *ori2* were unsuccessful [13]. We reasoned that such an exchange of *oriC* to *ori2* should be possible in general based on the findings outlined above. Indeed, we were able to replace the *oriC* sequence in *E. coli* strain MG1655 with the full *V. cholerae ori2* sequence, including the flanking genes *rctB* and *parAB* (Strain NZ138, see Figure 7A and Methods section for details). Successful *oriC* replacement was confirmed by the inability of a Δ*dam* allele to be transferred by P1 transduction to the constructed strain, similar to what was found for strain #16 above. A comparison of a wt *oriC*-strain, to this new *oriC* to *ori2* exchange strain (NZ138) revealed a slight increase of doubling time (21.6 vs. 22.6 respectively;

Figure 7B). The strain with the ectopic *ori2* insertion (NZ90) grew slower (27 min doubling time). DNA contents, as measured by flow cytometry were lower for both *ori2* strains compared to the *oriC* wt strain (Figure 7B, middle panel). The protein content as measure of the cell size varied slightly with cells of strain NZ90 being smallest on average and NZ138 being the largest cells (Figure 7B, right panel). In summary, characteristics of the newly constructed stain NZ138 differ from those of strain NZ90 and are more similar to a wt *E. coli* with *oriC*-driven replication. We believe that this *E. coli ori2* strain NZ138 will be of great help to derive new insights into *ori2*-dependent replication and screen for new *V. cholerae* specific replication inhibitors in the future.

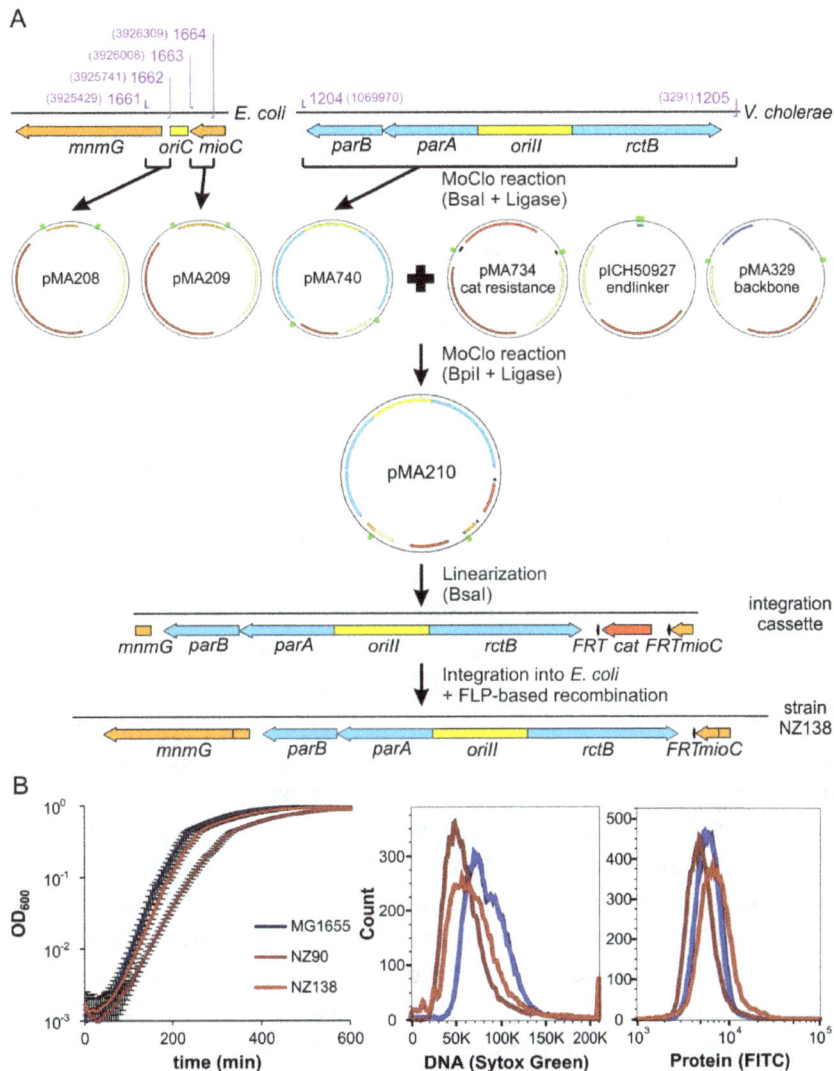

Figure 7. Construction and characterization of strain NZ138. (**A**) Scheme of NZ138 construction. Genes are indicated by arrows, origins of replication and the truncated end of *mnmG* by blocks. Genes of *V. cholerae* are colored blue, genes of *E. coli* orange, resistance genes red, FRT-sites black and origins of replication yellow. Green rectangles indicate BsaI and BpiI restriction sites. Binding sites of oligonucleotides are indicated in purple, numbers in brackets are genome positions of 5'-ends of the binding sites. Genomic and linearized DNA is indicated by grey lines, plasmids by circles. (**B**) Growth, DNA content and protein content of NZ138 compared to MG1655 and NZ90. All strains were grown in LB medium. For growth curves, five replicates for each strain were grown in a 96-well plate at 37 °C. For determination of DNA and protein content, samples were taken in exponential phase and fixed with ethanol. The samples were split, stained with SYTOX Green (DNA) or FITC (protein) and analyzed by flow cytometry.

3. Discussion

DNA replication is an attractive target for the development of antimicrobials. However, engineered systems are needed to be able to search specifically for chemicals targeted against the replication mechanism of interest. Such engineering approaches have for example used expression of hyperactive mutant proteins that kill the cells unless a chemical component suppresses their action [39]. The replication system of the secondary *V. cholerae* chromosome is especially interesting in respect to the development of antimicrobials because it is unique in the Vibrionaceae. The replication origin *ori2* can be studied in *E. coli* regarding general functionality and drug development using so-called minichromosomes [5,35]. These are plasmid-like replicons carrying a chromosomal replication origin and usually a conditional plasmid origin to be able to construct the replicons in the first place [40]. Minichromosomes are an important tool to, for example, identify the minimal region of a chromosome that functions as its origin of replication. Due to their easier genetic manipulation, they are also used frequently to characterize replication origins further—for example, in identification of the role of individual DNA motifs, as demonstrated with the DnaA box in *ori2* above (Figure 5). However, minichromosome-based studies also have drawbacks in both their small size and their competition with the chromosomal replication origin. *OriC*-minichromosomes have high copy numbers due to a lack of an equipartition mechanism [41]. The competition can lead to integration of minichromosomes into the primary chromosome [42]. An alternative to minichromosomes is the substitution of native chromosomal replication origins with the *ori* of interest. For instance, such an approach was instrumental in order to study the role of Dam methyltransferase and SeqA for *V. cholerae ori1* based replication [13,14]. However, while it is easy to see if a certain mutation is rendering a replication origin non-functional when using minichromosomes, investigating replication origins driving replication of the primary chromosome is not straightforward, as replication here is an essential process. One solution to this problem is the insertion of an additional plasmid origin which can be switched off, by, for example, repression of its initiator protein [43]. If depletion of an inducer leads to cell death, the origin of interest must be non-functional [43]. An alternative to this approach is the analysis of chromosomes carrying two functional replication origins which, for example, allow conclusions on their replication timing to be drawn by comparison with their MFA profiles [29]. The study showed that *E. coli oriC* and *V. cholerae ori2* can coexist on the chromosome and both be active [29]. This is consistent with many studies using *ori2*-based minichromosomes to study *V. cholerae* replication in *E. coli*. It was thus surprising that an *oriC*-minichromosome could not be transferred to an *E. coli* strain with chromosomal replication based on *V. cholerae ori2* (Figure 4A). We propose three possible reasons to explain this phenomenon; (i) the *oriC*-minichromosome leads to *ori2*-based over-replication of the chromosome, (ii) the *oriC*-minichromosome leads to *ori2*-based under-replication of the chromosome, and (iii) the interference of *oriC* and *ori2* hinders *oriC*-dependent minichromosome replication. Regarding the first possibility, over-replication is a commonly observed phenomenon caused by different mutations that might be tolerated in some cases and leading to cell death in others [44–47]. The differentiation between the other two hypotheses is related to the question of which origin can compete better for factors needed for replication initiation at both *oriC* and *ori2*. Three known protein factors are relevant in this context; SeqA, Dam and DnaA. SeqA is a negative regulator of initiation at both replication origins and competition should therefore lead to more initiations but never to a blocking of replication [13,48,49]. The role of Dam is to methylate the GATCs which occur at both replication origins, but the speed of the methylation process is so fast that a changed *ori2* methylation due to an increased number of GATCs on the *oriC* minichromosome is unlikely. These considerations leave DnaA remaining as the factor required by both *ori2* and *oriC*. It is well conceivable that *oriC* would win a competition for DnaA against *ori2* since it comprises multiple DnaA binding sites, while *ori2* has only a single one. Even more DnaA is directed away from *ori2* when the *oriC* on the minichromosome occurs in multiple copies [38,41]. A single *oriC* copy on the chromosome could also inhibit *ori2*-driven replication initiation, but perhaps only to a minor extent. Interestingly, this seems to be the case in practice, as copy numbers of *ori2* in *E. coli* strains that carry the native *oriC* are lower than *oriC* or similar. This is the case for *ori2* minichromosomes as well as ectopic *ori2* insertions [29,33,38]. This is remarkable, since *ori2* itself was shown to lead to over-initiation and higher chromosomal copy numbers without a competing *oriC* in the cell (Figure 1). These findings suggested that the availability of DnaA limits initiation at *ori2*. However, replication of Chr2 in *V. cholerae* did not increase with over-expression of DnaA while Chr1 copies were amplified [7]. One possible explanation for this discrepancy is that it is not the amount of DnaA per se that is important, but the availability of ATP vs. ADP-bound versions of this protein. Our data seem to suggest that DnaA-ATP is actually functional at *ori2*, based on our finding that lower affinity DnaA boxes can replace the native DnaA box (Figure 5B,E). These sites are able to bind ATP-DnaA but not ADP-DnaA [50]. The exact role of DnaA in replication initiation at *ori2* remains to be uncovered but mutational analyses of *ori2*-based minichromosomes presented here and in a previous study provide first insights (Figure 5) [19].

It appears that DnaA may add just another layer of regulation to the regulation of Chr2 replication in *V. cholerae* alongside SeqA, Dam methylation, and the recently found *crtS* site. The latter was found here to increase the copy number of an *ori2*-minichromosome when it was itself located on the *E. coli* chromosome (Figure 3). If a slight increase in the number of initiation events at *ori2* is the general effect of *crtS*, it is hard to find an explanation for the result where an F-plasmid-origin-based replicon carrying a *crtS* site could not be transformed into the *ori2 E. coli* strain (Figure 4). Notably, we were also not able to transfer the chromosomal *crtS* insertion into the *ori2*-strain. We suggest that *crtS* and *ori2* are actually regulated in a way that adjusts their copy numbers to be similar. This is what was found in *V. cholerae*, where copy numbers of Chr2 increased when the *crtS* was moved closer to *ori1*, coinciding with an increased copy number of *crtS*. Comparison to previous studies on *crtS* in *E. coli* are difficult because they used a three plasmid system with *ori2*, *rctB* and *crtS* each on an extra replicon [20]. Certainly, further research is needed to fully understand the mechanistic *crtS*-to-*ori2* interrelation. Nevertheless, we consider the heterologous *E. coli* system with chromosomal insertions of *ori2* and *crtS* presented here to be highly valuable in the study of the complex replication regulation system of *V. cholerae* in a simplified synthetic system. *Ori2* was used previously to search for replication inhibitors specific for *V. cholerae* and we anticipate that corresponding studies might be extended to the *crtS* site mechanism potentially with the experimental system presented here and its further development [35].

We have used the *ori2*-test system established here to investigate the activity of the chemical compound 3-(3,4-dichlorophenyl)cyclopropane-1,1,2,2-tetracarbonitrile, designated as "vibrepin" (for *Vibrio* replication inhibitor). Our results confirm the inhibition of *V. cholerae* growth that was found previously (Figure 6C) [35]. Surprisingly, vibrepin did not inhibit growth of *E. coli* strain NZ90 with *ori2*-driven chromosome replication more than that of a wt *E. coli* strain with *oriC*-based replication. This finding contradicts previous results showing that RctB is specifically inhibited by vibrepin both in vivo and in vitro [35]. This conclusion was also based on a plasmid-based *ori2*-system in *E. coli* similar to our minichromosome approach (Figure 6B) [35]. However, one difference of our replicon to the previously used one is the inclusion of the *parAB2* operon, encoding the partitioning proteins. Also, the *E. coli* strains with *ori2*-driven replication of the primary chromosome studied here, encode the *parAB2* operon. Notably, ParB2 was shown to participate in regulation of initiation at *ori2* [51]. One possibility to explain the contradicting results might thus be linked to the role of ParB2 in DNA replication initiation. It could, for example, be that ParB2 counteracts the activity of vibrepin against RctB in a yet unknown fashion yet to be discovered. Interestingly, the previous study suggested that vibrepin might have other targets in addition to RctB within *V. cholerae*. This note supports the need for heterologous systems as established in the project presented here to be able to determine specificities of inhibitors.

4. Materials and Methods

4.1. Bacterial Strains, Plasmids, Oligonucleotides, and Culture Conditions

Strains, plasmids and oligonucleotides are listed in Table S1–S3. Pre-cultures of *E. coli* were grown in 3 mL LB medium. Antibiotics and inducer were used with the following concentrations if not indicated otherwise: ampicillin (100 µg/mL), kanamycin (35 µg/mL), chloramphenicol (35 µg/mL). Growth curves were measured in 96-well plates in a microplate reader (Victor X3 Multilabel plate reader, PerkinElmer or Infinite M200pro multimode microplate reader, Tecan, Männedorf, Switzerland) at 37 °C. The 150 µL of main culture was inoculated 1:1000 and covered with 70 µL of mineral oil. Optical density was measured in 5 or 6-minute intervals.

4.2. P1 Transduction

P1*vir* transduction was carried out as described [52]. Equal cell numbers of strains #1 and NZ90 were incubated with the same P1*vir* lysate diluted 1:10 in steps to 10^{-3}. Cells were plated after a 1 h recovery, plated on selective medium and incubated overnight. Colonies resulting from transduction with P1*vir* lysate dilution of 10^{-2} were considered for all experiments with colony numbers ranging from 0 to 300.

4.3. Conjugation

The donor and acceptor strains were grown overnight and cell numbers adjusted to OD_{600} 3.0. 100 µL of cells were washed three times in LB medium supplemented with 300 µM DAP to remove antibiotics. 50 µL of both cell suspensions were mixed and 50 µL of the mix spotted on an LB-agar plate containing DAP. Conjugations were incubated for 5 h at 37 °C and about 1/3 of the drop scratched off the plate and re-suspended in 1 mL LB medium. Cells were washed three times in 1 mL LB and finally re-suspended in 100 µL of dilution buffer. Suspensions were diluted stepwise 1:10 until 10^{-9} and 20 µL of each dilution plated on LB with selection for the transconjugants (LB-amp without DAP) and the acceptor cells (LB without DAP), respectively. Plates with colony numbers suitable for counting were selected after overnight incubation and the ratio between transconjugants and acceptor calculated as measure of conjugation rate.

4.4. Quantification of Replicon Copy Numbers by qPCR

In exponential growth phase, 1 mL culture of the *E. coli* strains NZ72 and NZ140 grown in LB-amp was harvested by centrifugation at $15,000 \times g$ for 4 min. The cells were stored at –20 °C. After thawing on ice, the sample were re-suspended in 1 mL water and incubated at 95 °C for 10 min. According to the formula OD_{600} 1 = 8×10^5 cells/µL, the samples were diluted to 1.25×10^4 cells/µL. The *E. coli* strain FSK18 was used as reference. It was grown in LB to early exponential growth phase and incubated with 150 µg/mL rifampicin and 10 µg/mL cephalexin at 37 °C for 3.5 h. Each reaction was carried out in triplicates of 10 µL. Primer sets for *oriC* (3921366fw, 3921366rv, 3921366pr) and *synVicII* (ori2fw, ori2rv, ori2probe) were used in separate reactions. Three biological replicates were analyzed three times each. Ratios of *synVicII* to *oriC* were calculated relative to strain FSK18 containing the genomic regions that are template for the *oriC* and *synVicII* primer sets (see above). qPCR reactions were composed of 5 µL KAPA Probe Fast qPCR mastermix Universal 2× (peqlab, Erlangen, Germany), 1 µL primer mix and 4 µL cell suspension. The 250 µL primer mix was prepared for each set of primer and contains 22.5 µL primer fw (100 pmol/µL), 22.5 µL primer rv (100 pmol/µL), 6.25 µL probe (5′-Fam/3′-Tamra, 100 pmol/µL), 50 µL Rox Reference Dye Low 50× (peqlab) and 148.75 µL water. qPCR reactions were performed in the real-time cycler qTower (Analytik Jena AG, Jena, Germany) with the following program: 1, 95 °C for 3 min; 2, 95 °C for 3 s; 3, 55 °C for 20 s; and 4, fluorescence read. Steps 2–4 were repeated 45 times. The determination of the CT-values was carried out with the software qPCRsoft (Analytik Jena AG, Jena, Germany) without using the rox reference.

4.5. Quantification of Replicon Copy Number via Antibiotic Sensitivity

Analysis of the copy-up effect of *crtS* was done as described in [33]. Cells were grown in LB medium with either 100 or 500 μg/ mL ampicillin at 37 °C in 96-well plates in a microplate reader (Infinite M200pro multimode microplate reader, Tecan). The main culture (150 μL) was inoculated 1:1000 and growth curves recorded for 15 h. For better visualization, 1 divided by the time needed to reach an OD_{600} of 0.1 was defined as measure of the copy number.

4.6. Comparative Genomic Hybridization

Exponentially growing cells in LB (OD_{600} = 0.15) were mixed in a 1:1 ratio with cold killing buffer. Strain #1 (wt MG1655 with an inserted to site) grown in AB Glu-CAA until stationary phase was used as a reference. All samples were centrifuged at 4 °C and cells were resuspended in 300 μL immunoprecipitation buffer. Cells were sonicated via Bioruptor® Plus (Diagenode Diagnosics) (48 cycles of 30 s with 30 s cooling) to receive DNA fragments of around 500 bp. The cell extract was centrifuged and the supernatant was transferred to a new reaction tube. TE buffer (300 μL) and 2 μL RNase A (10 mg/mL) were added, and samples were incubated at 65 °C for 90 min. DNA was extracted with phenol/chloroform. DNA (400 ng; 20 ng/mL in 20 μL) was labeled with Cy3-dCTP (sample) or Cy5-dCTP (reference), mixed and hybridized to whole genome microarrays from Agilent (8 × 15 k) as described [53]. Arrays were scanned on an Agilent SureScan High Resolution Scanner. Spot intensities were extracted via AgilentScan Control software. Ratios of dye intensities were calculated and normalized to the array-wide average using R. A Loess fitting was applied to the microarray data to obtain a locally weighted average (shown as the colored line in CGH plot). For this average line, we detected maxima and minima. The maximal and minimal positions were used to dissect the data set in subsets delimited by the extrema. For these subsets, a linear regression line was determined, and the coordinates of the intersection points were taken as final maxima and minima.

4.7. Flow Cytometry

To generate Rif/Ceph run out samples, cells were grown in LB-medium [with Ohly® yeast extract] and treated with 150 μg/mL rifampicin and 10 μg/mL cephalexin in the early exponential phase for more than three generations (2–3 h), allowing them to finish ongoing rounds of replication [54]. For exponential phase samples, cells were grown in LB until the early exponential phase. The cells were harvested and washed twice in TBS (0.1 M Tris-HCl pH 7.5, 0.75 M NaCl). They were fixed in 100 μL TBS and 1 mL 77% ethanol and stored at least overnight at 4 °C. For run-out experiments, cell samples were washed and diluted in 0.1 M phosphate buffer, pH 9.0 (PB buffer). Proteins were stained overnight with 3 μg/mL FITC solution (PB buffer) at 4 °C. Afterwards, cells were stained with Hoechst 33,258 as has been outlined before [38]. They were analyzed on LSR II flow cytometer (BD Biosciences) and flow cytometry measurements were carried out as described [55]. *E. coli* MG1655 cells grown exponentially in AB-acetate and stained with Hoechst only served as an internal standard and were added to every sample. For DNA-stained exponential grown cells, the samples were washed in 0.5 M sodium-citrate and treated with 5 ng/mL RNase A in 0.5 M sodium-citrate for 4 h at 50 °C. They were stained with 250 nM SYTOX® Green Nucleic Acid Stain (Thermo Fisher Scientific, Waltham, MA, USA) and analyzed on Fortessa Flow Cytometer (BD Biosciences, San Jose, CA, USA). The SYTOX® Green fluorescence was measured through a 530/30 nm bandpass filter. *E. coli* MG1655 cells grown exponentially in AB-acetate and stained with SYTOX® Green served as standard. For protein-stained exponential grown cells, samples were treated with FITC as described above. The cells were washed with TBS and analyzed on Fortessa Flow Cytometer (BD Biosciences). The FITC fluorescence was measured through a 530/30 nm bandpass filter. Data was processed with the software FlowJo (Treestar, Ashland, OR, USA).

4.8. Fluorescence Microscopy and Data Evaluation

Cells were grown in AB glucose CAA to OD_{450} ~0.15. 1 mL of the culture was harvested by centrifugation and cells re-suspended in 25 μL fresh AB glucose CAA. Cells (2 μL) were transferred to 1% agarose pads containing 1% TAE. Fluorescence microscopy was performed with a Nikon Eclipse Ti-E microscope with a phase-contrast Plan Apo l oil objective (100; numerical aperture, 1.45) with the AHF HC filter set F36-528 YFP (excitation band pass [ex bp] 500/24-nm, beam splitter [bs] 515-nm, and emission [em] bp 535/30-nm filters) and an Argon Ion Laser (Melles Griot, Rochester, NY, USA). Images were acquired with an Andor iXon3 885 electron-multiplying charge-coupled device (EMCCD) camera. For quantification of fluorescence foci, 20 images were taken for every strain and the first 700 cells were used for further analyses. Images were analyzed by Fiji using the MircobeJ plugin [56].

4.9. Plasmid Construction

Plasmid pMA200 was constructed by the cutting of pMA308 with I-SceI and insertion of the *crtS* site amplified with primers 1593 and 1613 with *V. cholerae* chromosomal DNA as the template, by Gibson assembly [57]. Plasmid pMA308 was constructed by cutting pMA135 with AscI and inserting *oriC* amplified with primers 1349 and 1350 with *E. coli* MG1655 DNA as the template. Plasmid pMA899 was constructed by cutting of pMA135 with AscI and insertion of *oriF*, amplified with primers 1487 and 1488 with pMA129 as the template. Plasmid pMA206 was constructed by cutting of pMA899 with I-SceI and insertion of the *crtS* site, amplified with primers 1593 and 1613 with *V. cholerae* chromosomal DNA as the template, by Gibson assembly. Plasmid pMA568 was constructed by cutting pMA132 with I-SceI and insertion of a NotI restriction site flanked *lacZ* cassette amplified using primers 1002 and 1004. Plasmid pMA208 was constructed by a MoClo-reaction (with BsaI) with plasmid pMA350 and a PCR fragment amplified with primers 1661 and 1662 with *E. coli* DNA as the template. MoClo was carried out as described [27,58]. Plasmid pMA209 was constructed by a MoClo-reaction with plasmid pMA353 and a PCR fragment amplified with primers 1663 and 1664 with *E. coli* DNA as template. Plasmid pMA740 was constructed by a MoClo reaction with plasmid pMA351 and a PCR fragment amplified with primers 1204 and 1205 and plasmid pMA650 as the template to amplify an *ori2* without bpiI or BsaI restriction sites. Plasmid pMA734 was constructed by a MoClo reaction with plasmid pMA352 and a chloramphenicol resistance cassette flanked by FRT sites generated by PCR with primers 703 and 704. Plasmid pMA210 was constructed in a MoClo reaction (with bpiI) including plasmids pMA208, pMA209, pMA329, pMA734, pMA740 and pICH50927. Plasmid pMA157 was constructed by a MoClo reaction with plasmid pMA349 (with BsaI) and a PCR fragment amplified with primers 1439 and 1440 and *V. cholerae* chromosomal DNA as template. Plasmid pMA431 was constructed by a MoClo reaction (BsaI) with plasmid pMA350 and a kanamycin resistance cassette flanked by FRT sites generated by PCR with primers 1455 and 1456. Plasmid pMA710 was constructed as described for pMA711 before with pMA351 as MoClo vector instead pMA352 [27]. Plasmid pMA207 was constructed in a MoClo reaction (with bpiI) including plasmids pMA709, pMA710, pMA327, pMA431, pMA157 and pICH50900. Minichromosomes pMA108–116 were constructed by Gibson Assembly [57]. Inserts were amplified from pMA87 by PCR with primers that contain homologous sequences to sequences on pMA90, which contains only half of the *ori2* sequences, with the part missing starting close to the DnaA box. Primers used are given in supplementary Table S4. The vector pMA90 was linearized with NotI before assembly with the PCR products. Chemically competent *E. coli* DH5αλpir cells, which can replicate these minichromosomes using their R2K origin [59], were transformed with the Gibson Assembly products. Colonies were screened by colony PCR with primers 14 and 16. Primer 16 is located in a sequence missing in pMA90 but present in minichromosomes with a full *ori2*. All constructs were verified by sequencing.

4.10. Strain Construction

Strain SM113 was constructed by introduction of the FROS array by P1 transduction and subsequent FRT recombination as described previously for strain SM112 [27]. To integrate *ori2* into *oriC* in *E. coli* we used a DNA fragment consisting of *ori2* and a chloramphenicol resistance cassette flanked by regions beside *oriC* (parts of *mioC* and *mnmG*) for homologous recombination (Figure 7). The subsequent DNA fragment was generated by releasing the insert of plasmid pMA210 by cutting with BsaI and transformed into strain AB330 for recombineering. Exchange of *oriC* for *ori2* was confirmed by PCR and flow cytometry and the respective strain designated NZ135. The *ori2* insertion was transferred to *E. coli* MG1655 wt by P1 transduction to give strain NZ134. Subsequently the CAT cassette was removed via pCP20-based recombination resulting in strain NZ138 [60]. Introduction of the *crtS* site into the chromosome was similar to *ori2* into *oriC* but using pMA207 instead of pMA210.

Acknowledgments: We are grateful to Sonja Messerschmidt, Neda Farmani and Joel Eichmann for contributions to the experiments described here and to Celine Zumkeller for help with preparation of the manuscript. Beatrice Schofield is acknowledged for careful reading and editing of the manuscript. We thank Shanmuga Sozhamanan for providing strain NSCV1 as well as Xiquan Liang and Federico Katzen for sending strains #1, #15 and #16. We acknowledge the Flow Cytometry Core Facility (ZTI, Marburg, Germany) for providing devices and help. This work was supported within the LOEWE program of the State of Hesse and a grant of the Deutsche Forschungsgemeinschaft (Grant No. WA 2713/4-1).

Author Contributions: N.S., S.M., D.S. and T.W. conceived and designed the experiments; N.S., S.M., T.S., M.B. and F.S.K. performed the experiments; N.S., S.M., T.S., M.B., F.S.K., D.S. and T.W. analyzed the data; T.W. wrote the paper.

References

1. Kuzminov, A. The precarious prokaryotic chromosome. *J. Bacteriol.* **2014**, *196*, 1793–1806. [CrossRef] [PubMed]

2. Jha, J.K.; Baek, J.H.; Venkova-Canova, T.; Chattoraj, D.K. Chromosome dynamics in multichromosome bacteria. *Biochim. Biophys. Acta* **2012**, *1819*, 826–829. [CrossRef] [PubMed]

3. Chen, C.W.; Huang, C.H.; Lee, H.H.; Tsai, H.H.; Kirby, R. Once the circle has been broken: Dynamics and evolution of *Streptomyces* chromosomes. *Trends Genet.* **2002**, *18*, 522–529. [CrossRef]

4. Val, M.E.; Soler-Bistue, A.; Bland, M.J.; Mazel, D. Management of multipartite genomes: The *Vibrio cholerae* model. *Curr. Opin. Microbiol.* **2014**, *22*, 120–126. [CrossRef] [PubMed]

5. Egan, E.S.; Waldor, M.K. Distinct replication requirements for the two *Vibrio cholerae* chromosomes. *Cell* **2003**, *114*, 521–530. [CrossRef]

6. Heidelberg, J.F.; Eisen, J.A.; Nelson, W.C.; Clayton, R.A.; Gwinn, M.L.; Dodson, R.J.; Haft, D.H.; Hickey, E.K.; Peterson, J.D.; Umayam, L.; et al. DNA sequence of both chromosomes of the cholera pathogen *Vibrio cholerae*. *Nature* **2000**, *406*, 477–483. [PubMed]

7. Duigou, S.; Knudsen, K.G.; Skovgaard, O.; Egan, E.S.; Lobner-Olesen, A.; Waldor, M.K. Independent control of replication initiation of the two *Vibrio cholerae* chromosomes by DnaA and RctB. *J. Bacteriol.* **2006**, *188*, 6419–6424. [CrossRef] [PubMed]

8. Duigou, S.; Yamaichi, Y.; Waldor, M.K. ATP negatively regulates the initiator protein of *Vibrio cholerae* chromosome II replication. *Proc. Natl. Acad. Sci. USA* **2008**, *105*, 10577–10582. [CrossRef] [PubMed]

9. Jha, J.K.; Ghirlando, R.; Chattoraj, D.K. Initiator protein dimerization plays a key role in replication control of *Vibrio cholerae* chromosome 2. *Nucleic Acids Res.* **2014**, *42*, 10538–10549. [CrossRef] [PubMed]

10. Orlova, N.; Gerding, M.; Ivashkiv, O.; Olinares, P.D.B.; Chait, B.T.; Waldor, M.K.; Jeruzalmi, D. The replication initiator of the cholera pathogen's second chromosome shows structural similarity to plasmid initiators. *Nucleic Acids Res.* **2017**, *45*, 3724–3737. [CrossRef] [PubMed]

11. Jha, J.K.; Li, M.; Ghirlando, R.; Miller Jenkins, L.M.; Wlodawer, A.; Chattoraj, D. The DnaK chaperone uses different mechanisms to promote and inhibit replication of *Vibrio cholerae* chromosome 2. *Mbio* **2017**, *8*. [CrossRef] [PubMed]

12. Venkova-Canova, T.; Chattoraj, D.K. Transition from a plasmid to a chromosomal mode of replication entails additional regulators. *Proc. Natl. Acad. Sci. USA* **2011**, *108*, 6199–6204. [CrossRef] [PubMed]

13. Demarre, G.; Chattoraj, D.K. DNA adenine methylation is required to replicate both *Vibrio cholerae* chromosomes once per cell cycle. *PLoS Genet.* **2010**, *6*. [CrossRef] [PubMed]

14. Koch, B.; Ma, X.; Lobner-Olesen, A. Replication of *Vibrio cholerae* chromosome I in *Escherichia coli*: Dependence on dam methylation. *J. Bacteriol.* **2010**, *192*, 3903–3914. [CrossRef] [PubMed]

15. Egan, E.S.; Lobner-Olesen, A.; Waldor, M.K. Synchronous replication initiation of the two *Vibrio cholerae* chromosomes. *Curr. Biol.* **2004**, *14*, R501–R502. [CrossRef] [PubMed]

16. Chao, M.C.; Pritchard, J.R.; Zhang, Y.J.; Rubin, E.J.; Livny, J.; Davis, B.M.; Waldor, M.K. High-resolution definition of the *Vibrio cholerae* essential gene set with hidden Markov model-based analyses of transposon-insertion sequencing data. *Nucleic Acids Res.* **2013**, *41*, 9033–9048. [CrossRef] [PubMed]

17. Kamp, H.D.; Patimalla-Dipali, B.; Lazinski, D.W.; Wallace-Gadsden, F.; Camilli, A. Gene fitness landscapes of *Vibrio cholerae* at important stages of its life cycle. *PLoS Pathog.* **2013**, *9*. [CrossRef] [PubMed]

18. Jha, J.K.; Demarre, G.; Venkova-Canova, T.; Chattoraj, D.K. Replication regulation of *Vibrio cholerae* chromosome II involves initiator binding to the origin both as monomer and as dimer. *Nucleic Acids Res.* **2012**, *40*, 6026–6038. [CrossRef] [PubMed]

19. Gerding, M.A.; Chao, M.C.; Davis, B.M.; Waldor, M.K. Molecular dissection of the essential features of the origin of replication of the second *Vibrio cholerae* chromosome. *Mbio* **2015**, *6*. [CrossRef] [PubMed]

20. Baek, J.H.; Chattoraj, D.K. Chromosome I controls chromosome II replication in *Vibrio cholerae*. *PLoS Genet.* **2014**, *10*. [CrossRef] [PubMed]

21. Val, M.E.; Marbouty, M.; de Lemos Martins, F.; Kennedy, S.P.; Kemble, H.; Bland, M.J.; Possoz, C.; Koszul, R.; Skovgaard, O.; Mazel, D. A checkpoint control orchestrates the replication of the two chromosomes of *Vibrio cholerae*. *Sci. Adv.* **2016**, *2*. [CrossRef] [PubMed]

22. Rasmussen, T.; Jensen, R.B.; Skovgaard, O. The two chromosomes of *Vibrio cholerae* are initiated at different time points in the cell cycle. *EMBO J.* **2007**, *26*, 3124–3131. [CrossRef] [PubMed]

23. Stokke, C.; Waldminghaus, T.; Skarstad, K. Replication patterns and organization of replication forks in *Vibrio cholerae*. *Microbiology* **2011**, *157*, 695–708. [CrossRef] [PubMed]

24. Val, M.E.; Kennedy, S.P.; Soler-Bistue, A.J.; Barbe, V.; Bouchier, C.; Ducos-Galand, M.; Skovgaard, O.; Mazel, D. Fuse or die: How to survive the loss of Dam in *Vibrio cholerae*. *Mol. Microbiol.* **2014**, *91*, 665–678. [CrossRef] [PubMed]

25. Liang, X.; Baek, C.H.; Katzen, F. *Escherichia coli* with two linear chromosomes. *ACS Synth. Biol.* **2013**, *2*, 734–740. [CrossRef] [PubMed]

26. Skarstad, K.; Steen, H.B.; Boye, E. Cell cycle parameters of slowly growing *Escherichia coli* B/r studied by flow cytometry. *J. Bacteriol.* **1983**, *154*, 656–662. [PubMed]

27. Schindler, D.; Milbredt, S.; Sperlea, T.; Waldminghaus, T. Design and assembly of DNA sequence libraries for chromosomal insertion in bacteria based on a set of modified moclo vectors. *ACS Synth. Biol.* **2016**, *5*, 1362–1368. [CrossRef] [PubMed]

28. Simmons, L.A.; Breier, A.M.; Cozzarelli, N.R.; Kaguni, J.M. Hyperinitiation of DNA replication in *Escherichia coli* leads to replication fork collapse and inviability. *Mol. Microbiol.* **2004**, *51*, 349–358. [CrossRef] [PubMed]

29. Milbredt, S.; Farmani, N.; Sobetzko, P.; Waldminghaus, T. DNA Replication in engineered *Escherichia coli* genomes with extra replication origins. *ACS Synth. Biol.* **2016**, *5*, 1167–1176. [CrossRef] [PubMed]

30. Julio, S.M.; Heithoff, D.M.; Provenzano, D.; Klose, K.E.; Sinsheimer, R.L.; Low, D.A.; Mahan, M.J. DNA adenine methylase is essential for viability and plays a role in the pathogenesis of *Yersinia pseudotuberculosis* and *Vibrio cholerae*. *Infect. Immun.* **2001**, *69*, 7610–7615. [CrossRef] [PubMed]

31. Uhlin, B.E.; Nordstrom, K. Plasmid incompatibility and control of replication: Copy mutants of the R-factor R1 in *Escherichia coli* K-12. *J. Bacteriol.* **1975**, *124*, 641–649. [PubMed]

32. Carleton, S.; Projan, S.J.; Highlander, S.K.; Moghazeh, S.M.; Novick, R.P. Control of pT181 replication II. Mutational analysis. *EMBO J.* **1984**, *3*, 2407–2414. [PubMed]

33. Messerschmidt, S.J.; Schindler, D.; Zumkeller, C.M.; Kemter, F.S.; Schallopp, N.; Waldminghaus, T. Optimization and characterization of the synthetic secondary chromosome synVicII in *Escherichia coli*. *Front. Bioeng. Biotechnol.* **2016**, *4*. [CrossRef] [PubMed]

34. Bates, D.B.; Asai, T.; Cao, Y.; Chambers, M.W.; Cadwell, G.W.; Boye, E.; Kogoma, T. The DnaA box R4 in the minimal *oriC* is dispensable for initiation of *Escherichia coli* chromosome replication. *Nucleic Acids Res.* **1995**, *23*, 3119–3125. [CrossRef] [PubMed]

35. Yamaichi, Y.; Duigou, S.; Shakhnovich, E.A.; Waldor, M.K. Targeting the replication initiator of the second *Vibrio* chromosome: Towards generation of vibrionaceae-specific antimicrobial agents. *PLoS Pathog.* **2009**, *5*. [CrossRef] [PubMed]

36. Val, M.E.; Skovgaard, O.; Ducos-Galand, M.; Bland, M.J.; Mazel, D. Genome engineering in *Vibrio cholerae*: A feasible approach to address biological issues. *PLoS Genet.* **2012**, *8*. [CrossRef] [PubMed]

37. Xie, G.; Johnson, S.L.; Davenport, K.W.; Rajavel, M.; Waldminghaus, T.; Detter, J.C.; Chain, P.S.; Sozhamannan, S. Exception to the rule: Genomic characterization of naturally occurring unusual *Vibrio cholerae* strains with a single chromosome. *Int. J. Genom.* **2017**. [CrossRef] [PubMed]

38. Messerschmidt, S.J.; Kemter, F.S.; Schindler, D.; Waldminghaus, T. Synthetic secondary chromosomes in *Escherichia coli* based on the replication origin of chromosome II in *Vibrio cholerae*. *Biotechnol. J.* **2015**, *10*, 302–314. [CrossRef] [PubMed]

39. Fossum, S.; De Pascale, G.; Weigel, C.; Messer, W.; Donadio, S.; Skarstad, K. A robust screen for novel antibiotics: Specific knockout of the initiator of bacterial DNA replication. *FEMS Microbiol. Lett.* **2008**, *281*, 210–214. [CrossRef] [PubMed]

40. Lobner-Olesen, A.; Atlung, T.; Rasmussen, K.V. Stability and replication control of *Escherichia coli* minichromosomes. *J. Bacteriol.* **1987**, *169*, 2835–2842. [CrossRef] [PubMed]

41. Lobner-Olesen, A. Distribution of minichromosomes in individual *Escherichia coli* cells: Implications for replication control. *EMBO J.* **1999**, *18*, 1712–1721. [CrossRef] [PubMed]

42. Skarstad, K.; Lobner-Olesen, A. Stable co-existence of separate replicons in *Escherichia coli* is dependent on once-per-cell-cycle initiation. *EMBO J.* **2003**, *22*, 140–150. [CrossRef] [PubMed]

43. Richardson, T.T.; Harran, O.; Murray, H. The bacterial DnaA-trio replication origin element specifies single-stranded DNA initiator binding. *Nature* **2016**, *534*, 412–416. [CrossRef] [PubMed]

44. Camara, J.E.; Breier, A.M.; Brendler, T.; Austin, S.; Cozzarelli, N.R.; Crooke, E. Hda inactivation of DnaA is the predominant mechanism preventing hyperinitiation of *Escherichia coli* DNA replication. *EMBO Rep.* **2005**, *6*, 736–741. [CrossRef] [PubMed]

45. Simmons, L.A.; Kaguni, J.M. The DnaAcos allele of *Escherichia coli*: Hyperactive initiation is caused by substitution of A184V and Y271H, resulting in defective ATP binding and aberrant DNA replication control. *Mol. Microbiol.* **2003**, *47*, 755–765. [CrossRef] [PubMed]

46. Yamaguchi, K.; Tomizawa, J. Establishment of *Escherichia coli* cells with an integrated high copy number plasmid. *Mol. Gen. Genet.* **1980**, *178*, 525–533. [CrossRef] [PubMed]

47. Hansen, E.B.; Yarmolinsky, M.B. Host participation in plasmid maintenance: Dependence upon *dnaA* of replicons derived from P1 and F. *Proc. Natl. Acad. Sci. USA* **1986**, *83*, 4423–4427. [CrossRef] [PubMed]

48. Waldminghaus, T.; Skarstad, K. The *Escherichia coli* SeqA protein. *Plasmid* **2009**, *61*, 141–150. [CrossRef] [PubMed]

49. Saint-Dic, D.; Kehrl, J.; Frushour, B.; Kahng, L.S. Excess SeqA leads to replication arrest and a cell division defect in *Vibrio cholerae*. *J. Bacteriol.* **2008**, *190*, 5870–5878. [CrossRef] [PubMed]

50. McGarry, K.C.; Ryan, V.T.; Grimwade, J.E.; Leonard, A.C. Two discriminatory binding sites in the *Escherichia coli* replication origin are required for DNA strand opening by initiator DnaA-ATP. *Proc. Natl. Acad. Sci. USA* **2004**, *101*, 2811–2816. [CrossRef] [PubMed]

51. Venkova-Canova, T.; Baek, J.H.; Fitzgerald, P.C.; Blokesch, M.; Chattoraj, D.K. Evidence for two different regulatory mechanisms linking replication and segregation of *Vibrio cholerae* chromosome II. *PLoS Genet.* **2013**, *9*. [CrossRef] [PubMed]

52. Miller, J.H. *A Short Course in Bacterial Genetics: A Laboratory Manual and Handbook for Escherichia coli and Related Bacteria*; Cold Spring Harbor Laboratory Press: Cold Spring Harbor, NY, USA, 1992.

53. Johnsen, L.; Flatten, I.; Morigen; Dalhus, B.; Bjoras, M.; Waldminghaus, T.; Skarstad, K. The G157C mutation in the *Escherichia coli* sliding clamp specifically affects initiation of replication. *Mol. Microbiol.* **2011**, *79*, 433–446. [CrossRef] [PubMed]

54. Boye, E.; Lobner-Olesen, A.; Skarstad, K. Timing of chromosomal replication in *Escherichia coli. Biochim. Biophys. Acta* **1988**, *951*, 359–364. [CrossRef]

55. Waldminghaus, T.; Weigel, C.; Skarstad, K. Replication fork movement and methylation govern SeqA binding to the *Escherichia coli* chromosome. *Nucleic Acids Res.* **2012**, *40*, 5465–5476. [CrossRef] [PubMed]

56. Jiang, C.; Brown, P.J.; Ducret, A.; Brun, Y.V. Sequential evolution of bacterial morphology by co-option of a developmental regulator. *Nature* **2014**, *506*, 489–493. [CrossRef] [PubMed]

57. Gibson, D.G.; Young, L.; Chuang, R.Y.; Venter, J.C.; Hutchison, C.A., III; Smith, H.O. Enzymatic assembly of DNA molecules up to several hundred kilobases. *Nat. Methods* **2009**, *6*, 343–345. [CrossRef] [PubMed]

58. Weber, E.; Engler, C.; Gruetzner, R.; Werner, S.; Marillonnet, S. A modular cloning system for standardized assembly of multigene constructs. *PLoS ONE* **2011**, *6*. [CrossRef] [PubMed]

59. Miller, V.L.; Mekalanos, J.J. A novel suicide vector and its use in construction of insertion mutations: Osmoregulation of outer membrane proteins and virulence determinants in *Vibrio cholerae* requires *toxR. J. Bacteriol.* **1988**, *170*, 2575–2583. [CrossRef] [PubMed]

60. Cherepanov, P.P.; Wackernagel, W. Gene disruption in *Escherichia coli*: TcR and KmR cassettes with the option of Flp-catalyzed excision of the antibiotic-resistance determinant. *Gene* **1995**, *158*, 9–14. [CrossRef]

14

Erythromycin Modification That Improves Its Acidic Stability while Optimizing It for Local Drug Delivery

Erika L. Cyphert [1], Jaqueline D. Wallat [2], Jonathan K. Pokorski [2] and Horst A. von Recum [1,*]

[1] Department of Biomedical Engineering, Case Western Reserve University, 10900 Euclid Avenue, Cleveland, OH 44106, USA; elc50@case.edu

[2] Department of Macromolecular Science and Engineering, Case Western Reserve University, 2100 Adelbert Road, Cleveland, OH 44106, USA; jdw114@case.edu (J.D.W.); jon.pokorski@case.edu (J.K.P.)

* Correspondence: horst.vonrecum@case.edu

Academic Editor: Naresh Kumar

Abstract: The antibiotic erythromycin has limited efficacy and bioavailability due to its instability and conversion under acidic conditions via an intramolecular dehydration reaction. To improve the stability of erythromycin, several analogs have been developed—such as azithromycin and clarithromycin—which decrease the rate of intramolecular dehydration. We set out to build upon this prior work by developing a conjugate of erythromycin with improved pH stability, bioavailability, and preferential release from a drug delivery system directly at the low pH of an infection site. To develop this new drug conjugate, adamantane-1-carbohydrazide was covalently attached to erythromycin via a pH-degradable hydrazone bond. Since *Staphylococcus aureus* infection sites are slightly acidic, the hydrazone bond will undergo hydrolysis liberating erythromycin directly at the infection site. The adamantane group provides interaction with the drug delivery system. This local delivery strategy has the potential of reducing off-target and systemic side-effects. This work demonstrates the synthesis of a pH-cleavable, erythromycin conjugate that retains the inherent antimicrobial activity of erythromycin, has an increased hydrophobicity, and improved stability in acidic conditions; thereby enhancing erythromycin's bioavailability while simultaneously reducing its toxicity.

Keywords: erythromycin; infection; pH-sensitive; pH-responsive; hydrophobic; adamantane; cyclodextrin; polymer

---

1. Introduction

Erythromycin (EM) is a macrolide antibiotic that is frequently used in the treatment of *Staphylococcus aureus* (*S. aureus*) infections and is a common alternative for patients with penicillin allergies [1,2]. Generally, EM has a low cytotoxicity; however, it has been reported to cause gastrointestinal problems as well as liver toxicity due to its instability and chemical conversion under acidic conditions [1,3]. To improve the acid-stability of macrolide antibiotics, different analogs have been developed such as azithromycin and clarithromycin [1]. While azithromycin and clarithromycin have an improved acidic stability compared to EM, all three macrolides nevertheless undergo an acid-mediated chemical conversion via the slow loss of cladinose sugar from the 14-membered aglycone ring [4,5]. We therefore set out to develop a modified, more acid-stable form of EM to minimize these toxicities as well as increase its hydrophobicity slightly to improve EM's overall bioavailability at an infection site, and which can be combined with a smart drug delivery system.

In an effort to improve the bioavailability and pharmacokinetic properties of antibiotics, a variety of chemical conjugations have been employed. Specifically, ciprofloxacin and vancomycin have been chemically modified with hydrolytic ((acyloxy)alkyl ester) and different aliphatic and aromatic linkers (cathelicidin-related antimicrobial peptides) in order to enable a targeted antibiotic delivery and to enhance the antibacterial activity (i.e., improved ability to penetrate the bacterial membrane) of the original drug [6,7]. Furthermore, several different analogs of clarithromycin and β-lactam antibiotics have been synthesized that are less susceptible towards developing resistance to certain bacterial strains [8,9]. Amino acid sequences have also been utilized to chemically modify antibiotics in order to increase the drug's hydrophobicity and concentration at the target delivery site [10].

Adamantane (AD) is a hydrophobic molecule that has frequently been used to chemically modify drugs to improve a variety of drug properties [11]. Specifically, AD has been conjugated to a variety of central nervous system drugs and antiviral agents in an effort to improve their hydrophobicity, drug stability, pharmacokinetics, and clinical efficacy [11]. In another application, AD has been conjugated to chemotherapeutic agents to maximize their therapeutic efficacy while minimizing their hepatic and cardiotoxicities [12–14]. Non-steroidal anti-inflammatory drugs (NSAIDs) and diacylglycerol acyltransferase 1 inhibitors (DGAT1) have also utilized AD modifications to increase the potency of NSAIDs and to create a novel DGAT1 inhibitor drug for more effective diabetic treatment [15,16]. Generally, when AD is conjugated to drugs, it functions to increase the drug's hydrophobicity which can enable the drug to bind to tissue more readily. With more drug binding to tissue, AD thereby increases the tissue residence time of the drug and its therapeutic effects [17,18]. Similar strategy can be used to retain the AD conjugated drugs in a drug delivery system.

Several methods have been used to improve the acidic stability and therapeutic efficacy of EM. When EM is in an acidic environment it degrades via an intramolecular dehydration reaction and forms the compound anhydroerythromycin A which is an inactive and more toxic form of the drug [19]. Several analogs of EM (azithromycin and clarithromycin) have been developed that have a chemical substitution at the location where internal dehydration is first initiated to prevent the degradation reaction from starting, resulting in slightly increased acidic stability and therapeutic efficacy [19–21]. However, these analogs are still susceptible to acid degradation. Several techniques have been used to improve the acid stability and bioavailability of the analogs. For clarithromycin, amorphous solid dispersions have been created using cellulose acetate adipate propionate that has a high affinity for hydrophobic drugs in order to enhance the clarithromycin's bioavailability [22]. Furthermore, alkalizers including MgO and Na$_2$CO$_3$ have been used to manipulate the microenvironment of clarithromycin to improve its stability and solubility when combined in a crystalline-solid dispersion system using polyvinylpyrrolidone and hydroxypropylmethylcellulose [23]. For EM, enteric coatings have been developed to create delayed-release tablets that 'shield' EM from acidic degradation while in the stomach [24]. Furthermore, pH-responsive polymers have also been used to improve the acidic stability of EM [25]. While these methods improve the efficacy and acidic stability of EM, none of the current studies have developed a form of EM capable of demonstrating increased acidic stability while simultaneously optimizing the drug to remain at the infection site, such as through drug delivery.

To create a more acid-stable form of EM, we chemically linked adamantane-1-carbohydrazide (AD) to EM via hydrazone chemistry [13] to create the modified drug AD-EM. Because *S. aureus* infection sites are slightly acidic [25] they would be able to cleave the acid-sensitive hydrazone bond and liberate unmodified EM. When administered locally, this would increase the residence time at the infection site, reduce availability to healthy tissues, and decrease EM's toxicity. Our further interest is in stimulus-responsive local delivery, so the AD-EM was tested to bind to our high-affinity cyclodextrin-based polymer delivery system at physiologically normal pH and to release free drug during infection in a pH-dependent manner.

To further elaborate, our primary motivation for developing a form of EM with a degradable linkage was to create a more stable form of EM that is able to return to its original active form when EM is liberated upon cleavage of the linkage. Further, we wanted to improve the tissue residence time of EM locally at the infection site by increasing its hydrophobicity and its affinity for our drug delivery system. With an increased hydrophobicity, the modified EM is able to remain in our drug delivery system and therefore in the tissue for a longer period of time (compared to normal EM), allowing the degradable linkage to be cleaved under the slightly acidic infection conditions and liberating the normal EM locally to the infection site.

In this paper, we have developed a synthesis procedure for adamantane-modified erythromycin (AD-EM), characterized AD-EM with Fourier transform infrared spectroscopy (FTIR), Nuclear Magnetic Spectroscopy (^{1}H NMR), and Matrix Assisted Laser Desorption Ionization (MALDI) mass spectrometry, determined the hydrophobicity and solubility of AD-EM in several solvents, and evaluated the stability of AD-EM in acidic conditions. We used a zone of inhibition assay against *S. aureus* to evaluate the antibacterial activity of AD-EM compared to EM and completed bacterial biofilm penetration/biofilm quantification studies using both drugs. We also completed a preliminary drug release study from our cyclodextrin-polymer drug delivery system using both AD-EM and EM in neutral and slightly acidic conditions.

2. Results and Discussion

2.1. Synthesis of Adamantane-Modified EM (AD-EM)

By chemically linking adamantane (AD) to the C-9 primary ketone of EM, a hydrazone bond is formed that is cleavable in slightly acidic environments (Figure 1) [13]. The chemical modification is specifically designed to improve the stability of EM in acidic conditions, since the AD is linked at the site where the intramolecular dehydration chemical conversion reaction of EM originates [19]. Because the hydrazone bond is cleaved in acidic conditions, the modified drug is optimized to preferentially respond to the acidic environments of infection. This is clinically relevant because *S. aureus* infections demonstrate a slightly lower pH compared to normal physiological conditions [26]. The hypothesis is that AD-EM will be capable of maximizing the antibiotic concentration of locally administered EM at the infection site, thereby reducing associated systemic toxicities and improving the therapeutic efficacy of EM. The AD moiety has previously been shown to have a high affinity (binding constant) and stably bind to cyclodextrin-based polymer systems [14,27], such as our drug delivery platform. The goal in designing the chemistry of AD-EM was to optimize the drug such that it had an improved stability while demonstrating a high affinity for cyclodextrin to facilitate a controlled pH-responsive release of EM directly at the infection site.

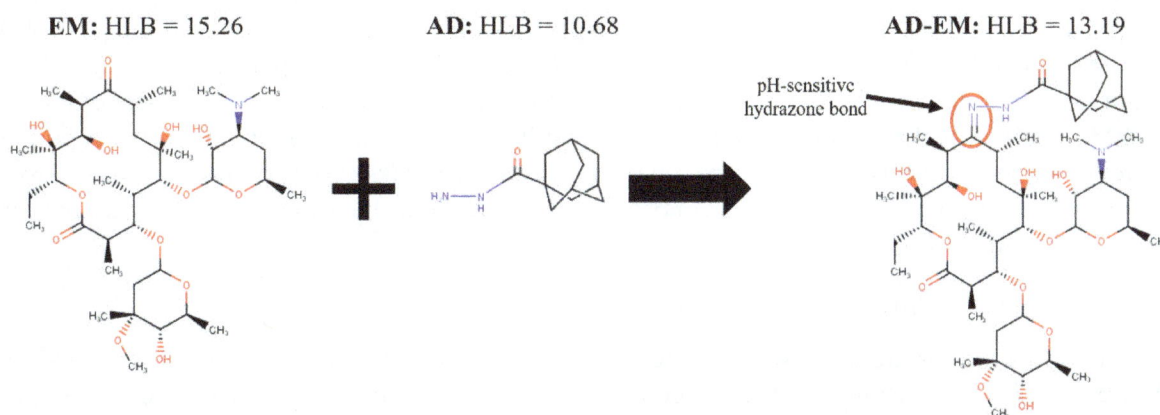

Figure 1. Schematic of the chemical structure and synthesis of adamantane-modified erythromycin (AD-EM). In the synthesis of AD-EM, adamantane (AD) is chemically linked to EM via a pH-sensitive hydrazone bond (C = N) at the site of the C-9 primary ketone on EM.

2.2. FTIR Spectrum of AD, EM, and AD-EM

FTIR spectra were generated for AD, EM, and AD-EM from 500–4000 cm^{-1}. The spectra were superimposed upon one another in order to evaluate whether the hydrazone bond was successfully created between AD and EM. The formation of the hydrazone bond is indicated by a peak over the span of 1560–1570 cm^{-1} on the AD-EM spectrum that is not present on the other spectra [14,28]. Figure 2 depicts the appearance of the hydrazone peak (1560–1570 cm^{-1}) on the spectrum of AD-EM validating the formation and presence of the hydrazone bond.

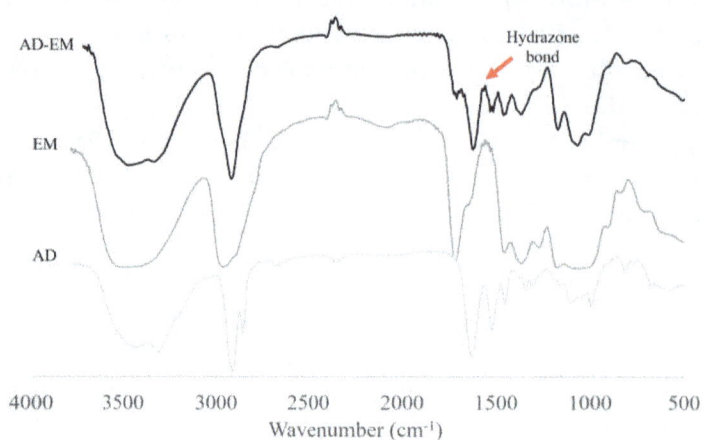

Figure 2. Fourier transform infrared spectroscopy (FTIR) spectra of AD-EM, EM, and AD superimposed. The chemical modification of EM to AD-EM was validated based upon the appearance of the pH-sensitive hydrazone bond peak at 1560–1570 cm^{-1} on the AD-EM FTIR spectrum that is not present in either of the spectra of AD or EM.

2.3. ^{1}H NMR of EM and AD-EM

^{1}H NMR was used to confirm the presence of AD in the AD-EM (Figure S1). Both EM and AD-EM were dissolved in deuterated dimethyl sulfoxide (DMSO-d$_6$) and spectra acquired. The spectra are in agreement with the reported literature spectra [29], thus we looked to see changes in the spectra following the conjugation reaction. The processed spectra of each species were compared to monitor structural differences between protons from EM and AD-EM. The AD-EM spectra confirms the presence of both AD and EM, as well as hydrazone formation, indicating successful reaction. In the NMR spectra of AD-EM, AD attachment is confirmed by the presence of two multiplet peaks at approximately 1.9 ppm and from 1.6–1.8 ppm, corresponding to protons from the fused cyclohexane rings of AD. In the spectra of the AD-EM, a singlet peak, corresponding to a hydrazone, appears at 9.0 ppm. These protons are attributed to AD-EM conjugate, since AD alone is completely insoluble in DMSO. Of note, AD-EM remained slightly insoluble in DMSO-d$_6$, resulting in minor peak shape distortions, poorer resolution of peak splitting and peak broadening, for resonance peaks corresponding to protons from EM. However, peak placement is consistent between AD-EM and EM, indicating the presence of both species in the AD-EM conjugate.

2.4. MALDI Mass Spectrometry of EM and AD-EM

MALDI mass spectrometry was used to elucidate the molecular mass of AD-EM. The MALDI spectra of AD-EM was compared to EM. From the MALDI spectra of AD-EM, two chemical species are present. One species corresponds to the mass of the conjugate (AD-EM) (910 m/z), while the other corresponds to the mass of the EM (733 m/z) (Figure S2). It is possible that the labile hydrazone bond fragments during ionization, hence the biomodal distribution [30,31]. To further probe if ionization was responsible for the two chemical species, thin layer chromatography of AD-EM was carried out and showed evidence of two species indicating incomplete conjugation (data not shown). Although hydrazones are relatively stable, they can undergo spontaneous hydrolytic cleavage which would afford free EM and AD [32]. Alternatively, it is possible that inefficient purification resulted in residual unreacted EM in the conjugate mixture.

2.5. Hydrophilic-Lipophilic Balance Calculations

The hydrophilic-lipophilic balance (HLB) numbers were calculated for AD, EM, and conjugated AD-EM using three different methods (ChemAxon, Davies, and Griffin) in ChemAxon MarvinSketch Version 16.10.31 software with the HLB Predictor plug-in (See Table S1). The reported HLB numbers for each molecule were calculated using the ChemAxon method, which is an optimized weighted combination of both the Davies and Griffin methods [33]. A larger HLB number indicates a more hydrophilic molecule. The conjugated AD-EM molecule was more hydrophobic than the unmodified EM (AD-EM = 13.19; EM = 15.26) due to the addition of the hydrophobic AD group (AD = 10.68). Similar patterns were observed when the Davies and Griffin methods were used to calculate the HLB numbers where the AD-EM molecule was more hydrophobic than unmodified EM (See Table S1). When the HLB values obtained through the software are compared to experimental results, they have been shown to correlate with an R^2 value of 0.79 [33]. Therefore, we believe that the HLB numbers that we obtained through this modeling software are a good representation of the anticipated experimental values of the HLB numbers.

2.6. Solubility Study

The solubility of AD-EM compared to EM was evaluated in several different aqueous buffers (i.e., PBS, Water, Acetate pH 5.0) and polar solvents (i.e., methanol, ethyl acetate, acetone). The solubility study presented in Table 1 further verifies that modified AD-EM is more hydrophobic than EM due to the addition of the hydrophobic AD group. AD-EM demonstrated a decrease in solubility in aqueous solutions compared to EM (PBS: AD-EM = 0.34 mg/mL, EM = 1.6 mg/mL; Water: AD-EM = 0.33 mg/mL, EM = 1.5 mg/mL), a decreased solubility in methanol, but showed comparable solubility to EM in several polar solvents (~40 mg/mL). This indicates that the increased hydrophobicity from the modification had a relatively large impact on its aqueous solubility, but the increase in hydrophobicity was not large enough to dramatically impact its solubility in some polar protic and aprotic solvents. The increased hydrophobicity of AD-EM is desirable to enhance its ability to bind to tissue, thereby increasing its tissue residence time and therapeutic activity.

Table 1. Relative solubility (n = 3) of EM and AD-EM in several different aqueous buffers and organic solvents.

Solvent	EM (mg/mL)	AD-EM (mg/mL)
Water	1.5 ± 0.2	0.33 ± 0.03
Phosphate Buffered Saline (PBS), pH 7.4	1.6 ± 0.4	0.34 ± 0.01
Acetate buffer, pH 5.0	15	1.39 ± 0.04
Methanol	>40	7.3 ± 0.2
Ethyl Acetate	>40	>40
Acetone	>40	37.5

2.7. Acidic Stability Spectral Scan Analysis

The stability of EM and AD-EM in slightly acidic conditions (pH 5.0) was analyzed by studying the absorbance signal of the drug solution over a range of wavelengths (Figure 3). This technique capitalizes on the differences in absorbance signal between active EM and the major inactive (but reversible) acid-conversion product of EM—anhydroerythromycin A—which has a lower absorbance signal than active EM [4,34]. Figure 3a validates the hypothesis that EM in an acidic solution has a lower absorbance signal (0.17) compared to the drug in a neutral solution (0.22). Further, it shows that when the acidic solution of EM is later neutralized, the absorbance signal is restored back to the absorbance value in neutral conditions (0.22), presumably due to the reversible nature of the anhydroerythromycin A conversion. This restoration of signal intensity further validates the predicted model where inactive anhydroerythromycin A is in equilibrium with active EM and can be converted back to active EM in a neutralized solution [4]. A noticeable acidic conversion of EM (Figure 3a) was observed over a period of several hours.

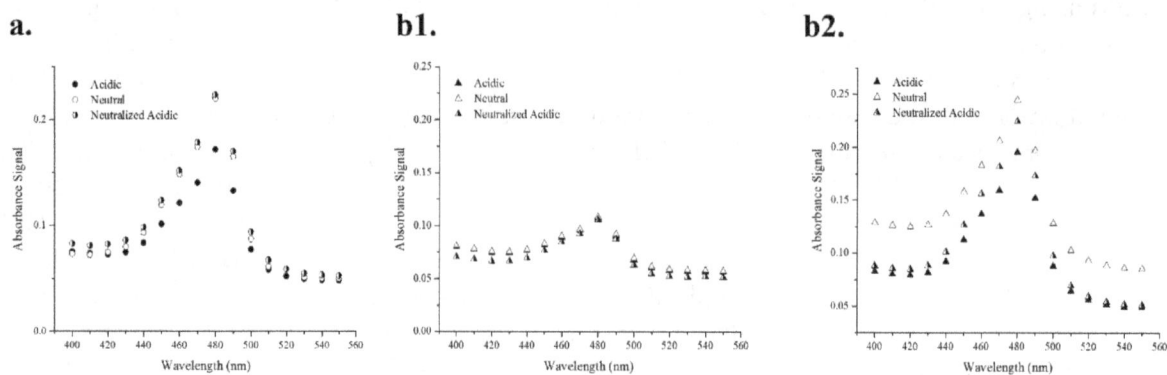

Figure 3. (**a**) Absorbance spectral scan of EM in acidic and neutral environments (t = several hours). (**b**) Absorbance spectral scan of AD-EM in acidic and neutral environments (t = several hours (**b1**); t = several days (**b2**)). In acidic conditions, EM is converted to an inactive form that demonstrates a lower absorbance signal than the original EM. When it is later placed in neutral conditions, the original absorbance signal in neutral conditions is restored.

The acidic stability of AD-EM was evaluated in Figure 3b1,b2. In Figure 3b1, the experiment was conducted over a period of several hours (the same amount of time in which a noticeable acidic conversion of EM was observed). There were no distinguishable differences observed in the absorbance patterns between the three solutions (AD-EM in acidic, neutral, and acidic later neutralized conditions) over the same period of time in which acidic conversion occurred in EM. The lack of acidic conversion in AD-EM over the same period of time as EM conversion demonstrates that AD-EM has an increased stability compared to EM in slightly acidic environments. We hypothesize that the increased acidic stability of AD-EM is due to the addition of the chemical modification at the location where the intramolecular dehydration reaction initially occurs in EM [4,34].

The same experiment as Figure 3b1 was also conducted over a longer period of time (i.e., several days instead of hours) (Figure 3b2). It was observed that, after several days, AD-EM in acidic conditions has a lower absorbance signal than in neutral conditions, demonstrating eventual loss of the adamantane and conversion of AD-EM into anhydroerythromycin A which has a lower absorbance signal in acidic conditions [34]. When AD-EM was first placed in an acidic solution and later neutralized, it showed an increased absorbance signal compared to the signal of AD-EM in acidic conditions, but was not equivalent to the original signal in neutral conditions. As stated above, this is most likely due to the reversible conversion through anhydroerythromycin A and back again. The signal of AD-EM under these conditions (i.e., initially acid and later neutralized), however, was not fully returned to the original signal of AD-EM in neutral conditions. We hypothesize that this is due to the irreversible transformation that AD-EM encounters under these conditions. Specifically, the acid cleavable linker (hydrazone bond) that was chemically added to EM to create AD-EM is irreversibly broken in acidic conditions to liberate active EM. Under neutral conditions this linker is not cleaved and the absorbance signal is higher. However, once this hydrazone bond is cleaved in acidic conditions, EM is liberated and the absorbance signal decreases (due to the intramolecular dehydration of EM). The initial absorbance signal in neutral conditions cannot be fully restored, even if EM is returned to its active form, since the bond between AD and EM cannot be re-formed.

The underlying hypothesis is that the acid-mediated conversion of AD-EM occurs over a longer period of time compared to EM, due to the addition of the linker at the location where intramolecular dehydration first occurs. While AD-EM ultimately is converted into anhydroerythromycin A in acidic conditions, the addition of the adamantane group delays the onset of acid-mediated conversion of EM. The improved acidic stability of AD-EM can help to reduce some of the toxicities and gastrointestinal side-effects that are commonly associated with the instability of EM in acidic conditions and enhance the bioavailability of active drug at a local injection site.

Colorimetric absorbance spectroscopy was determined to be the optimal and efficient method to track the acid-stability of EM and AD-EM. Once EM is reacted with concentrated sulfuric acid (27 N), the sugar groups are hydrolyzed and a yellow chromophore results that can be detected with absorbance spectroscopy [35–37].

2.8. Zone of Inhibition Antibacterial Study

A zone of inhibition study against *S. aureus* was conducted for approximately two weeks using EM and AD-EM loaded into insoluble cyclodextrin polymer disks to evaluate whether the chemical modification altered the intrinsic antimicrobial activity of EM (Figure 4). Both AD-EM and EM demonstrated comparable activity to inhibit the growth of *S. aureus* during the duration of the study. It is possible that the slight decrease in antibacterial activity after 8 days in AD-EM (compared to EM) can be attributed to the presence of both species in the final AD-EM composition. However, despite the presence of both species in AD-EM, we concluded that the chemical modification to EM did not significantly affect the antibacterial activity of EM.

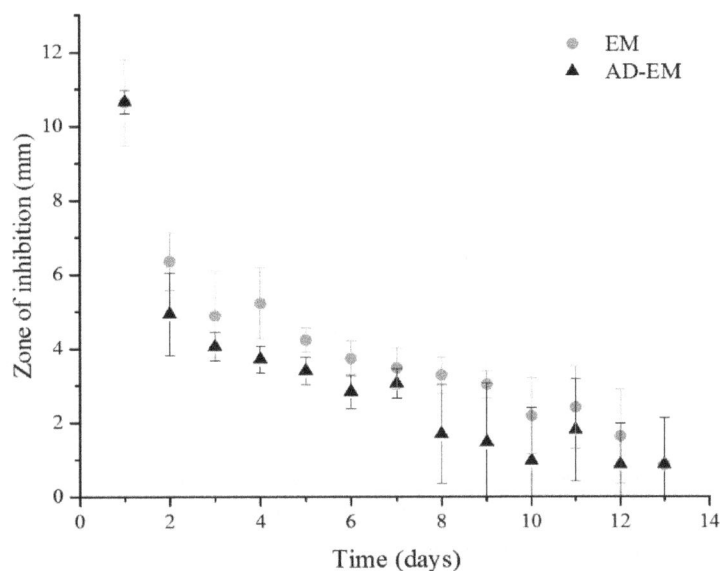

Figure 4. Zone of inhibition study of AD-EM and EM against *S. aureus*. AD-EM and EM demonstrated comparable activity against the growth of *S. aureus* for nearly 2 weeks. Therefore, the chemical modification did not alter the intrinsic antibacterial activity of EM.

2.9. Bacterial Biofilm Penetration Studies

Through the bacterial (*S. aureus*) biofilm penetration studies using both the modified (AD-EM) and EM, we observed that both the modified and unmodified drug were capable of achieving a comparable penetration through the bacterial biofilm. The ability to penetrate through the biofilm is related to the number of bacteria remaining in the biofilm after exposure to a drug compared to the control condition (90% PBS/10% DMSO). The control condition was set-up in such a way that the biofilm coated cyclodextrin polymer was placed in a solution under the same conditions used to make the drug-containing solutions. The colonies remaining in the biofilms after 1, 7, and 24 h after being treated with AD-EM, EM, or the control solution are reported in Table 2, where the remaining colonies from drug-treated biofilms are compared to the number of colonies in a control solution. After only 1 h of exposure to the drug (AD-EM or EM), nearly 30% of the original colonies in the biofilm were eradicated, and after 7 h of drug (AD-EM or EM) exposure >85% of the original colonies were killed. Interestingly, after 24 h of exposure to the drug only a small amount of additional killing occurred (~2%) compared to the 7 h time point. We hypothesize that this could be due to presence of planktonic bacteria naturally resistant to antibiotic effect, as well as the development of drug-resistant bacteria that are unable to be fully eradicated even after extended periods of exposure time to the drug. This latter hypothesis was further validated when we carried out the same experiment to 48 and 72 h using non-modified EM and approximately the same number of colonies remained even after 72 h of exposure to EM (data not shown). Given the relative comparable activity of each drug (AD-EM and EM) against *S. aureus* in the mature biofilms combined with the zone of inhibition data, we further confirm that the chemical modification to EM did not alter the intrinsic antibacterial activity of EM and that both drugs (AD-EM and EM) are capable of penetrating and killing the majority of the bacteria in a mature biofilm within 7 h. High variability in the studies reflects both the inconsistent nature of the biofilm as well as difficulty recovering bacteria to make accurate counts.

Table 2. Quantification of bacterial colonies remaining in mature (72 h) *S. aureus* biofilms after exposure to AD-EM, EM, or a control solution (90% PBS/10% DMSO), calculated as a percentage of the colonies remaining from the control solution at each time point.

Drug Incubation Time (Hours)	AD-EM (% Control Colonies * Remaining)	EM (% Control Colonies * Remaining)
1	62.7% ± 22.1%	71.6% ± 40.2%
7	14.8% ± 13.7%	10.5% ± 6.8%
24	11.7% ± 7.9%	8.3% ± 6.6%

* Control colonies quantified after 1, 7, and 24 h incubation in PBS with 10% DMSO.

2.10. pH-Dependent Drug Release Study

As a proof-of-concept to evaluate the acid-labile modification, AD-EM and unmodified EM were loaded into insoluble cyclodextrin polymer disks, and drug release studies were conducted in both neutral and slightly acidic conditions to simulate both normal physiological conditions and the microenvironment of an infection. The slightly acidic conditions were necessary to provide the pH-stimulus required to cleave the hydrazone bond of AD-EM. Over a period of approximately 40 days, AD-EM loaded disks demonstrated a slightly increased release profile in acidic conditions compared to neutral conditions, which is attributed to the addition of the pH-sensitive linker (Figure 5). Conversely, the EM loaded polymer disks demonstrated comparable and consistent release profiles in both acidic and neutral conditions. Since EM lacked the pH-sensitive hydrazone bond, the release profiles were similar regardless of the pH condition, unlike release from AD-EM loaded disks. As we had anticipated for a pH-responsive drug delivery system, we observed an accelerated release rate of AD-EM in acidic conditions and a much slower release in neutral (presumably non-infection) conditions. This further maximizes (in addition to improved drug stability and tissue residence) the therapeutic delivery of EM at the acidic infection site when compared to delivery to pH neutral non-infected tissues.

While the difference in release rate between the AD-EM in acidic and neutral conditions may not be large, there is a more noticeable difference in the AD-EM release rates compared to the EM in both pH conditions. We hypothesize that the limited difference in release rate between AD-EM in neutral and acidic conditions is due to the relatively high binding energy of even the unmodified erythromycin for beta-cyclodextrin (−9.0 kcal/mol) [38]. Due to the high binding energy between the drug and polymer without the additional high-affinity AD moiety, it is hypothesized that with the addition of this group there is no longer a 1:1 binding interaction between the drug and polymer, but potentially a 2:1 binding interaction with the higher binding energy of that complex. Therefore, due to this complex interaction, a large amount of drug may still be trapped in the matrix of the polymer even after an extended period of time and the release results shown in Figure 5 may only demonstrate a release of the drug from the surface of the polymer. Additionally, it is possible that the mixed (2 species) composition of AD-EM also contributed to the small difference in acidic release conditions. Yet, even with the mixed composition of AD-EM, we were still able to observe slight differences in release in acidic conditions. Furthermore, due to an uncertain amount of drug still remaining in the polymer after the nearly 40 day release study, it is challenging to determine the total amount of drug initially loaded into the polymer necessary to construct a plot of total percent of drug released from the polymer.

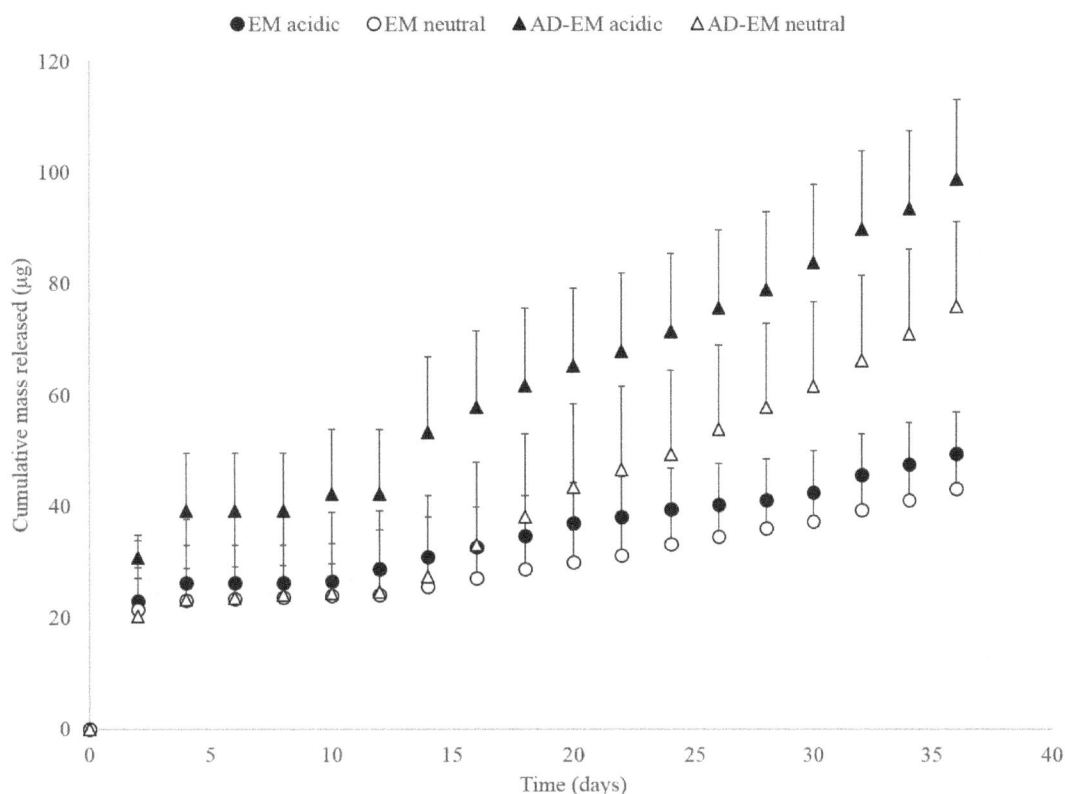

Figure 5. Cumulative mass of AD-EM and EM released in both acidic (pH 5.0) and neutral (pH 7.4) conditions.

Overall, our proof-of-concept release study demonstrates a small difference in these release rates as initially hypothesized. However, future release studies are planned that will work to optimize the release conditions and that take the large binding energy into account with the goal of demonstrating a more statistically significant difference in the release rate of AD-EM in acidic and neutral conditions.

Through Figure 5, we were also able to conclude that we were able to achieve higher levels of drug loading into the polymers with AD-EM compared to EM. This observation was consistent between the drugs released in each pH condition. We hypothesize that, with AD-EM, we can drive higher levels of drug loading into the insoluble cyclodextrin polymers due to the extra high-affinity AD group that unmodified EM lacks. To treat long-term infections clinically, it may be desirable to load a large amount of drug into the polymers to prolong the drug release time and minimize the need for additional antibiotic doses. Therefore, since AD-EM is capable of achieving increased loading over EM into our polymers it is a promising candidate for long-term antibacterial therapeutic applications.

3. Materials and Methods

3.1. Synthesis of Adamantane-Modified EM (AD-EM)

The process for synthesizing AD-EM was based upon a published protocol previously used to synthesize adamantane-modified doxorubicin but slightly modified for working with EM [13]. Specifically, 67 mg of adamantane-1-carbohydrazide (Matrix Scientific, Columbia, SC, USA) and 100 mg of erythromycin (Fisher Scientific, Pittsburgh, PA, USA) were dissolved in 50 mL methanol. Afterwards, 50 µL of trifluoroacetic acid (TFA) was used to catalyze the reaction and the solution was refluxed in an oil bath at 50 °C for 48 h in the darkness. The methanol was evaporated off using rotary evaporation and the precipitate was covered in foil and allowed to cool overnight. A mixture of 60:40% hexane:ethyl acetate solvent was used to precipitate out the unreacted AD. The solution was poured through a vacuum filter to remove the unreacted AD. The solvent mixture was evaporated off of the dissolved AD-EM with a rotary evaporator. The final AD-EM was washed with 100% hexane and vacuum filtered to remove the TFA. The purified drug was dried under vacuum and transferred to storage in a cool and dark environment.

3.2. FTIR Study

Small samples (<1 mg) of dried AD-EM, EM, and AD were each ground into a fine powder with a mortar and pestle. Dried potassium bromide (KBr, 0.1 g) was added to the powdered drug sample and ground into a fine powder. Each sample was placed in a 13 mm die and pressed with a force of 10 metric tons for 10 min. Each pellet was removed from the die and scanned in an Excaliber Series-BioRad FTS3000MX spectrometer. Then, 200 background and 400 sample scans were collected from 500–4000 cm^{-1}. Varian Resolution Pro Software was used to transform the data using ratio and transmittance transformations. A boxcar function was used to smooth out each plot.

3.3. ^1H NMR of EM and AD-EM

EM (approximately 40 mg) and AD-EM (approximately 40 mg) were dissolved in 500 μL of DMSO-d$_6$, and sonication was used to promote dissolution. Samples were analyzed on a 600 MHz Varian Nuclear Magnetic Resonance Spectrometer, using 128 scans and a 45 degree pulse angle. Spectra were analyzed using MesReNova software using the residual solvent peak from DMSO-d$_6$ as the reference.

3.4. MALDI of EM and AD-EM

EM (0.5 mg) and AD-EM (0.5 mg) were dissolved in 100 μL of acetonitrile. A saturated solution of alpha-cyano-4-hydroxy-cinnamic acid (CHCA) in acetonitrile was prepared. MALDI samples were prepared according to a three-layer method [39]: 1 μL of CHCA solution was cast onto the MALDI plate and allowed to dry; once dry, 1 μL of EM and AD-EM were cast atop the CHCA matrix and allowed to dry; once dry, an additional 1 μL of CHCA was added. MALDI was conducted on a Bruker Autoflex III operated in linear positive ion mode.

3.5. Hydrophilic-Lipophilic Balance Calculations

The hydrophilic-lipophilic balance (HLB) numbers of AD, EM, and the conjugate drug AD-EM were determined using ChemAxon MarvinSketch modeling software (Version 16.10.31, ChemAxon, 2016). The chemical structure of each molecule was drawn in the program and the HLB numbers were calculated using the HLB predictor plug-in using three different methods (ChemAxon, Davies, and Griffin; data for each method reported in Table S1). The larger the HLB number, the more hydrophilic the molecule. The ChemAxon method is an optimized weighted combination of the Davies and Griffin method [33]. In the Davies method, the computation is based upon different group numbers that are assigned to hydrophilic or lipophilic structural groups in a molecule [40,41]. The following equation is used in the calculation: HLB = 7 + Σ(hydrophilic group numbers) + Σ(lipophilic group numbers) [40,41]. With this method alone, it can be challenging to calculate the HLB if a group number is not assigned to a particular structural group [41]. In the Griffin method, the computation is based upon saponification (measure of fatty acids; S) and acid (A) indices of different structural groups; HLB = $20\left(1 - \frac{S}{A}\right)$ [42,43].

3.6. Solubility Study

Small samples of both EM and AD-EM (1–3 mg samples for aqueous solvents (water, PBS (pH 7.4), and acetate buffer (pH 5.0)); 10 mg samples for methanol, ethyl acetate, and acetone) were placed in individual vials. Each solvent was gradually added to either the EM or AD-EM samples in 50–100 µL increments until the drug sample was completely dissolved and the solution was homogeneous [44,45]. Three trials were completed for each drug in each solvent and the results are reported as an average of these three trials. The solubility limit of each drug was determined to be the minimum amount of volume of each solvent where the drug was completely soluble.

3.7. Acidic Conversion Spectral Scans

Small samples of EM were dissolved in 2 separate solutions: neutral phosphate buffered saline (PBS) and acetate pH 5.0 buffer. The PBS solution was diluted to a concentration of 70 µM and concentrated sulfuric acid (27 N) was added to the solution in a volume equal to that of the total volume of the initial 70 µM solution to elicit a color change detectable with absorbance spectroscopy [34]. Two separate solutions were initially created with the acetate buffer. One solution was diluted to 70 µM and allowed to sit for several hours at room temperature. The other acetate solution was diluted to a slightly higher concentration, sat for 1 h at room temperature, was neutralized with sodium hydroxide (0.1 N) (such that the concentration of the solution was 70 µM), and sat for several more hours at room temperature. Both acetate solutions were treated with equal volumes of sulfuric acid to elicit a color change. After the addition of sulfuric acid, all solutions had a final concentration of 35 µM and were immediately scanned with absorbance spectroscopy (Biotek[TM] 96 well plate reader, H1; Winooski, VT, USA) over the wavelength range of 300–700 nm in steps of 10 nm. Similar scans were collected for EM without sulfuric acid and of AD-EM over the same and a longer time frame with sulfuric acid (i.e., hours and days).

3.8. Synthesis of Insoluble Cyclodextrin Polymer Disks and Antibiotic Loading

Synthesis of insoluble cyclodextrin polymer disks was carried out according to a previously published protocol by Thatiparti et al. [46]. Briefly, 1 g cyclodextrin (CycloLab, Budapest, Hungary) was dissolved in 4 mL dimethylformamide (DMF) and stirred. The solution was cross-linked with hexamethylene diisocyanate (HDI; Sigma Aldrich, St. Louis, MO, USA) in a molar ratio of 1:0.16 (glucose residue: HDI). The solution was cured at 70 °C for 45 min and punched into 8 mm disks. Disks were washed to removed unreacted products over several days in 100% DMF, 50:50 DMF:water, and 100% water before use. Six disks were placed in a solution of 1.25 mg/mL AD-EM in DMF or a solution of EM in the same concentration. Solutions were covered in foil and placed on a laboratory shaker for 96 h. Loaded disks were removed from the solutions and air-dried at room temperature for later use.

3.9. Zone of Inhibition Antibacterial Study

The antibacterial activity of EM and AD-EM loaded insoluble cyclodextrin polymer disks was evaluated against *S. aureus* (GFP labeled *S. aureus* kindly provided by Ed Greenfield, Case Western Reserve University, Cleveland, OH, USA) according to the protocol outlined by Thatiparti et al. [46]. Briefly, fresh 70 µL fresh *S. aureus* culture was spread on a Trypticase soy agar plate. Each antibiotic loaded disk was placed in the center of a freshly seeded *S. aureus* plate and incubated overnight at 37 °C. After 24 h, the zone of inhibition (clearance) around each disk was measured using calipers and averaged. Each disk was transferred onto a freshly seeded *S. aureus* plate and placed in the incubator. This process was repeated for approximately 2 weeks, when the zones of inhibition were <2 mm.

3.10. Bacterial Biofilm Penetration Study

5 mm insoluble cyclodextrin polymer disks were placed in 3 mL solutions of 2× Trypticase soy broth with 30 μL of freshly cultured GFP-labeled *S. aureus*. Solutions were incubated at 37 °C for 72 h to form a mature biofilm. Each condition was set-up in triplicate. Following incubation, polymer disks were removed from the bacterial culture, excess broth removed, and placed in a 1.25 mg/mL drug solution of either EM or AD-EM dissolved in PBS with 10% DMSO. As a control, biofilm coated disks were also placed in a solution of just PBS and 10% DMSO. Each solution was placed in a laboratory shaker at 37 °C for either 1, 7, or 24 h. After this time, disks were removed from the drug solution, dried off, and placed in 4 mL of sterile Trypticase soy broth and homogenized for 30 s with an Omni TH homogenizer. Then, 70 μL of each solution was spread in duplicate on Trypticase soy agar plates and incubated overnight. Bacterial colonies were then counted and averaged using ImageJ software. Bacterial eradication was calculated as the percentage of colonies remaining in drug treated samples after different time points compared to the control colonies at that time point.

3.11. Proof-of-Concept Drug Release Study

Firstly, 5 mg samples of AD-EM and EM were each dissolved in 4 mL DMF. Six insoluble cyclodextrin disks were added to each solution and the samples were covered in foil and placed on an agitator for 96 h. Each drug loaded disk was washed with MilliQ water and dried at room temperature overnight. Dried disks were transferred into individual vials containing either 1 mL PBS (pH 7.4) or acetate (pH 5.0). All four conditions were set-up in triplicate. Every 48 h, all of the solution surrounding each loaded disk was removed and replenished with fresh buffer to maintain infinite sink conditions. The acidic release samples were neutralized with 0.1 N sodium hydroxide and allowed to sit overnight. To elicit a colorimetric change in the drug and enable it to be detected using absorbance spectroscopy, a volume of 27 N sulfuric acid (equal amount to the volume of the release sample) was added to each solution (acidic and neutral solutions). Aliquots of the release solution were scanned with absorbance spectroscopy using a Biotek™ microplate reader at 480 nm. This process was continued for a period of 36 days. Standard curves were created with known amounts of EM and AD-EM under all of the test conditions (with NaOH and sulfuric acid). All of the dilutions (neutralization with NaOH and addition of sulfuric acid) were accounted for in the calculation of the concentration of the drug at each time point during the release study.

4. Conclusions

In this paper, we have created a chemically-modified, more acid stable, hydrophobic form of EM (AD-EM) that demonstrates comparable antibacterial activity against *S. aureus* as unmodified EM. Due to its increased hydrophobicity, we hypothesize that AD-EM has an increased resident time in both our cyclodextrin polymers and in tissues enabling us to capitalize on its degradable linkage which, when cleaved, liberates free EM locally at the acidic (i.e., infection) site. Given that the addition of the degradable linkage to EM does not affect the antibacterial activity of EM both in conjugated (AD-EM) and liberated (EM) form, our future work includes developing a modified form of EM with a non-degradable linkage. We believe a non-degradable linkage may ultimately be a more desirable form of EM to minimize the potential toxicity concerns with non-drug molecules that may result following the cleavage of the linkage and liberation of EM.

Acknowledgments: The authors would like to thank the Case Alumni Association and the office of Support of Undergraduate Creative Research & Endeavors (SOURCE, Case Western Reserve University) for assisting with the funding for this project.

Author Contributions: All authors conceived and designed the experiments; Erika L. Cyphert and Jaqueline D. Wallat performed the experiments, all authors analyzed the data; Horst A. von Recum and Jonathan K. Pokorski contributed reagents/materials/analysis tools; all authors wrote the paper.

References

1. Alvarez-Elcoro, S.; Enzler, M.J. The macrolides: Erythromycin, clarithromycin, and azithromycin. *Mayo Clin. Proc.* **1999**, *74*, 613–634. [CrossRef] [PubMed]

2. White, R.J. Why use erythromycin? *Thorax* **1994**, *49*, 944–945. [CrossRef] [PubMed]

3. Braun, P. Hepatotoxicity of erythromycin. *J. Infect. Dis.* **1969**, *119*, 300–306. [CrossRef] [PubMed]

4. Hassanzadeh, A.; Barber, J.; Morris, G.A.; Gorry, P.A. Mechanism for the degradation of erythromycin A and erythromycin A 2'-ethyl succinate in acidic aqueous solution. *J. Phys. Chem. A* **2007**, *111*, 10098–10104. [CrossRef] [PubMed]

5. Noguchi, S.; Takiyama, K.; Fujiki, S.; Iwao, Y.; Miura, K.; Itai, S. Polymorphic transformation of antibiotic clarithromycin under acidic condition. *J. Pharm. Sci.* **2014**, *103*, 580–586. [CrossRef] [PubMed]

6. Zheng, T.; Nolan, E.M. Evaluation of (acyloxy)alkyl ester linkers for antibiotic release from siderophore-antibiotic conjugates. *Bioorganic Med. Chem. Lett.* **2015**, *25*, 4987–4991. [CrossRef] [PubMed]

7. Mishra, N.M.; Briers, Y.; Lamberigts, C.; Steenackers, H.; Robijns, S.; Landuyt, B.; Vanderleyden, J.; Schoofs, L.; Lavigne, R.; Luyten, W.; et al. Evaluation of the antibacterial and antibiofilm activities of novel CRAMP-vancomycin conjugates with diverse linkers. *Org. Biomol. Chem.* **2015**, *13*, 7477–7486. [CrossRef] [PubMed]

8. Zhu, D.; Xu, Y.; Liu, Y.; Chen, X.; Zhao, Z.; Lei, P. Synthesis of 4″-O-desosaminyl clarithromycin derivatives and their anti-bacterial activities. *Bioorganic Med. Chem. Lett.* **2013**, *23*, 6274–6279. [CrossRef] [PubMed]

9. Lewandowski, E.M.; Skiba, J.; Torelli, N.J.; Rajnisz, A.; Solecka, J.; Kowalski, K.; Chen, Y. Antibacterial properties and atomic resolution X-ray complex crystal structure of a ruthenocene conjugated β-lactam antibiotic. *Chem. Commun.* **2015**, *51*, 6186–6189. [CrossRef] [PubMed]

10. Ibrahim, M.A.; Panda, S.S.; Birs, A.S.; Serrano, J.C.; Gonzalez, C.F.; Alamry, K.A.; Katritzky, A.R. Synthesis and antibacterial evaluation of amino acid-antibiotic conjugates. *Bioorganic Med. Chem. Lett.* **2014**, *24*, 1856–1861. [CrossRef] [PubMed]

11. Wanka, L.; Iqbal, K.; Schreiner, P.R. The lipophilic bullet hits the targets: Medicinal chemistry of adamantane derivatives. *Chem. Rev.* **2013**, *113*, 3516–3604. [CrossRef] [PubMed]

12. Zefirova, O.N.; Nurieva, E.V.; Shishov, D.V.; Baskin, I.I.; Fuchs, F.; Lemcke, H.; Schröder, F.; Weiss, D.G.; Zefirov, N.S.; Kuznetsov, S.A. Synthesis and SAR requirements of adamantane-colchicine conjugates with both microtubule depolymerizing and tubulin clustering activities. *Bioorganic Med. Chem.* **2011**, *19*, 5529–5538. [CrossRef] [PubMed]

13. Luo, G.F.; Xu, X.D.; Zhang, J.; Yang, J.; Gong, Y.H.; Lei, Q.; Jia, H.Z.; Li, C.; Zhuo, R.X.; Zhang, X.Z. Encapsulation of an adamantane-doxorubicin prodrug in pH-responsive polysaccharide capsules for controlled release. *ACS Appl. Mater. Interfaces* **2012**, *4*, 5317–5324. [CrossRef] [PubMed]

14. Cyphert, E.L.; Fu, A.S.; von Recum, H.A. Chemotherapeutic delivery using pH-responsive, affinity-based release. *Exp. Biol. Med.* **2017**, *242*, 692–699. [CrossRef] [PubMed]

15. Kouatly, O.; Geronikaki, A.; Kamoutsis, C.; Hadjipavlou-Litina, D.; Eleftheriou, P. Adamantane derivatives of thiazolyl-N-substituted amide, as possible non-steroidal anti-inflammatory agents. *Eur. J. Med. Chem.* **2009**, *44*, 1198–1204. [CrossRef] [PubMed]

16. Pagire, S.H.; Pagire, H.S.; Lee, G.B.; Han, S.J.; Kwak, H.J.; Kim, J.Y.; Kim, K.Y.; Rhee, S.D.; Ryu, J.I.; Song, J.S.; et al. Discovery and optimization of adamantane carboxylic acid derivatives as potent diacylglycerol acyltransferase 1 inhibitors for the potential treatment of obesity and diabetes. *Eur. J. Med. Chem.* **2015**, *101*, 716–735. [CrossRef] [PubMed]

17. Creel, C.J.; Lovich, M.A.; Edelman, E.R. Arterial paclitaxel distribution and deposition. *Circ. Res.* **2000**, *86*, 879–884. [CrossRef] [PubMed]

18. Copeland, R.A. The drug-target residence time model: A 10-year retrospective. *Nat. Rev. Drug Discov.* **2016**, *15*, 87–95. [CrossRef] [PubMed]

19. Fiese, E.F.; Steffen, S.H. Comparison of the acid stability of azithromycin and erythromycin A. *J. Antimicrob. Chemother.* **1990**, *25*, 39–47. [CrossRef] [PubMed]

20. Hill, D.R. 9-Hydrazone and 9-Azine Erythromycin Derivatives and a Process for Making the Same. U.S. Patent RE39,531 E, 27 March 2007.

21. Whitman, M.S.; Tunkel, A.R. Azithromycin and clarithromycin: Overview and comparison with erythromycin. *Infect. Control Hosp. Epidemiol.* **1992**, *13*, 357–368. [CrossRef] [PubMed]

22. Pereira, J.M.; Mejia-Ariza, R.; Ilevbare, G.A.; McGettigan, H.E.; Sriranganathan, N.; Taylor, L.S.; Davis, R.M.; Edgar, K.J. Interplay of degradation, dissolution and stabilization of clarithromycin and its amorphous solid dispersions. *Mol. Pharm.* **2013**, *10*, 4640–4653. [CrossRef] [PubMed]

23. Park, J.-B.; Park, Y.-J.; Kang, C.-Y.; Lee, B.-J. Modulation of microenvironmental pH and utilization of alkalizers in crystalline solid dispersions for enhanced solubility and stability of clarithromycin. *Arch. Pharm. Res.* **2015**, *38*, 839–848. [CrossRef] [PubMed]

24. Ogwal, S.T.U.X. Bioavailability and stability of erythromycin delayed release tablets. *Afr. Health Sci.* **2001**, *1*, 90–96. [PubMed]

25. Zhang, H.; Wu, H.; Fan, L.; Li, F.; Gu, C.; Jia, M. Preparation and characteristics of pH-sensitive derivated dextran hydrogel nanoparticles. *Polym. Compos.* **2009**, *30*, 1243–1250. [CrossRef]

26. Bronner, S.; Monteil, H.; Prévost, G. Regulation of virulence determinants in *Staphylococcus aureus*: Complexity and applications. *FEMS Microbiol. Rev.* **2004**, *28*, 183–200. [CrossRef] [PubMed]

27. Granadero, D.; Bordello, J.; Perez-Alvite, M.J.; Novo, M.; Al-Soufi, W. Host-guest complexation studied fluorescence correlation spectroscopy: Adamantane-cyclodextrin inclusion. *Int. J. Mol. Sci.* **2010**, *11*, 173–188. [CrossRef] [PubMed]

28. Belskaya, N.P.; Dehaen, W.; Bakulev, V.A. Synthesis and properties of hydrazones bearing amide, thioamide, and amidine functions. *Online J. Org. Chem.* **2010**, *1*, 275–332.

29. Everett, J.R.; Tyler, J.W. An analysis of the ^{1}H and ^{13}C N.M.R. spectra of erythromycin a using two-dimensional methods. *J. Chem. Soc. Perkin Trans.* **1985**, *1*, 2599–2603. [CrossRef]

30. Crisalli, P.; Hernández, A.R.; Kool, E.T. Fluorescence quenchers for hydrazone and oxime orthoganol bioconjugation. *Bioconjug. Chem.* **2012**, *23*, 1969–1980. [CrossRef] [PubMed]

31. Carpenter, C.A.; Kenar, J.A.; Price, N. Preparation of saturated and unsaturated fatty acid hydrazides and long chain C-glycoside ketohydrazones. *Green Chem.* **2010**, *12*, 2012–2018. [CrossRef]

32. Kalia, J; Raines, R.T. Hydrolytic stability of hydrazones and oximes. *Agnew. Chem. Int. Ed. Engl.* **2008**, *47*, 7523–7526. [CrossRef] [PubMed]

33. Szisz, D. HLB Predictor. *ChemAxon Docs.* 2015. Available online: https://docs.chemaxon.com/display/docs/HLB+Predictor (accessed on 11 November 2016).

34. Van den Bossche, L.; Lodi, A.; Schaar, J.; Shaakov, S.; Zorzan, M.; Tranquillini, M.E.; Overballe-Petersen, C.; Hoogmartens, J.; Adams, E. An interlaboratory study on the suitability of a gradient LC-UV method as a compendial method for the determination of erythromycin and its related substances. *J. Pharm. Biomed. Anal.* **2010**, *53*, 109–112. [CrossRef] [PubMed]

35. Ford, J.H.; Prescott, G.C.; Hinman, J.W.; Caron, E.L. Colorimetric determination of erythromycin. *Anal. Chem.* **1953**, *25*, 1195–1197. [CrossRef]

36. Danielson, N.D.; Holeman, J.A.; Bristol, D.C.; Kirzner, D.H. Simple methods for the qualitative identification and quantitative determination of macrolide antibiotics. *J. Pharm. Biomed. Anal.* **1993**, *11*, 121–130. [CrossRef]

37. Gallagher, P.A.; Danielson, N.D. Colorimetric determination of macrolide antibiotics using ferric ion. *Talanta* **1995**, *42*, 1425–1432. [CrossRef]

38. Rivera-Delgado, E.; Ward, E.; von Recum, H.A. Providing sustained transgene induction through affinity-based drug delivery. *J. Biomed. Mater. Res. A* **2016**, *104*, 1135–1142. [CrossRef] [PubMed]

39. Keller, B.O.; Li, L. Three-layer matrix/sample preparation method for MALDI MS analysis of low nanomolar protein samples. *J. Am. Soc. Mass Spectrom.* **2006**, *17*, 780–785. [CrossRef] [PubMed]

40. Davies, J.T. A quantitative kinetic theory of emulsion type, I. Physical chemistry of the emulsifying agent. In Proceedings of the Second International Congress of Surface Activity; Butterworths: London, UK, 1957; pp. 426–438.

41. Guo, X.; Rong, Z.; Ying, X. Calculation of hydrophile-lipophile balance for polyethoxylated surfactants by group contribution method. *J. Colloid Interface Sci.* **2006**, *298*, 441–450. [CrossRef] [PubMed]

42. Griffin, W.C. Calculation of HLB values of non-ionic surfactants. *J. Soc. Cosmet. Chem.* **1954**, *5*, 249–256.

43. Kabri, T.; Arab-Tehrany, E.; Belhaj, N.; Linder, M. Physico-chemical characterization of nano-emulsions in cosmetic matrix enriched on omega-3. *J. Nanobiotechnol.* **2011**, *9*. [CrossRef] [PubMed]

44. Manna, P.K.; Kumaran, V.; Mohanta, G.P.; Manvalan, R. Preparation and evaluation of a new erythromycin derivative-erythromycin taurate. *Acta Pharm.* **2004**, *54*, 231–242. [PubMed]

45. Varanda, F.; Pratas de Melo, M.J.; Caço, A.I.; Dohrn, R.; Makrydaki, F.A.; Voutsas, E.; Tassios, D.; Marrucho, I.M. Solubility of antibiotics in different solvents. 1. Hydrochloride forms of tetracycline, moxifloxacin, and ciprofloxacin. *Ind. Eng. Chem. Res.* **2006**, *45*, 6368–6374. [CrossRef]

46. Thatiparti, T.R.; von Recum, H.A. Cyclodextrin complexation for affinity-based antibiotic delivery. *Macromol. Biosci.* **2010**, *10*, 82–90. [CrossRef] [PubMed]

15

Streptomyces Differentiation in Liquid Cultures as a Trigger of Secondary Metabolism

Ángel Manteca and Paula Yagüe * (ID)

Área de Microbiología, Departamento de Biología Funcional IUOPA, Facultad de Medicina, Universidad de Oviedo, 33006 Oviedo, Spain; mantecaangel@uniovi.es
* Correspondence: paula.yague@gmail.com

Abstract: *Streptomyces* is a diverse group of gram-positive microorganisms characterised by a complex developmental cycle. *Streptomycetes* produce a number of antibiotics and other bioactive compounds used in the clinic. Most screening campaigns looking for new bioactive molecules from actinomycetes have been performed empirically, e.g., without considering whether the bacteria are growing under the best developmental conditions for secondary metabolite production. These screening campaigns were extremely productive and discovered a number of new bioactive compounds during the so-called "golden age of antibiotics" (until the 1980s). However, at present, there is a worrying bottleneck in drug discovery, and new experimental approaches are needed to improve the screening of natural actinomycetes. *Streptomycetes* are still the most important natural source of antibiotics and other bioactive compounds. They harbour many cryptic secondary metabolite pathways not expressed under classical laboratory cultures. Here, we review the new strategies that are being explored to overcome current challenges in drug discovery. In particular, we focus on those aimed at improving the differentiation of the antibiotic-producing mycelium stage in the laboratory.

Keywords: *streptomyces*; screening; antibiotics; secondary metabolism; differentiation; elicitors; morphology; liquid cultures

1. Introduction

The *Streptomyces* genus includes an important group of biotechnological bacteria. They produce two-thirds of the antibiotics of medical and agricultural interest, several antitumor agents, antifungals, and a great number of eukaryotic cell differentiation effectors, such as apoptosis inducers and inhibitors [1]. Drug discovery from *streptomycetes* fell considerably after initial screenings where the most common compounds were discovered. Antibiotic resistance is increasing dramatically, and new antibiotics are urgently required in the clinic. Alternative methods, such as the exploration of chemical libraries and combinatorial chemistry, have provided limited yields. Screening from nature has resumed through methods such as exploring new environments, looking for elicitors, accessing the metagenome, etc.

One of the most important characteristics of *Streptomyces* is its complex life cycle, which is closely related to secondary metabolite production [2] (outlined in Figure 1). In solid sporulating cultures, development starts with spore germination and the rapid development of compartmentalised hyphae into the medium (early substrate mycelium or MI) [3]. After that, programmed cell death (PCD) occurs (red cellular segments in Figure 1) which triggers the differentiation of the multinucleated (MII) antibiotic-producing hyphae (late substrate mycelium, early MII) [3,4]. Then, the mycelium starts to grow into the air forming the aerial mycelium (late MII). At the end of the cycle, there is a second round of PCD, and most of the remaining viable hyphae undergo a process of compartmentalisation that culminates in the formation of unigenomic spores [5].

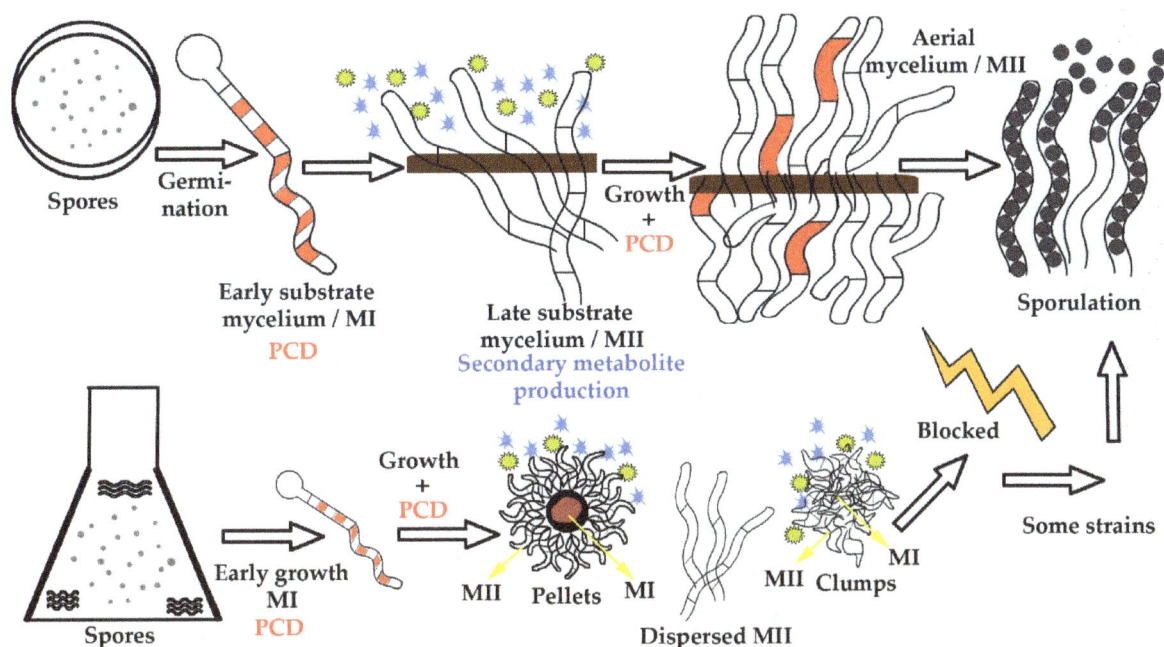

Figure 1. *Streptomyces* growth in solid cultures (**upper panels**) and liquid cultures (**lower panels**). In solid cultures (petri plates), spores germinate developing a compartmentalised mycelium (early substrate mycelium, MI) with 1 μm average cross-membrane spacing [6]. Some of the MI cells suffer a first round of programmed cell death PCD (red segments). The remaining viable segments start to grow as a multinucleated mycelium with sporadic septa (early MII, late substrate mycelium) [6]. The mycelium substrate suffers a second round of PCD (red segments) and differentiates into a mycelium that starts to grow into the air (the medium/agar border is indicated by a brown line) (late MII, aerial mycelium). Part of the aerial hyphae form spore chains (black circles). In liquid cultures, there is germination, MI development, PCD (in the centre of the mycelial pellets) and MII differentiation (in the periphery of the pellets). In most species, there is no aerial mycelium formation or sporulation, and hyphae form pellets and clumps [2]. Secondary metabolites (outlined as yellow circles and blue starts) are produced by the MII hyphae.

Most *streptomycetes* do not sporulate in liquid cultures. Therefore, it was previously assumed that under these conditions, there was no differentiation. However, industrial antibiotic production is mostly performed in liquid cultures (flasks and bioreactors). Currently, it is known that in liquid cultures, differentiation is comparable to that observed in solid cultures (Figure 1). In liquid cultures, there is a first mycelium stage (MI), PCD and the differentiation of a secondary metabolite, producing mycelium (MII). However, in most *Streptomyces* strains, aerial mycelium formation and sporulation are blocked [6] (Figure 1). *S. coelicolor* proteomic and transcriptomic studies have shown that physiological differentiation in liquid and solid cultures is comparable [6,7]. MII expresses/translates the genes/proteins involved in secondary metabolism in both solid and liquid cultures [6,7].

Surprisingly, *Streptomyces* differentiation as a trigger for antibiotic production remains almost unexplored. The absence of a developmental model to describe differentiation in liquid cultures has inhibited the understanding of the relationship between macroscopic morphology (pellet and clump formation) and differentiation. Pellet and clump formation has been classically correlated with secondary metabolite production, but the relationship between both processes remains obscure. Most authors have affirmed that pellets and clumps are fundamental for secondary metabolite production (e.g., retamycin in *S. olindensis* [8], nikkomycins in *S. tendae* [9], hybrid antibiotics in *S. lividans* [10]), while some authors have affirmed that pellet and clump formation reduces antibiotic production (e.g., nystatin in *S. noursei* [11], tylosin in *S. fradiae* [12]). More recently, our group demonstrated that one of the key events in the activation of secondary metabolite production in

Streptomyces liquid cultures is the differentiation of MII (e.g., actinorhodin/undecylprodigiosin production in *S. coelicolor* [2,13], microbial transglutaminase production in *S. mobarensis* [14], apigenin and luteolin production in *S. albus* [15]). The differentiation of this mycelium is conditioned by PCD of the vegetative hyphae (MI) [2], which, in liquid cultures, depends on the growth rate of the strain and hypha aggregation (pellet/clump formation) [2,7,14–16]. However, secondary metabolism has additional regulations (elicitors activate specific biosynthetic pathways) [17], and most *Streptomyces* strains do not display all their potential secondary metabolites under standard developmental laboratory conditions, even if they are differentiated at the MII stage [7].

Each *Streptomyces* strain can harbour up to 30 secondary metabolite pathways, but only a few of these are active in usual screening processes [18]. Activating these pathways in the lab will be crucial in the process of screening for new secondary metabolites from actinomycetes. Here, we review the most important strategies that are being explored to activate cryptic pathways and/or those that are being explored to enhance secondary metabolites production.

2. Screening for New Secondary Metabolites from *Streptomycetes*

The search for new actinomycetes in unexplored niches or from the screening of strains that have not been previously cultivated is useful, but usually leads to the rediscovery of already known compounds [19]. New screening strategies are necessary to overcome the current challenges of discovering new bioactive compounds [19]. In 2013, Arryn Craney et al. [20] summarised the new strategies that are being used to enhance secondary metabolite production and activate cryptic pathways, dividing them into unselective and selective methods [20]. Unselective methods are non-specific methods that are used to screen for new activities, whereas selective methods are biosynthetic cluster-specific methods that are used to improve the production of already known molecules [20].

Non-specific methods were largely used during "the golden age of antibiotics", and they are still useful. These methods include classical strategies, such as changing media components, increasing general precursors (metabolic engineering), inducing stress responses (with heat/ethanol/salt/acid shock, nutrient limitations) [21], and obtaining strains that overproduce secondary metabolites by random mutagenesis [22–24]. More novel non-specific methods include ribosomal engineering (the alteration of ribosomal proteins to activate cryptic secondary metabolites in *streptomycetes*) [20,25] and the use of small molecules as elicitors of secondary metabolism [20,26] (Table 1). Differentiation of the antibiotic producer mycelium (MII) as a non-specific method to activate antibiotic production remains almost unexplored. There has been no previous analysis of the frequency of *Streptomyces* strains that do not produce secondary metabolites because they are not differentiated at the MII stage in the laboratory.

Biosynthetic cluster-specific methods include self-resistance engineering (upregulation of self-resistance genes), regulatory engineering (overexpression of activators or elimination of repressors) and genome mining to search for new biosynthetic pathways [20] (Table 2). One of the most important biosynthetic cluster-specific methods is heterologous expression. Heterologous expression has been used to express *Streptomyces* industrial enzymes, such as laccases, in microorganisms with simpler developmental cycles than *Streptomyces*, such as *E. coli* [27]. However, the complex biosynthetic pathways of *Streptomyces* rarely can be expressed in simple expression hosts, such as *E. coli* or *Bacillus*. Thus, other *streptomycetes*, such as *S. lividans*, *S. albus*, *S. coelicolor* or *S. avermitilis*, are commonly used as expression hosts [28]. The activation of cryptic metabolites through the expression of the *Streptomyces coelicolor* pleiotropic regulator, *Afs*Q, in other *streptomycetes* [29] has been successfully achieved. Combinatorial biosynthesis, chemical modification of existing molecules, has been largely developed over the last 20 years, in particular, progress has been made in the last few years thanks to genome mining and synthetic biology [30–32]. Differentiation of *Streptomyces* MII was successfully used to enhance the production of various products [2,13–15] through its role as a trigger for antibiotic production (described in Section 2.3).

2.1. Streptomyces Differentiation Strategies Based on Elicitors

In the last few years, effort has been made to elucidate the mechanism by which some small molecules (elicitors) affect differentiation and secondary metabolite production in *Streptomyces* strains. Elicitors can be defined as diffusible signals that are able to induce cryptic pathways and/or differentiation in *Streptomyces* cultures [17]. Some elicitors act as signals for interspecies interaction [33]. Thus, subinhibitory concentrations of certain antibiotics produced by a given *Streptomyces* strain accelerate differentiation and antibiotic production in other *Streptomyces* strains through "pseudo" gamma-butyrolactone receptors [33]. Another good strategy is the use of random chemical probes (natural or synthetic) as elicitors (reviewed in [21]).

One of the most common strategies used to activate secondary metabolism and differentiation is mimicking the ecological environment through co-cultures of different microbes [17,34]. This methodology typically uses species that have symbiotic relationships with *Streptomyces* in nature [35,36] or pathogen partners that activate the production of antimicrobial compounds [37–39]. For instance, fungal elicitors (complex mix of cell walls and filtered cultures) positively affect the production of natamycin [40], bacterial and yeast elicitors improve valinomycin production [41], nutrients such as glucose and xylose repress the production of actinorhodin [42,43], and small molecules, such as GlcNAc or phosphate, can trigger differentiation and antibiotic production in *S. coelicolor* through the activation of *act*II-ORF4/*red*Z genes [44].

Pimentel-Elardo et al. [45] developed an activity-independent screening method based on the use of elicitors, to prevent the rediscovery of the most active/abundant compounds. In addition, cheminformatics techniques are used to identify the putative biological activities of identified compounds [45]. The use of elicitors increases the production of low-abundant compounds which were undetected in the classical activity dependent screening. The chemical elicitor "CI-ARC" has been identified as being responsible for triggering several cryptic biosynthetic genes [45].

2.2. Differentiation Strategies Based on Macroscopic Morphology

2.2.1. The Genetic Control of Aggregation and Macroscopic Morphology in Liquid Cultures

Large-scale antibiotic production is mostly performed in liquid cultures. It is almost unanimously accepted that the macroscopic morphology of the mycelium (pellets and clump formation) is correlated with the production of secondary metabolites. However, it was not until recently that the genes controlling pellet and clump formation have been characterised. The *S. coelicolor mat* gene cluster [46] and the *cslA*, *glxA*, *dtpA* genes [47–49] are responsible for mycelial aggregation and pellet formation. These genes could be a great tool for controlling the morphology in industrial fermentation.

The *Streptomyces* life cycle in liquid cultures starts with the germination of spores. Awakening from the dormant spore state depends on the level of AMPc in the cultures [50] and involves the small hydrophobic protein NepA, [51]. The expression of several sigma factors involved in osmotic and oxidative stress (SigH, SigB, SigI, SigJ) undergoes remarkable changes during germination, indicating that germination evokes stress-like cell responses [52]. Several genes encoding proteins involved in lipid metabolism and membrane transport are overexpressed during germination [52]. The conservation of D-alanyl-D-alanine carboxypeptidase (SCO4439) contributes to the swelling phase of germination [53]. Cell wall hydrolases participate in germination [54]. SsgA protein marks the germinative tube emission points [55]. Recently it was described that during germination, spores aggregate due to extracellular glycans synthesized by the MatA, MatB [46,56] and the CslA/GlxA/DtpA proteins [56]. These aggregates determine the macroscopic morphology (pellets and clumps) of the culture [56] which triggers PCD and the physiological differentiation of the antibiotic producer, mycelium MII [2].

Another issue that influence secondary metabolite production is sporulation. Several *streptomycetes* are able to sporulate in liquid cultures [57] and some strains, that normally do not sporulate are also able to sporulate in bioreactors due to the stress generated in the fermenter [13]. Sporulation stops metabolism, including secondary metabolite production. Consequently, in industrial fermentations and during screening for new secondary metabolites, it is important to avoid sporulation to increase and maintain secondary metabolism for as long as possible [13].

2.2.2. Monitoring of *Streptomyces* Macroscopic Morphology and Differentiation in Liquid Cultures

Pellet and clump formation led to differentiation and secondary metabolism [2]. Consequently, new methodologies to monitor macroscopic morphology have been developed. Laser diffraction has been used to measure pellet size [58]. Flow cytometry has been used to establish pellet size distribution of culture populations [59,60]. Recently, a useful algorithm was developed as a plug-in for the open-source software, ImageJ, to characterize the morphology of filamentous microorganisms in liquid cultures [61]. Mathematical models have been performed to predict the behaviour of *Streptomyces* liquid cultures based on pellet/clump morphology [62,63].

Biophysical parameters (e.g., pH, viscosity, agitation, dissolved oxygen levels and surface tension, among others) directly affect morphology and differentiation [13,64]. These parameters must be considered when scaling up production to industrial conditions [65]. Interestingly, a recent study downscaled liquid cultures to the 100 μL scale in microtiter plates [66], reproducing the same range of production and morphology as large-scale bioreactors, making screening easier and facilitating further upscaling.

2.2.3. Macroscopic Morphology Conditions, Programmed Cell Death and Second Mycelium Differentiation in Liquid Cultures

PCD is the key event that triggers the differentiation of the antibiotic producer, mycelium (MII), in liquid and solid cultures [2]. However, the specific signals derived from cell death are not yet known. The production of *N*-acetylglucosamine from peptidoglycan dismantling accelerates development and antibiotic production [67,68] and might be one of the signals released during PCD.

A simple methodology based on fluorometric measures of cultures stained with SYTO9 and propidium iodide was designed to quantify PCD in liquid cultures [69]. This method allows the efficiency of antibiotic production to be predicted based on the level of PCD [69].

Strains showing dispersed growth take a long time to suffer PCD, and sometimes, PCD does not occur. Modify the developmental conditions to enhance PCD and MII differentiation, leads to an improvement in secondary metabolite production. This approach was recently applied to enhance flavonoid production in a strain of *Streptomyces albus* [15] and to enhance microbial transglutaminase production from *Streptomyces mobaraensis* [14]. The "PCD-MII" approach complements other approaches well; there is no secondary metabolite production without differentiation of MII, but there are biosynthetic pathways that in addition to MII differentiation, need specific elicitors to become active [70].

2.3. L-Forms

An interesting alternative that would avoid the problems of mycelial growth in industry, is the use of L-forms, which are individual cells without cell walls [71]. However, until now, the antibiotic levels reached by *Streptomyces* L-forms have been quite minor compared to those reached by the regular form. Therefore, future research should explore whether L-forms could offer an industrial alternative.

2.4. Other Strategies

A big challenge in screening for new secondary metabolites is exploring non-cultivated bacteria. The scientific community is aware of the huge quantity of microorganisms that are not cultivated under laboratory conditions. Next Generation Sequencing revealed the big pharmacological potential of uncultured bacteria. Innovative culturing techniques, such as the isolation chip (iChip), are being used successfully in combination with co-cultures to grow previously uncultured bacteria [72]. The study of unexplored niches to look for new Actinomycetes is another strategy that enables the discovery of new species and compounds [73–75]. The combination of these two methods is a promising strategy to identify new compounds.

One of the newest strategies focusses on primary metabolism and vegetative growth. Very recently, work by Schniete et al. [76] showed how genetic redundancy within actinobacterial genomes allows functional specialization of two pyruvate kinases in *Streptomyces* under different life cycle stages and environmental conditions. Genetic redundancy within actinobacteria genomes as being a key to understanding how the plasticity of this microorganism enhances the production of clinically useful molecules. Furthermore, Cihak et al. [77] recently described the production of secondary metabolites during germination in *Streptomyces coelicolor*. The germination stage was ignored in most secondary metabolite screening campaigns and constitutes a potential source of bioactive compounds to be explored [77].

Table 1. Non-specific methods and some successful examples of their enforcement. "Enhance" means an improvement in production; "cryptic" means activation of the expression of cryptic pathways.

Methods	Microorganism	Product	Effect	Ref.
Media manipulation	*S. roseosporus*	Daptomycin	Enhance	[78]
Stress Response	*S. venezuelae*	Jadomycin B	Enhance	[79]
	S. hygroscopicus	Validamycin A	Enhance	[21]
	S. parvulus	Manumycin family	Cryptic	[80]
	S. coelicolor	Ectoine, 5-hydroxyectoine	Enhance	[81]
	S. coelicolor	Methylenomycin	Enhance	[82]
One Strain Many Compounds (OSMAC)	*S. parvulus*	20 cryptic compounds	Cryptic	[80]
Random Mutagenesis	*S. clavuligerus*	Clavulanic acid	Enhance	[83]
	S. hygroscopicus	Rapamycin	Enhance	[84]
	S. coelicolor	Actinorhodin, Undecylprodigiosin	Enhance	[22]
Ribosomal Engineering	*S. coelicolor*	Actinorhodin	Enhance	[85]
Engineering Global Regulation	*S. coelicolor*	Actinorhodin, Prodigiosin, Calcium-Dependent Antibiotic	Enhance	[86]
	S. griseus	Streptomycin	Enhance	[86]
	S. griseochromogenes	Blasticidin S	Enhance	[86]
Elicitors	*S. coelicolor*	Actinorhodin	Enhance	[87]
	S. pristinaespiralis	Desferrioxamine B/E	Enhance	[20]
	S. peucetius	Doxorubicin, Baumycin	Enhance	[20]
	S. coelicolor	Actinorhodin, Undecylprodigiosin	Enhance	[68]
	S. lividans	Prodiginine	Enhance	[88]
	S. griseus	Streptomycin	Enhance	[21]
	S. natalensis	Pimaricin	Enhance	[89]
	29 strains	Cryptic compounds	Cryptic	[45]
Metabolic Engineering	*S. clavuligerus*	FK606	Enhance	[90]
	S. coelicolor	Actinorhodin	Enhance	[90]
	S. rimosus	Oxytetracycline	Enhance	[91]
Co-cultures	*S. rimosus* MY02	Antifungal activity	Enhance	[36]
	S. coelicolor	Actinorhodin	Enhance	[37]
	S. fradiae 007	Phenolic polyketides	Enhance	[38]
	Marine *streptomycetes*	See tables in reference	Cryptic	[39]
Conditioning Morphology (PCD + MII)	*S. cattleya*	Tienamycin	Enhance	[92]
	S. cinereoruber	Rodomycin	Enhance	
	Saccharopolyspora erythraea	Erithromycin	Enhance	
	S. coelicolor	Actinorhodin	Enhance	

Table 2. Biosynthetic cluster specific methods and some successful examples of their enforcement.

Methods	Microorganism	Product	Effect	Ref.
Engineering Self-Resistance	S. peucetius	Doxorubicin, Daunorubicin	Enhance	[93]
	S. avermitilis	Avermectin,	Enhance	[94]
	S. coelicolor	Actinorhodin	Enhance	[95]
Regulatory Engineering				
Delete repressor AbsA2~P	S. coelicolor	Actinorhodin, Undecylprodigiosin, Calcium-dependent antibiotic	Enhance	[96]
Overexpress AverR/StrR	S. avermitilis	Avermectin	Enhance	[97]
Overexpress AverR/StrR	S. griseous	Streptomycin	Enhance	[98]
Overexpress SamR0484	S. ambofaciens	Stambomicin A-D	Cryptic	[99]
Delete repressor cmmRII	S. griseus	Chromomycin	Enhance	[100]
Delete repressor AlpW	S. ambofaciens	Alpomycin	Enhance	[101]
Heterologous Expression	S. avermitilis	Streptomycin	Enhance	[102]
	S. coelicolor	Chloramphenicol	Enhance	[103]
	S. coelicolor	Congocidine	Enhance	[103]
	S. cyaneus	CECT 3335 laccase	Enhance	[27]
	S. lividans TK24	Mithramycin A	Enhance	[104]
	Streptomyces sp.	Neothioviridamide	Cryptic	[105]
	Several wild-type	Siamycin-I	Cryptic	[29]
Combinatorial Biosynthesis	S. albus J1074	Novel paulomycin	Cryptic	[31]
	See table 1 in ref.			[30]
Conditioning Morphology (PCD + MII)	S. albus	Apigenin, Luteolin	Enhance	[15]
	S. mobarensis	Microbial transglutaminase	Enhance	[14]

3. Conclusions

We generally face the great challenge of fighting antibiotic resistance, which is growing much faster than our capacity to find new antimicrobials and new strategies to face this problem. The *Streptomyces* genus is still a huge source of natural bioactive compounds, but we need to form new strategies to avoid rediscovering compounds. There is not a single methodology to trigger differentiation, activate cryptic secondary metabolism pathways and improve the discovery of new bioactive compounds. However, the multidisciplinary biosynthetic cluster specific and non-specific approaches discussed in this manuscript, will be key to improving the screening for new secondary metabolites from *streptomycetes*.

Author Contributions: P.Y. planned the topic of the review and searched the information; A.M. and P.Y. wrote the manuscript.

Acknowledgments: We thank the Spanish "Ministerio de Economía y Competitividad" (MINECO; BIO2015-65709-R) for financial support.

References

1. Worrall, J.A.; Vijgenboom, E. Copper mining in *streptomyces*: Enzymes, natural products and development. *Nat. Prod. Rep.* **2010**, *27*, 742–756. [CrossRef] [PubMed]

2. Manteca, A.; Alvarez, R.; Salazar, N.; Yague, P.; Sanchez, J. Mycelium differentiation and antibiotic production in submerged cultures of *Streptomyces coelicolor*. *Appl. Environ. Microbiol.* **2008**, *74*, 3877–3886. [CrossRef] [PubMed]

3. Yague, P.; Willemse, J.; Koning, R.I.; Rioseras, B.; Lopez-Garcia, M.T.; Gonzalez-Quinonez, N.; Lopez-Iglesias, C.; Shliaha, P.V.; Rogowska-Wrzesinska, A.; Koster, A.J.; et al. Subcompartmentalization by cross-membranes during early growth of *streptomyces* hyphae. *Nat. Commun.* **2016**, *7*, 12467. [CrossRef] [PubMed]

4. Manteca, A.; Fernandez, M.; Sanchez, J. A death round affecting a young compartmentalized mycelium precedes aerial mycelium dismantling in confluent surface cultures of *streptomyces* antibioticus. *Microbiology* **2005**, *151*, 3689–3697. [CrossRef] [PubMed]

5. Flardh, K. Growth polarity and cell division in *streptomyces*. *Curr. Opin. Microbiol.* **2003**, *6*, 564–571. [CrossRef] [PubMed]

6. Manteca, A.; Jung, H.R.; Schwammle, V.; Jensen, O.N.; Sanchez, J. Quantitative proteome analysis of *Streptomyces coelicolor* nonsporulating liquid cultures demonstrates a complex differentiation process comparable to that occurring in sporulating solid cultures. *J. Proteome Res.* **2010**, *9*, 4801–4811. [CrossRef] [PubMed]

7. Yague, P.; Rodriguez-Garcia, A.; Lopez-Garcia, M.T.; Rioseras, B.; Martin, J.F.; Sanchez, J.; Manteca, A. Transcriptomic analysis of liquid non-sporulating *Streptomyces coelicolor* cultures demonstrates the existence of a complex differentiation comparable to that occurring in solid sporulating cultures. *PLoS ONE* **2014**, *9*, e86296. [CrossRef] [PubMed]

8. Giudici, R.; Pamboukian, C.R.; Facciotti, M.C. Morphologically structured model for antitumoral retamycin production during batch and fed-batch cultivations of streptomyces olindensis. *Biotechnol. Bioeng.* **2004**, *86*, 414–424. [CrossRef] [PubMed]

9. Vecht-Lifshitz, S.E.; Sasson, Y.; Braun, S. Nikkomycin production in pellets of streptomyces tendae. *J. Appl. Bacteriol.* **1992**, *72*, 195–200. [CrossRef] [PubMed]

10. Sarra, M.; Casas, C.; Godia, F. Continuous production of a hybrid antibiotic by *Streptomyces lividans* TK21 pellets in a three-phase fluidized-bed bioreactor. *Biotechnol. Bioeng.* **1997**, *53*, 601–610. [CrossRef]

11. Jonsbu, E.; McIntyre, M.; Nielsen, J. The influence of carbon sources and morphology on nystatin production by streptomyces noursei. *J. Biotechnol.* **2002**, *95*, 133–144. [CrossRef]

12. Park, Y.; Tamura, S.; Koike, Y.; Toriyama, M.; Okabe, M. Mycelial pellet intrastructure visualization and viability prediction in a culture of streptomyces fradiae using confocal scanning laser microscopy. *J. Ferment. Bioeng.* **1997**, *84*, 483–486. [CrossRef]

13. Rioseras, B.; Lopez-Garcia, M.T.; Yague, P.; Sanchez, J.; Manteca, A. Mycelium differentiation and development of *Streptomyces coelicolor* in lab-scale bioreactors: Programmed cell death, differentiation, and lysis are closely linked to undecylprodigiosin and actinorhodin production. *Bioresour. Technol.* **2014**, *151*, 191–198. [CrossRef] [PubMed]

14. Treppiccione, L.; Ottombrino, A.; Luongo, D.; Maurano, F.; Manteca, A.; Lombó, F.; Rossi, M. Development of gluten with immunomodulatory properties using mTG-active food grade supernatants from *Streptomyces mobaraensis* cultures. *J. Funct. Foods* **2017**, *34*, 390–397. [CrossRef]

15. Marin, L.; Gutierrez-Del-Rio, I.; Yague, P.; Manteca, A.; Villar, C.J.; Lombo, F. De novo biosynthesis of apigenin, luteolin, and eriodictyol in the actinomycete *Streptomyces albus* and production improvement by feeding and spore conditioning. *Front. Microbiol.* **2017**, *8*, 921. [CrossRef] [PubMed]

16. Zhang, L.; Zhang, L.; Han, X.; Du, M.; Zhang, Y.; Feng, Z.; Yi, H.; Zhang, Y. Enhancement of transglutaminase production in *Streptomyces mobaraensis* as achieved by treatment with excessive MgCl$_2$. *Appl. Microbiol. Biotechnol.* **2012**, *93*, 2335–2343. [CrossRef] [PubMed]

17. Onaka, H. Novel antibiotic screening methods to awaken silent or cryptic secondary metabolic pathways in actinomycetes. *J. Antibiot.* **2017**, *70*, 865–870. [CrossRef] [PubMed]

18. Genilloud, O. The re-emerging role of microbial natural products in antibiotic discovery. *Antonie Van Leeuwenhoek* **2014**, *106*, 173–188. [CrossRef] [PubMed]

19. Genilloud, O. Actinomycetes: Still a source of novel antibiotics. *Nat. Prod. Rep.* **2017**, *34*, 1203–1232. [CrossRef] [PubMed]

20. Craney, A.; Ahmed, S.; Nodwell, J. Towards a new science of secondary metabolism. *J. Antibiot.* **2013**, *66*, 387–400. [CrossRef] [PubMed]

21. Yoon, V.; Nodwell, J.R. Activating secondary metabolism with stress and chemicals. *J. Ind. Microbiol. Biotechnol.* **2014**, *41*, 415–424. [CrossRef] [PubMed]

22. Xu, Z.; Wang, Y.; Chater, K.F.; Ou, H.Y.; Xu, H.H.; Deng, Z.; Tao, M. Large-scale transposition mutagenesis of *Streptomyces coelicolor* identifies hundreds of genes influencing antibiotic biosynthesis. *Appl. Environ. Microbiol.* **2017**, *83*, e02889-16. [CrossRef] [PubMed]

23. Khaliq, S.; Akhtar, K.; Afzal Ghauri, M.; Iqbal, R.; Mukhtar Khalid, A.; Muddassar, M. Change in colony morphology and kinetics of tylosin production after UV and gamma irradiation mutagenesis of streptomyces fradiae NRRL-2702. *Microbiol. Res.* **2009**, *164*, 469–477. [CrossRef] [PubMed]

24. Korbekandi, H.; Darkhal, P.; Hojati, Z.; Abedi, D.; Hamedi, J.; Pourhosein, M. Overproduction of clavulanic acid by UV mutagenesis of *Streptomyces clavuligerus. Iran. J. Pharm. Res.* **2010**, *9*, 177–181. [CrossRef] [PubMed]

25. Hosaka, T.; Ohnishi-Kameyama, M.; Muramatsu, H.; Murakami, K.; Tsurumi, Y.; Kodani, S.; Yoshida, M.; Fujie, A.; Ochi, K. Antibacterial discovery in actinomycetes strains with mutations in RNA polymerase or ribosomal protein S12. *Nat. Biotechnol.* **2009**, *27*, 462–464. [CrossRef] [PubMed]

26. Ahmed, S.; Craney, A.; Pimentel-Elardo, S.M.; Nodwell, J.R. A synthetic, speciesspecific activator of secondary metabolism and sporulation in *Streptomyces coelicolor. Chembiochem* **2013**, *14*, 83–91. [CrossRef] [PubMed]

27. Ece, S.; Lambertz, C.; Fischer, R.; Commandeur, U. Heterologous expression of a *Streptomyces cyaneus* laccase for biomass modification applications. *AMB Express* **2017**, *7*, 86. [CrossRef] [PubMed]

28. Baltz, R.H. Streptomyces and saccharopolyspora hosts for heterologous expression of secondary metabolite gene clusters. *J. Ind. Microbiol. Biotechnol.* **2010**, *37*, 759–772. [CrossRef] [PubMed]

29. Daniel-Ivad, M.; Hameed, N.; Tan, S.; Dhanjal, R.; Socko, D.; Pak, P.; Gverzdys, T.; Elliot, M.A.; Nodwell, J.R. An engineered allele of afsQ1 facilitates the discovery and investigation of cryptic natural products. *ACS Chem. Biol.* **2017**, *12*, 628–634. [CrossRef] [PubMed]

30. Olano, C.; Mendez, C.; Salas, J.A. Post-PKS tailoring steps in natural product-producing actinomycetes from the perspective of combinatorial biosynthesis. *Nat. Prod. Rep.* **2010**, *27*, 571–616. [CrossRef] [PubMed]

31. González, A.; Rodríguez, M.; Braña, A.F.; Méndez, C.; Salas, J.A.; Olano, C. New insights into paulomycin biosynthesis pathway in *Streptomyces albus* j1074 and generation of novel derivatives by combinatorial biosynthesis. *Microb. Cell Fact.* **2016**, *15*. [CrossRef] [PubMed]

32. Baltz, R.H. Synthetic biology, genome mining, and combinatorial biosynthesis of NRPS-derived antibiotics: A perspective. *J. Ind. Microbiol. Biotechnol.* **2017**. [CrossRef] [PubMed]

33. Wang, W.; Ji, J.; Li, X.; Wang, J.; Li, S.; Pan, G.; Fan, K.; Yang, K. Angucyclines as signals modulate the behaviors of *Streptomyces coelicolor. Proc. Natl. Acad. Sci. USA* **2014**, *111*, 5688–5693. [CrossRef] [PubMed]

34. Marmann, A.; Aly, A.H.; Lin, W.; Wang, B.; Proksch, P. Co-cultivation—A powerful emerging tool for enhancing the chemical diversity of microorganisms. *Mar. Drugs* **2014**, *12*, 1043–1065. [CrossRef] [PubMed]

35. Piel, J. Metabolites from symbiotic bacteria. *Nat. Prod. Rep.* **2004**, *21*, 519–538. [CrossRef] [PubMed]

36. Yu, J.; Liu, Q.; Chen, C.; Qi, X. Antifungal activity change of streptomyces rimosus MY02 mediated by confront culture with other microorganism. *J. Basic Microbiol.* **2017**, *57*, 276–282. [CrossRef] [PubMed]

37. Perez, J.; Munoz-Dorado, J.; Brana, A.F.; Shimkets, L.J.; Sevillano, L.; Santamaria, R.I. *Myxococcus Xanthus* induces actinorhodin overproduction and aerial mycelium formation by *Streptomyces coelicolor. Microb. Biotechnol.* **2011**, *4*, 175–183. [CrossRef] [PubMed]

38. Wang, Y.; Wang, L.; Zhuang, Y.; Kong, F.; Zhang, C.; Zhu, W. Phenolic polyketides from the co-cultivation of marine-derived *Penicillium* sp. Wc-29-5 and *Streptomyces fradiae* 007. *Mar. Drugs* **2014**, *12*, 2079–2088. [CrossRef] [PubMed]

39. Sung, A.A.; Gromek, S.M.; Balunas, M.J. Upregulation and identification of antibiotic activity of a marine-derived *Streptomyces* sp. Via co-cultures with human pathogens. *Mar. Drugs* **2017**, *15*, 250. [CrossRef] [PubMed]

40. Wang, D.; Yuan, J.; Gu, S.; Shi, Q. Influence of fungal elicitors on biosynthesis of natamycin by streptomyces natalensis HW-2. *Appl. Microbiol. Biotechnol.* **2013**, *97*, 5527–5534. [CrossRef] [PubMed]

41. Sharma, R.; Jamwal, V.; Singh, V.P.; Wazir, P.; Awasthi, P.; Singh, D.; Vishwakarma, R.A.; Gandhi, S.G.; Chaubey, A. Revelation and cloning of valinomycin synthetase genes in streptomyces lavendulae acr-da1 and their expression analysis under different fermentation and elicitation conditions. *J. Biotechnol.* **2017**, *253*, 40–47. [CrossRef] [PubMed]

42. Gubbens, J.; Janus, M.M.; Florea, B.I.; Overkleeft, H.S.; van Wezel, G.P. Identification of glucose kinase-dependent and -independent pathways for carbon control of primary metabolism, development and antibiotic production in *Streptomyces coelicolor* by quantitative proteomics. *Mol. Microbiol.* **2017**, *105*, 175. [CrossRef] [PubMed]

43. Park, S.S.; Yang, Y.H.; Song, E.; Kim, E.J.; Kim, W.S.; Sohng, J.K.; Lee, H.C.; Liou, K.K.; Kim, B.G. Mass spectrometric screening of transcriptional regulators involved in antibiotic biosynthesis in *Streptomyces coelicolor* A3(2). *J. Ind. Microbiol. Biotechnol.* **2009**, *36*, 1073–1083. [CrossRef] [PubMed]

44. Liu, G.; Chater, K.F.; Chandra, G.; Niu, G.; Tan, H. Molecular regulation of antibiotic biosynthesis in streptomyces. *Microbiol. Mol. Biol. Rev.* **2013**, *77*, 112–143. [CrossRef] [PubMed]

45. Pimentel-Elardo, S.M.; Sorensen, D.; Ho, L.; Ziko, M.; Bueler, S.A.; Lu, S.; Tao, J.; Moser, A.; Lee, R.; Agard, D.; et al. Activity-independent discovery of secondary metabolites using chemical elicitation and cheminformatic inference. *ACS Chem. Biol.* **2015**, *10*, 2616–2623. [CrossRef] [PubMed]

46. Van Dissel, D.; Claessen, D.; Roth, M.; van Wezel, G.P. A novel locus for mycelial aggregation forms a gateway to improved streptomyces cell factories. *Microb. Cell Fact.* **2015**, *14*, 44. [CrossRef] [PubMed]

47. Chaplin, A.K.; Petrus, M.L.; Mangiameli, G.; Hough, M.A.; Svistunenko, D.A.; Nicholls, P.; Claessen, D.; Vijgenboom, E.; Worrall, J.A. Glxa is a new structural member of the radical copper oxidase family and is required for glycan deposition at hyphal tips and morphogenesis of *Streptomyces lividans*. *Biochem. J.* **2015**, *469*, 433–444. [CrossRef] [PubMed]

48. Petrus, M.L.; Vijgenboom, E.; Chaplin, A.K.; Worrall, J.A.; van Wezel, G.P.; Claessen, D. The dyp-type peroxidase dtpa is a tat-substrate required for glxa maturation and morphogenesis in streptomyces. *Open Biol.* **2016**, *6*, 150149. [CrossRef] [PubMed]

49. Petrus, M.L.; Claessen, D. Pivotal roles for streptomyces cell surface polymers in morphological differentiation, attachment and mycelial architecture. *Antonie Van Leeuwenhoek* **2014**, *106*, 127–139. [CrossRef] [PubMed]

50. Susstrunk, U.; Pidoux, J.; Taubert, S.; Ullmann, A.; Thompson, C.J. Pleiotropic effects of camp on germination, antibiotic biosynthesis and morphological development in *Streptomyces coelicolor*. *Mol. Microbiol.* **1998**, *30*, 33–46. [CrossRef] [PubMed]

51. De Jong, W.; Manteca, A.; Sanchez, J.; Bucca, G.; Smith, C.P.; Dijkhuizen, L.; Claessen, D.; Wosten, H.A. Nepa is a structural cell wall protein involved in maintenance of spore dormancy in *Streptomyces coelicolor*. *Mol. Microbiol.* **2009**, *71*, 1591–1603. [CrossRef] [PubMed]

52. Bobek, J.; Strakova, E.; Zikova, A.; Vohradsky, J. Changes in activity of metabolic and regulatory pathways during germination of *S. coelicolor*. *BMC Genomics* **2014**, *15*, 1173. [CrossRef] [PubMed]

53. Rioseras, B.; Yague, P.; Lopez-Garcia, M.T.; Gonzalez-Quinonez, N.; Binda, E.; Marinelli, F.; Manteca, A. Characterization of SCO4439, a D-alanyl-D-alanine carboxypeptidase involved in spore cell wall maturation, resistance, and germination in *Streptomyces coelicolor*. *Sci. Rep.* **2016**, *6*, 21659. [CrossRef] [PubMed]

54. Sexton, D.L.; St-Onge, R.J.; Haiser, H.J.; Yousef, M.R.; Brady, L.; Gao, C.; Leonard, J.; Elliot, M.A. Resuscitation-promoting factors are Cell wall-lytic enzymes with important roles in the germination and growth of *Streptomyces coelicolor*. *J. Bacteriol.* **2015**, *197*, 848–860. [CrossRef] [PubMed]

55. Noens, E.E.; Mersinias, V.; Willemse, J.; Traag, B.A.; Laing, E.; Chater, K.F.; Smith, C.P.; Koerten, H.K.; van Wezel, G.P. Loss of the controlled localization of growth stage-specific cell-wall synthesis pleiotropically affects developmental gene expression in an ssga mutant of *Streptomyces coelicolor*. *Mol. Microbiol.* **2007**, *64*, 1244–1259. [CrossRef] [PubMed]

56. Zacchetti, B.; Willemse, J.; Recter, B.; van Dissel, D.; van Wezel, G.P.; Wosten, H.A.; Claessen, D. Aggregation of germlings is a major contributing factor towards mycelial heterogeneity of *streptomyces*. *Sci. Rep.* **2016**, *6*, 27045. [CrossRef] [PubMed]

57. Girard, G.; Traag, B.A.; Sangal, V.; Mascini, N.; Hoskisson, P.A.; Goodfellow, M.; van Wezel, G.P. A novel taxonomic marker that discriminates between morphologically complex actinomycetes. *Open Biol.* **2013**, *3*, 130073. [CrossRef] [PubMed]

58. Ronnest, N.P.; Stocks, S.M.; Lantz, A.E.; Gernaey, K.V. Comparison of laser diffraction and image analysis for measurement of *Streptomyces coelicolor* cell clumps and pellets. *Biotechnol. Lett.* **2012**, *34*, 1465–1473. [CrossRef] [PubMed]

59. Van Veluw, G.J.; Petrus, M.L.; Gubbens, J.; de Graaf, R.; de Jong, I.P.; van Wezel, G.P.; Wosten, H.A.; Claessen, D. Analysis of two distinct mycelial populations in liquid-grown streptomyces cultures using a flow cytometry-based proteomics approach. *Appl. Microbiol. Biotechnol.* **2012**, *96*, 1301–1312. [CrossRef] [PubMed]

60. Petrus, M.L.; van Veluw, G.J.; Wosten, H.A.; Claessen, D. Sorting of streptomyces cell pellets using a complex object parametric analyzer and sorter. *J. Vis. Exp.* **2014**, e51178. [CrossRef] [PubMed]

61. Willemse, J.; Buke, F.; van Dissel, D.; Grevink, S.; Claessen, D.; van Wezel, G.P. Sparticle, an algorithm for the analysis of filamentous microorganisms in submerged cultures. *Antonie Van Leeuwenhoek* **2017**, 171–182. [CrossRef]

62. Celler, K.; Cristian, P.; van Loosdrecht, M.C.; van Wezel, G.P. Structured morphological modeling as a framework for rational strain design of streptomyces species. *Antonie Van Leeuwenhoek* **2012**, *102*, 409–423. [CrossRef] [PubMed]

63. Nieminen, L.; Webb, S.; Smith, M.C.; Hoskisson, P.A. A flexible mathematical model platform for studying branching networks: Experimentally validated using the model actinomycete, *Streptomyces coelicolor*. *PLoS ONE* **2013**, *8*, e54316. [CrossRef] [PubMed]

64. Van Dissel, D.; Claessen, D.; van Wezel, G.P. Morphogenesis of streptomyces in submerged cultures. *Adv. Appl. Microbiol.* **2014**, *89*, 1–45. [PubMed]

65. Ha, S.; Lee, K.J.; Lee, S.I.; Gwak, H.J.; Lee, J.H.; Kim, T.W.; Choi, H.J.; Jang, J.Y.; Choi, J.S.; Kim, C.J.; et al. Optimization of herbicidin a production in submerged culture of streptomyces scopuliridis m40. *J. Microbiol. Biotechnol.* **2017**, *27*, 947–955. [CrossRef] [PubMed]

66. Van Dissel, D.; van Wezel, G.P. Morphology-driven downscaling of streptomyces lividans to micro-cultivation. *Antonie Van Leeuwenhoek* **2017**, 457–469. [CrossRef]

67. Rigali, S.; Nothaft, H.; Noens, E.E.; Schlicht, M.; Colson, S.; Müller, M.; Joris, B.; Koerten, H.K.; Hopwood, D.A.; Titgemeyer, F.; van Wezel, G.P. The sugar phosphotransferase system of *Streptomyces coelicolor* is regulated by the gntr-family regulator dasr and links n-acetylglucosamine metabolism to the control of development. *Mol. Microbiol.* **2006**, *61*, 1237–1251. [CrossRef] [PubMed]

68. Rigali, S.; Titgemeyer, F.; Barends, S.; Mulder, S.; Thomae, A.W.; Hopwood, D.A.; van Wezel, G.P. Feast or famine: The global regulator dasr links nutrient stress to antibiotic production by streptomyces. *EMBO Rep.* **2008**, *9*, 670–675. [CrossRef] [PubMed]

69. Yague, P.; Manteca, A.; Simon, A.; Diaz-Garcia, M.E.; Sanchez, J. New method for monitoring programmed cell death and differentiation in submerged streptomyces cultures. *Appl. Environ. Microbiol.* **2010**, *76*, 3401–3404. [CrossRef] [PubMed]

70. Yague, P.; Lopez-Garcia, M.T.; Rioseras, B.; Sanchez, J.; Manteca, A. Pre-sporulation stages of streptomyces differentiation: State-of-the-art and future perspectives. *FEMS Microbiol. Lett.* **2013**, *342*, 79–88. [CrossRef] [PubMed]

71. Innes, C.M.; Allan, E.J. Induction, growth and antibiotic production of streptomyces viridifaciens l-form bacteria. *J. Appl. Microbiol.* **2001**, *90*, 301–308. [CrossRef] [PubMed]

72. Kealey, C.; Creaven, C.A.; Murphy, C.D.; Brady, C.B. New approaches to antibiotic discovery. *Biotechnol. Lett.* **2017**, *39*, 805–817. [CrossRef] [PubMed]

73. Bai, L.; Liu, C.; Guo, L.; Piao, C.; Li, Z.; Li, J.; Jia, F.; Wang, X.; Xiang, W. *Streptomyces formicae* sp. Nov., a novel actinomycete isolated from the head of *Camponotus japonicus* mayr. *Antonie Van Leeuwenhoek* **2016**, *109*, 253–261. [CrossRef] [PubMed]

74. Sarmiento-Vizcaino, A.; Brana, A.F.; Gonzalez, V.; Nava, H.; Molina, A.; Llera, E.; Fiedler, H.P.; Rico, J.M.; Garcia-Florez, L.; Acuna, J.L.; et al. Atmospheric dispersal of bioactive *Streptomyces albidoflavus* strains among terrestrial and marine environments. *Microb. Ecol.* **2016**, *71*, 375–386. [CrossRef] [PubMed]

75. Sarmiento-Vizcaino, A.; Gonzalez, V.; Brana, A.F.; Palacios, J.J.; Otero, L.; Fernandez, J.; Molina, A.; Kulik, A.; Vazquez, F.; Acuna, J.L.; et al. Pharmacological potential of phylogenetically diverse actinobacteria isolated from deep-sea coral ecosystems of the submarine aviles canyon in the cantabrian sea. *Microb. Ecol.* **2017**, *73*, 338–352. [CrossRef] [PubMed]

76. Schniete, J.K.; Cruz-Morales, P.; Selem-Mojica, N.; Fernandez-Martinez, L.T.; Hunter, I.S.; Barona-Gomez, F.; Hoskisson, P.A. Expanding primary metabolism helps generate the metabolic robustness to facilitate antibiotic biosynthesis in streptomyces. *MBio* **2018**, *9*. [CrossRef] [PubMed]

77. Cihak, M.; Kamenik, Z.; Smidova, K.; Bergman, N.; Benada, O.; Kofronova, O.; Petrickova, K.; Bobek, J. Secondary metabolites produced during the germination of *Streptomyces coelicolor*. *Front. Microbiol.* **2017**, *8*, 2495. [CrossRef] [PubMed]

78. Yu, G.; Jia, X.; Wen, J.; Lu, W.; Wang, G.; Caiyin, Q.; Chen, Y. Strain improvement of streptomyces roseosporus for daptomycin production by rational screening of he-ne laser and NTG induced mutants and kinetic modeling. *Appl. Biochem. Biotechnol.* **2011**, *163*, 729–743. [CrossRef] [PubMed]

79. Jakeman, D.L.; Graham, C.L.; Young, W.; Vining, L.C. Culture conditions improving the production of jadomycin b. *J. Ind. Microbiol. Biotechnol.* **2006**, *33*, 767–772. [CrossRef] [PubMed]

80. Bode, H.B.; Bethe, B.; Hofs, R.; Zeeck, A. Big effects from small changes: Possible ways to explore nature's chemical diversity. *Chembiochem* **2002**, *3*, 619–627. [CrossRef]

81. Bursy, J.; Kuhlmann, A.U.; Pittelkow, M.; Hartmann, H.; Jebbar, M.; Pierik, A.J.; Bremer, E. Synthesis and uptake of the compatible solutes ectoine and 5-hydroxyectoine by *Streptomyces coelicolor* A3(2) in response to salt and heat stresses. *Appl. Environ. Microbiol.* **2008**, *74*, 7286–7296. [CrossRef] [PubMed]

82. Hayes, A.; Hobbs, G.; Smith, C.P.; Oliver, S.G.; Butler, P.R. Environmental signals triggering methylenomycin production by *Streptomyces coelicolor* A3(2). *J. Bacteriol.* **1997**, *179*, 5511–5515. [CrossRef] [PubMed]

83. Medema, M.H.; Alam, M.; Breitling, R.; Takano, E. The future of industrial antibiotic production: From random mutagenesis to synthetic biology. *Bioeng. Bugs.* **2011**, 230–233. [CrossRef]

84. Cheng, Y.R.; Huang, J.; Qiang, H.; Lin, W.L.; Demain, A.L. Mutagenesis of the rapamycin producer streptomyces hygroscopicus FC904. *J. Antibiot.* **2001**, *54*, 967–972. [CrossRef] [PubMed]

85. Wang, G.; Hosaka, T.; Ochi, K. Dramatic activation of antibiotic production in *Streptomyces coelicolor* by cumulative drug resistance mutations. *Appl. Environ. Microbiol.* **2008**, *74*, 2834–2840. [CrossRef] [PubMed]

86. McKenzie, N.L.; Thaker, M.; Koteva, K.; Hughes, D.W.; Wright, G.D.; Nodwell, J.R. Induction of antimicrobial activities in heterologous streptomycetes using alleles of the *Streptomyces coelicolor* gene absa1. *J. Antibiot.* **2010**, *63*, 177–182. [CrossRef] [PubMed]

87. Foley, T.L.; Young, B.S.; Burkart, M.D. Phosphopantetheinyl transferase inhibition and secondary metabolism. *FEBS J.* **2009**, *276*, 7134–7145. [CrossRef] [PubMed]

88. Onaka, H. Biosynthesis of indolocarbazole and goadsporin, two different heterocyclic antibiotics produced by actinomycetes. *Biosci. Biotechnol. Biochem.* **2009**, *73*, 2149–2155. [CrossRef] [PubMed]

89. Recio, E.; Colinas, A.; Rumbero, A.; Aparicio, J.F.; Martin, J.F. Pi factor, a novel type quorum-sensing inducer elicits pimaricin production in streptomyces natalensis. *J. Biol. Chem.* **2004**, *279*, 41586–41593. [CrossRef] [PubMed]

90. Mo, S.; Ban, Y.H.; Park, J.W.; Yoo, Y.J.; Yoon, Y.J. Enhanced FK506 production in *Streptomyces clavuligerus* ckd1119 by engineering the supply of methylmalonyl-coa precursor. *J. Ind. Microbiol. Biotechnol.* **2009**, *36*, 1473–1482. [CrossRef] [PubMed]

91. Liu, Z.; Guo, M.; Qian, J.; Zhuang, Y.; Zhang, S. Disruption of ZWF2 gene to improve oxytetraclyline biosynthesis in streptomyces rimosus M4018. *Wei Sheng Wu Xue Bao* **2008**, *48*, 21–25. [PubMed]

92. Yagüe, P.; Manteca, A. Optimization of the antibiotic producction in different Streptomyces strains by conditioning the MII differentiation. **2018**. Unpublished results.

93. Malla, S.; Niraula, N.P.; Liou, K.; Sohng, J.K. Self-resistance mechanism in streptomyces peucetius: Overexpression of drra, drrb and drrc for doxorubicin enhancement. *Microbiol. Res.* **2010**, *165*, 259–267. [CrossRef] [PubMed]

94. Qiu, J.; Zhuo, Y.; Zhu, D.; Zhou, X.; Zhang, L.; Bai, L.; Deng, Z. Overexpression of the abc transporter avtab increases avermectin production in streptomyces avermitilis. *Appl. Microbiol. Biotechnol.* **2011**, *92*, 337–345. [CrossRef] [PubMed]

95. Xu, Y.; Willems, A.; Au-Yeung, C.; Tahlan, K.; Nodwell, J.R. A two-step mechanism for the activation of actinorhodin export and resistance in *Streptomyces coelicolor*. *MBio* **2012**, *3*, e00191-12. [CrossRef] [PubMed]

96. McKenzie, N.L.; Nodwell, J.R. Phosphorylated absa2 negatively regulates antibiotic production in *Streptomyces coelicolor* through interactions with pathway-specific regulatory gene promoters. *J. Bacteriol.* **2007**, *189*, 5284–5292. [CrossRef] [PubMed]

97. Guo, J.; Zhao, J.; Li, L.; Chen, Z.; Wen, Y. Li, J. The pathway-specific regulator aver from *Streptomyces avermitilis* positively regulates avermectin production while it negatively affects oligomycin biosynthesis. *Mol. Genet. Genomics* **2010**, *283*, 123–133. [CrossRef] [PubMed]

98. Retzlaff, L.; Distler, J. The regulator of streptomycin gene expression, strr, of streptomyces griseus is a DNA binding activator protein with multiple recognition sites. *Mol. Microbiol.* **1995**, *18*, 151–162. [CrossRef] [PubMed]

99. Laureti, L.; Song, L.; Huang, S.; Corre, C.; Leblond, P.; Challis, G.L.; Aigle, B. Identification of a bioactive 51-membered macrolide complex by activation of a silent polyketide synthase in *Streptomyces ambofaciens*. *Proc. Natl. Acad. Sci. USA* **2011**, *108*, 6258–6626. [CrossRef] [PubMed]

100. Menendez, N.; Brana, A.F.; Salas, J.A.; Mendez, C. Involvement of a chromomycin abc transporter system in secretion of a deacetylated precursor during chromomycin biosynthesis. *Microbiology* **2007**, *153*, 3061–3070. [CrossRef] [PubMed]

101. Bunet, R.; Song, L.; Mendes, M.V.; Corre, C.; Hotel, L.; Rouhier, N.; Framboisier, X.; Leblond, P.; Challis, G.L.; Aigle, B. Characterization and manipulation of the pathway-specific late regulator alpw reveals *Streptomyces ambofaciens* as a new producer of kinamycins. *J. Bacteriol.* **2010**. [CrossRef] [PubMed]

102. Gomez-Escribano, J.P.; Bibb, M.J. Engineering *Streptomyces coelicolor* for heterologous expression of secondary metabolite gene clusters. *Microb. Biotechnol.* **2011**, *4*, 207–215. [CrossRef] [PubMed]

103. Komatsu, M.; Uchiyama, T.; Omura, S.; Cane, D.E.; Ikeda, H. Genome-minimized streptomyces host for the heterologous expression of secondary metabolism. *Proc. Natl. Acad. Sci. USA* **2010**, *107*, 2646–2651. [CrossRef] [PubMed]

104. Novakova, R.; Nunez, L.E.; Homerova, D.; Knirschova, R.; Feckova, L.; Rezuchova, B.; Sevcikova, B.; Menendez, N.; Moris, F.; Cortes, J.; et al. Increased heterologous production of the antitumoral polyketide mithramycin a by engineered streptomyces lividans TK24 strains. *Appl. Microbiol. Biotechnol.* **2018**, *102*, 857–869. [CrossRef] [PubMed]

105. Kawahara, T.; Izumikawa, M.; Kozone, I.; Hashimoto, J.; Kagaya, N.; Koiwai, H.; Komatsu, M.; Fujie, M.; Sato, N.; Ikeda, H.; et al. Neothioviridamide, a polythioamide compound produced by heterologous expression of a *Streptomyces* sp. Cryptic ripp biosynthetic gene cluster. *J. Nat. Prod.* **2018**, 264–269. [CrossRef] [PubMed]

16

Interplay between Colistin Resistance, Virulence and Fitness in *Acinetobacter baumannii*

Gabriela Jorge Da Silva [1,2,]* and Sara Domingues [1,2]

1   Faculty of Pharmacy, University of Coimbra, 3000-548 Coimbra, Portugal; saradomingues@ff.uc.pt
2   Centre for Neurosciences and Cell Biology, University of Coimbra, 3000-548 Coimbra, Portugal
*   Correspondence: gjsilva@ci.uc.pt

Abstract: *Acinetobacter baumannii* is an important opportunistic nosocomial pathogen often resistant to multiple antibiotics classes. Colistin, an "old" antibiotic, is now considered a last-line treatment option for extremely resistant isolates. In the meantime, resistance to colistin has been reported in clinical *A. baumannii* strains. Colistin is a cationic peptide that disrupts the outer membrane (OM) of Gram-negative bacteria. Colistin resistance is primarily due to post-translational modification or loss of the lipopolysaccharide (LPS) molecules inserted into the outer leaflet of the OM. LPS modification prevents the binding of polymyxin to the bacterial surface and may lead to alterations in bacterial virulence. Antimicrobial pressure drives the evolution of antimicrobial resistance and resistance is often associated with a reduced bacterial fitness. Therefore, the alterations in LPS may induce changes in the fitness of *A. baumannii*. However, compensatory mutations in clinical *A. baumannii* may ameliorate the cost of resistance and may play an important role in the dissemination of colistin-resistant *A. baumannii* isolates. The focus of this review is to summarize the colistin resistance mechanisms, and understand their impact on the fitness and virulence of bacteria and on the dissemination of colistin-resistant *A. baumannii* strains.

Keywords: *Acinetobacter baumannii*; colistin; polymyxin; antimicrobial resistance; multidrug resistance; lipopolysaccharide; lipid A; biological cost; virulence; two-component systems

---

1. Introduction

Acinetobacter baumannii is an opportunistic Gram-negative pathogen recognized worldwide as a significant concern. Many isolates express diverse mechanisms of resistance that lead to the difficulty of treatment of infections caused by this microorganism. Most of the infections are in the forms of ventilator-associated pneumonia and septicaemia, especially in patients from intensive care units [1,2]. In the 1970s it was considered a low-virulence pathogen. The increased use of antibiotics and invasive methods of treatment and diagnostics in the last decades have led to the development of multidrug resistance and a rise in the frequency and severity of *A. baumannii* infections [3]. Carbapenems represent one of the last therapeutic choices for the treatment of infections due to multidrug-resistant (MDR) *A. baumannii*. Nevertheless, carbapenem-resistant isolates have been emerging [2]. Indeed, in 2017 the World Health Organization published a report where carbapenem-resistant *A. baumannii* was classified in the group of "priority 1 for research of new antibiotics" and considered as a "critical" pathogen [4]. The emergence of extensively drug-resistant (XDR) strains led to the human clinical use of an "old" antibiotic from the 1960s, colistin, which was abandoned in human therapy due to its nephrotoxicity and neurotoxicity, at a time where new antibiotics were emerging that still showed good antibacterial efficacy and less toxic effects. Since then, colistin has been mostly used in topical formulations. Nonetheless, the emergence of XDR strains has forced clinicians to use colistin as one of the last therapeutic options to fight these infections. Since the re-introduction of colistin in human clinical practice, the appearance of colistin-resistant strains has been reported [5–7]. Colistin resistance can be chromosomally or plasmid encoded, with the latter described recently in enterobacteria from food animals for the first time [8]. Since then, the plasmidic colistin-resistance genes *mcr*-1 to -5 have been reported worldwide in Gram-negative bacteria from human, animal, and environmental samples [7,9–14], but not in *A. baumannii*. So far, the reported mechanisms of resistance in *A. baumannii* are chromosomally encoded [15,16]. Nonetheless, the number of cases of of polymyxin-resistant *A. baumannii* strains has been increasing worldwide [16], leading to a global concern on the treatment of these infections. The majority of resistance mechanisms to colistin rely on alterations of the lipopolysaccharide (LPS), the primary target of colistin and an important virulence factor in Gram-negative bacteria. Many virulence factors have been identified in *A. baumannii* [3,17], but fundamental knowledge on virulence gene regulation and infection biology is still poorly understood [3,18].

The outcome of infections caused by drug-resistant bacteria is a complex relationship between the bacterial pathogenicity, biological cost of the resistance mutations in bacteria, host factors, and antibiotic therapy. Mutations that lead to antimicrobial resistance may modulate bacterial fitness and virulence potential. The comprehension of how antimicrobial resistance drives the biology of resistant bacterial pathogens is important to understand the outcome of an infection and the dissemination of drug resistance. Considering the clinical relevance of *A. baumannii*, some studies have been performed to evaluate the fitness cost of colistin-resistant strains.

The purpose of this review is to summarize the resistance mechanisms of *A. baumannii* to colistin and to focus on the interplay of colistin resistance, virulence, and fitness cost of the bacteria to better understand the consequences of the mutations associated with colistin resistance and the biological response of the pathogen.

2. Mechanism of Action of Colistin

Colistin, a bactericidal polycationic lipopeptide also known as polymyxin E, is composed of a cyclic decapeptide bound to a fatty acid chain. Its initial cellular target is the polyanionic LPS, a component of the Gram-negative bacterial outer membrane (OM). The amphiphilic feature of colistin is crucial for its interaction with the hydrophobic lipid A, a component of LPS. Lipid A has a crucial role in the control of cell permeability [19]. The electrostatic interaction between the positively-charged α,γ-diaminobutyric acid (Dab) residues of colistin and the negatively-charged phosphate groups of lipid A leads to the displacement of divalent cations Ca^{2+} and Mg^{2+}, which destabilize the molecule. The alteration of the three-dimensional structure triggers the permeability of some areas of the OM, facilitating the passage of colistin through a self-promoted uptake mechanism [20]. Colistin destroys the bacterial membrane, leading to the leakage of the cytoplasmatic content and cell death [19].

Lipid A is considered an endotoxin in Gram-negative bacteria since it induces the inflammatory response with the initial release of cytokines (TNF-α) and IL-8 [21]. The anti-endotoxin effect is considered another mechanism of action of colistin by the neutralization of the LPS molecule [22].

More recently, it was reported that colistin inhibited the vital respiratory enzyme NADH-quinone oxidoreductase in the cytoplasmic membrane, although this is seen as a secondary mechanism [23].

3. Mechanisms of Resistance in *A. baumannii*

In *A. baumannii*, two main mechanisms of acquired resistance have been described: the modification of lipid A by adding phosphoetanolamine (PEtN) as a consequence of mutations in the *pmrA/pmrB* two-component system; and the complete loss of the LPS due to impaired lipid A synthesis. However, other genes that affect the biosynthesis of LPS and the structure of lipid A are also being described. Efflux pumps might also be involved in colistin resistance.

3.1. LPS Modification Mediated by the Two-Component System pmrA/pmrB

The most common mechanism of resistance to colistin is the modification of LPS by substitution of the phosphate groups by molecules that confer a positive charge to LPS, preventing the binding of colistin. In *A. baumannii*, the mutations in the *pmrA* and/or *pmrB* genes (more common in *pmrB*) may induce the constitutive expression of *pmrA* that leads to the up-regulation of the *pmrCAB* operon, and subsequent synthesis and addition of PEtN to the 4'-phosphate or 1'-phosphate of lipid A [24–29].

The resistant phenotype can be reverted to a susceptible one due to compensatory mutations in the *pmr locus*, decreasing the hyper-activation of the *pmrCAB* operon, or the *pmr* gene may change to its non-mutated form [26,27]. However, some strains can maintain the *pmrB* mutation, with no additional compensatory mutations. Moreover, a study reported that six out of 30 colistin-resistant *A. baumannii* strains did not evidence any mutations in the *pmrA/pmrB* locus. This finding suggests that other genes might be involved in the acquisition of colistin resistance, leading to the overexpression of the PmrAB two-component system. Increased expression of both genes seems to be essential for colistin resistance, in contrast with amino acid changes [30].

Other alterations of the lipid A structure were found in clinical and laboratory colistin-resistant strains that have a diphosphoryl hepta-acylated lipid A structure with both pEtN and galactosamine (GalN) modifications [31]. Hepta-acylation of lipid A promotes protection against cationic antimicrobial polipeptides, including polymyxins. In *Escherichia coli* and *Salmonella* spp. the LPS portion of the OM barrier is reinforced by the increased production of the OM acyltransferase PagP, resulting in the formation of protective hepta-acylated lipid A. *A. baumannii* does not possess the gene *pagP*, and developed a PagP-independent mechanism to synthesize the protective hepta-acylated lipid A. Two putative acyltransferases (designated LpxLAb and LpxMAb) were characterized, and transfer one and two lauroyl (C12:0) acyl chains, respectively, during lipid A biosynthesis. The LpxMAb-dependent acylation of lipid A was also shown to be essential to the survival of *A. baumannii* strains in desiccation conditions [32].

3.2. Loss of LPS

LPS is synthesised in the cytoplasm through the Lpx pathway and it is translocated to the OM by the Lpt pathway. Mutations by nucleotide substitution, deletion, or insertional inactivation by the insertion sequence IS*Aba11* in the genes *lpxA*, *lpbxC* and *lpxD*, which are involved in the lipid A biosynthesis, have been described in colistin-resistant *A. baumannii* strains, leading to the complete loss of LPS [33,34]. Additional mutations of the *lpsB* gene, encoding a glycosyltransferase, and involved in the synthesis of the LPS core, have also been associated to colistin resistance. The absence of lipid A, the initial target of colistin, results in high resistance to colistin [35,36]. Also, LPS may not be present in the OM due to mutations in the gene that encodes the outer membrane protein LptD, responsible for the final translocation of the LPS molecule after its synthesis [37]. The LPS-deficient bacteria alter the activation of the host innate immune inflammatory response [38].

A recent study compared the metabolome of polymyxin-susceptible and polymyxin-resistant *A. baumannii* strains, showing three quite different metabolic profiles: (1) alterations in specific amino acid and carbohydrate metabolites, particularly from the pentose phosphate pathway (PPP) and tricarboxylic acid (TCA) cycle intermediates; (2) nucleotide levels lower in the LPS-deficient strain; and (3), increased abundance of short-chain lipids compared to the parent polymyxin-susceptible ATCC 19606 (ATCC is international (American Type Culture Collection)) [39].

3.3. Genes Involved in the Outer-Membrane Asymmetry

Mutations in genes other than *pmrAB* and *lpxACD* may also be responsible for the change of antimicrobial susceptibility to colistin. The asymmetric distribution of lipids in the OM of Gram-negative bacteria is essential for its function as a barrier and integrity of the cell. The accumulation of phospholipids in the outer leaflet of the OM disrupts the LPS organization and increases the cell lability to small toxic molecules. The OM lipoprotein VacJ is part of the Vps-VacJ ABC transporter system responsible for maintaining the phospholipids in the OM inner leaflet and the LPS in the outer leaflet of the membrane (OM asymmetry) [40]. The activity of PldA, a phospholipase, is increased in bacteria cells with destabilized membrane and it seems to remove phospholipids from the outer leaflet of the OM to maintain asymmetry [41]. Recently, it was suggested that both *vacJ* and *pldA* genes, where mutations were identified, may play a role on the *A. baumannii* colistin resistance due to their association to the maintenance of OM asymmetry [42].

3.4. Efflux Pumps

A few studies suggest that efflux pumps may be involved in the colistin resistance phenotype in *A. baumannii*. Eighteen genes encoding putative efflux transporters were shown to be upregulated in response to physiological concentration of NaCl, resulting in a tolerance to diverse antibiotics, including colistin [43]. More recently, another study showed that the use of efflux inhibitors like cyanide 3-chlorophenylhydrazone (CCCP) may reduce significantly the minimal inhibitor concentrations for colistin, strongly suggesting the involvement of efflux pumps in the colistin resistance phenotype [44].

4. Fitness and Virulence

The biological cost conferred to the host by a resistance trait is considered a key parameter in the spread and stability of resistant bacteria. Resistance mutations typically change and/or impair targets with essential functions, and are usually associated with a fitness cost. Nonetheless, cells can often ameliorate the cost of the resistance due to compensatory mutations. The amelioration of resistance can result in the stabilization of the resistance in the bacterial population [45,46]. Fitness is usually evaluated by measurement of growth rates and/or pairwise competition experiments.

The pathogenic potential of a bacteria reflects its virulence, which is usually measured by the mortality or the host reproduction rates associated with a strain. Changes in virulence (increased or decreased) have been detected in resistant strains belonging to different species [47,48]. Some of the virulence factors that have been identified in *A. baumannii* include the outer membrane protein OmpA, phospholipases, efflux pumps, penicillin-binding proteins, and outer membrane vesicles [49,50].

Although fitness and virulence are different concepts, studies often evaluate both. Therefore, fitness and virulence will be discussed together and we will attempt to relate these traits with genetic mutations associated with colistin resistance. Some studies test clinical isolates while others expose ATCC strains to increased concentrations of colistin to generate different resistant isolates.

4.1. Colistin Resistance Due to Mutations in pmr Genes

Clinical *A. baumannii* isolates often acquire colistin resistance during treatment with this antibiotic [26,51–53]. Two clinical *A. baumannii* strains, which acquired colistin resistance after treatment with this polymyxin, were shown to have different clinical outcomes. *A. baumannii* ABIsac_ColiR [25] showed impaired virulence, as seen by loss of clinical signs of infection in the human patient [51] and in a rat model of acute pneumonia [52], while *A. baumannii* CR17 did not lose its infecting capacity [54]. Both strains were later further explored and colistin resistance was associated with *pmrA* mutations: *A. baumannii* ABIsac_ColiR with *pmrA* E8D [25] and *A. baumannii* CR17 with *pmrA* M12K [55]. Strain ABIsac_ColiR was also shown to have lost a prophage, which could contribute to or explain the loss of virulence in this strain [25]. A decreased in vitro and in vivo fitness has also been observed [52]. Although strain CR17 remained infectious, it was also associated with a decreased virulence and fitness, as compared with the initial susceptible strain CS01 [55]. The levels of virulence vary between *A. baumannii* strains [56], and the retention of the capacity to infect of CR17 strain might be related with the initial high virulence of the susceptible strain [55].

Four clinical *A. baumannii* strains showed an in vitro fitness cost, seen as the decreased growth rates of the resistant strains. The in vivo fitness cost was evidenced by the loss of resistance after treatment cessation. Although mutations in different genes were observed, all resistant isolates carried *pmrB* mutations which also varied, including P233S, R263C, M145I, T13A, or indel AAT at position 69. These mutations could be associated with the overexpression of the PmrC phosphoethanolamine transferase, with a consequent increase of the *pmr* operon transcript. Return to susceptibility to colistin occurred by different mechanisms. In two patients, there was re-emergence of the susceptible strain.

In another patient, the resistant strain was lost, but unexpectedly, the apparent susceptible strain was detected to be also present during colistin treatment. This strain carried a L271R mutation in *pmrB*, associated with a low fitness cost and in vivo stability in the absence of colistin. In the fourth patient, with the resistant isolate carrying the *pmrB* P233S mutation, a compensatory mutation in *pmrA* (L206P) was observed, making the future re-acquisition of colistin resistance highly unlikely [26]. In a different study, the same *pmrB* P233S mutation present in other clinical colistin-resistant *A. baumannii* strains (Ab4451 and Ab4452) was not associated with loss of virulence or reduced fitness; compensatory mutations in the *pmrCAB* locus were also not detected. Despite the fact that in vitro and in vivo fitness costs were not observed in Ab4451 and Ab4452, resistance to colistin was lost after colistin was withdrawn [57]. In a recent study, the *pmrB* P233S mutation was not associated with a fitness cost, but had an impact on the in vitro virulence, as evaluated by attenuated proteolytic activity and siderophore production, of the clinical strain C440 [58]. While the study by Snitkin and colleagues showed mutations in other genes usually not specifically related with colistin resistance [26], Durante-Mangoni et al. only sequenced the *pmrCAB* and *lpxACD* loci [57]. Whether compensatory mutations in non-analysed genes, post-translational modifications, or physiological changes could explain the different study outcomes remains to be determined.

Two different clinical strains acquired colistin resistance after patient treatment with colistin. Ab249 and Ab347 harboured *pmrB* P233S and P170L mutations, respectively. Both strains showed a reduced in vitro fitness and in vitro and in vivo decreased virulence [53,59]. The reduced virulence could be associated with a diminished initial cell adhesion with consequent reduced ability of the resistant strains to produce biofilm. Additionally, Ab249 carried a mutation in *lpsB* (*241K), and Ab347 lost several genes while carrying a mutation in CarO (A19fs), which has been previously associated with biofilm production [59].

In contrast, decreased in vitro fitness and virulence was not observed in a clinical *A. baumannii* strain with a deletion of one amino acid in PmrB (ΔI19) [58]. In another study, where clinical strains were exposed to sub-MIC concentrations of colistin, while *pmrB* S17R mutant showed a slight decrease in fitness and virulence, these changes were not observed in strains with *pmrB* 17_26dup or T235I [60].

An in vitro-induced colistin-resistant derivative of *A. baumannii* ATCC 19606, called RC64, showed an increased in vitro [61] and in vivo fitness cost as well as impaired virulence [62]. The decreased fitness in the resistant strain has been associated with the down-regulation of several proteins, including outer membrane proteins, chaperones, protein biosynthesis factors, and metabolic enzymes [61]. The mutations R134C and A227V have been identified in the *pmrB* of this strain [62]. Low-iron conditions, such as those found in the human serum, were related with the decrease in vitro fitness [63] of strain RC64 [62] and also clinical colistin-resistant strains [64] with different *pmrB* mutations, which were not directly correlated with the reduced growth phenotype [63]. Another colistin-resistant derivative of *A. baumannii* ATCC 19606, with A227V *pmrB*, showed decreased in vitro and in vivo fitness, as well as attenuated virulence, although this was not observed in all tested models [65].

A slight decrease of the in vitro fitness of a colistin-resistant derivative of *A. baumannii* ATCC 17978 was associated with *pmrB* G272D [46].

Colistin-resistant clinical strains recovered during colistin therapy revealed a reduced in vitro fitness as determined by the growth rates and by pairwise competitions assays with their susceptible counterparts. These strains presented mutations in *pmrB* S17R, T232I, R263L, Y116H and/or *pmrA1* E8D, with the highest fitness decrease associated with co-presence of *pmrB* Y116H and *pmrA1* E8D [24,66]. Some of the strains, collected from the same patient over the course of colistin treatment (which has its bactericidal effect due to production of hydroxyl radicals) were further studied; the study included the susceptible parental strain as well as five resistant strains. Both in vitro and in vivo assays revealed that, after an initial loss of fitness and virulence, colistin-resistant isolates progressively increase their fitness as well as virulence under oxidative stress. This study also shows that in vitro results do not necessarily correlate with the in vivo outcome [66].

4.2. Colistin Resistance Due to Mutations in lpx Genes

Fewer studies report on the fitness and virulence of colistin-resistant *A. baumannii* due to mutations in the *lpxACD* locus. In one of the studies, in vitro and in vivo fitness costs were detected in the *lpx* mutants, with the Δ*lpxD* mutant showing the highest in vitro fitness cost, as compared with the wild-type *A. baumannii* ATCC 19606. Virulence was also evaluated in A549 human alveolar cells and in a mouse model, and in *Caenorhabditis elegans*, with the *lpx* mutants showing decreased virulence, seen as decreased mortality rate or reduced inhibition of fertility, respectively [65]. In another study, Wand and colleagues showed that single mutations in the *lpxA* (E216*), *lpxC* (I253N, F191L or A82E), or *lpxD* (K318fs) genes, or inactivation of *lpxC* (*lpxC*::IS*Aba1*), obtained after colistin exposure to clinical *A. baumannii* strains, were associated with a reduced fitness and avirulence in *Galleria mellonella* [60]. As described above, these studies also evaluated the biological costs and effect on virulence associated with mutations in the *pmrB* gene. Comparing the results, the influence of mutations in the fitness and virulence was more pronounced in the *lpx* mutants [60,65].

Mu and colleagues showed that mutation *lpxA* I76K and disruption of *lpxC* or *lpxD* by IS*Aba1* confer fitness costs to colistin-resistant derivatives of *A. baumannii* ATCC 17978, but additional mutations in other genes, such as *hepA* or *rsfS*, contributed to an increased resistance to colistin, as well as a (partially or completely) compensated fitness cost of these mutants. Additional costs were observed when mutants were grown in serum [46].

Table 1 summarizes the outcome of fitness and virulence assays in *A. baumannii* strains with mutations in known colistin-resistance genes.

Table 1. Studies showing mutations present in well-known colistin-resistance genes and fitness cost and virulence observed in isolates.

Source of Resistance	Gene	Mutation (Amino Acid Level)	Fitness Cost In Vitro	Fitness Cost In Vivo	Impaired Virulence	Reference
Clinical	*pmrA*	E8D	Yes	Yes	Yes	[25,51,52]
Clinical	*pmrA*	M12K	Yes	Yes	Yes [b]	[54,55]
Clinical	*pmrA1*	E8D	Yes	-	-	[24]
Clinical	*pmrB* + *pmrA1*	Y116H + E8D	Yes	-	-	[24]
Lab acquired	*pmrB*	R134C and A227V	Yes	Yes	yes	[61,62]
Lab acquired	*pmrB*	G272D	Yes [a]	-	-	[46]
Clinical	*pmrB*	T13A; indel AAT at 69; M145I; P233S; R263C	Yes	Yes		[26]
Clinical	*pmrB*	L271R	-	Yes [a]	-	[26]
Clinical	*pmrB*	P233S	No	No	No	[57]
Clinical	*pmrB*	P233S	No	-	Yes	[58]
Clinical	*pmrB*	P233S; P170L	Yes	-	Yes	[53,59]
Clinical	*pmrB*	ΔI19	No	-	No	[58]
Clinical	*pmrB*	S17R; T232I; R263L	Yes	-	-	[24]
Lab acquired	*pmrB*	S17R	-	Yes [a]	Yes [b]	[60]
Lab acquired	*pmrB*	17_26dup; T235I	-	No	No	[60]
Lab acquired	*pmrB*	A227V	Yes	Yes	Yes [b]	[65]
Lab acquired	*lpxACD*	Δ*lpxA*; Δ*lpxC*; Δ*lpxD*	Yes	Yes	Yes	[65]
Lab acquired	*lpxA*	E216 *	-	Yes	Yes	[60]
Lab acquired	*lpxA*	I76K	Yes	-	-	[46]
Lab acquired	*lpxC*	I253N; F191L; A82E; Δ*lpxC*	-	Yes	Yes	[60]
Lab acquired	*lpxC*	Δ*lpxC*	Yes	-	-	[46]
Lab acquired	*lpxD*	K318fs	-	Yes	Yes	[60]
Lab acquired	*lpxD*	Δ*lpxD*	Yes	-	-	[46]

[a] A slight cost was observed; [b] Although reduced virulence was observed, the strains did not become avirulent; * Stop codon.

5. Conclusions

Most of the studies report a fitness cost and a decreased virulence of colistin-resistant *A. baumannii*. However, this seems to be dependent on several factors, such as the mutated gene, the specific mutation, and the tested strain. The loss of LPS (*lpx* mutants) has a higher impact on the strain fitness and virulence in comparison with those that only have modifications of the LPS (*pmr* mutants). This is comprehensible since *lpx* mutants lack the endotoxic LPS and the cells lose the wall integrity.

Numerous mutations in the same gene are associated with colistin resistance. Diverse mutations might be associated with different outcomes, especially if they differently influence the protein structure or function [58,62]. At the same time, the same mutation might have different effects on the fitness and the virulence of the strain, which can also be associated with the existence of compensatory mutations in other genes. The plasticity of the *A. baumannii* regulation systems can also potentially affect the influence of colistin resistance on virulence [58], as well as post-translational modifications or physiological changes [66].

Another factor that can influence the fitness and virulence results is the different genetic backgrounds of the tested strains. Clinical strains are highly variable, belong to different sequence types, and carry different virulence genes, which can impact the overall virulence and fitness of each strain. Different ATCC strains also produce different outcomes [46]. To overcome this limitation, the different genes involved in colistin resistance, carrying different mutations, should be tested in the same genetic background.

The reported studies use different methods, which can also influence the result. Additionally, as recently observed, in vitro results might not correlate well with the in vivo outcome [66]. Therefore, more in vivo studies are needed.

The high fitness costs associated with colistin resistance, especially in mutants that lose LPS, may limit the spread of these isolates in clinical environment and could explain the sporadic nature of colistin-resistant *A. baumannii* outbreaks [6,64,67,68]. Nonetheless, recent evidence shows that compensatory mutations can ameliorate the biology cost triggered by colistin resistance, which can increase survival and spread in these environments. At the same time, there is some confidence in the successful treatment of colistin-resistant *A. baumannii* infections, as colistin-resistant mutants have an increased susceptibility to several antibiotics [46,69,70]. Nonetheless, this trait does not seem to be universal [24,53].

In conclusion, *A. baumannii* shows a remarkable genetic plasticity that allows a quick adaption to environmental conditions. The old paradigm that there is a trade-off between resistance and virulence might not always apply, even in colistin-resistant strains where LPS is lost or modified. The interplay between genetic virulence regulation and antimicrobial resistance is complex and seems to be highly strain-dependent. More in depth and fundamental studies are needed to fully comprehend the interaction of resistance and bacteria biology that could help in the development of interventions to control the dissemination of colistin-resistant strains.

Acknowledgments: Faculty of Pharmacy of the University of Coimbra and Center for Neurosciences and Cell Biology through "Fundação para a Ciência e a Tecnologia, projecto Estratégico: UID/NEU/04539/2013".

Author Contributions: The authors contribute equally to the manuscript.

References

1. Dijkshoorn, L.; Nemec, A.; Seifert, H. An increasing threat in hospitals: Multidrug-resistant *Acinetobacter baumannii*. *Nat. Rev. Microbiol.* **2007**, *5*, 939–951. [CrossRef] [PubMed]
2. Lee, C.R.; Lee, J.H.; Park, M.; Park, K.S.; Bae, I.K.; Kim, Y.B.; Cha, C.J.; Jeong, B.C.; Lee, S.H. Biology of *Acinetobacter baumannii*: Pathogenesis, antibiotic resistance mechanisms, and prospective treatment options. *Front. Cell. Infect. Microbiol.* **2017**, *7*, 55. [CrossRef] [PubMed]
3. Wong, D.; Nielsen, T.B.; Bonomo, R.A.; Pantapalangkoor, P.; Luna, B.; Spellberg, B. Clinical and pathophysiological overview of *Acinetobacter* infections: A century of challenges. *Clin. Microbiol. Rev.* **2017**, *30*, 409–447. [PubMed]
4. World Health Organization. Global Priority List of Antibiotic-Resistant Bacteria to Guide Research, Discovery, and Development of New Antibiotics. Available online: http://www.who.int/medicines/publications/WHO-PPL-Short_Summary_25Feb-ET_NM_WHO.pdf (accessed on 2 October 2017).

5. Mavroidi, A.; Likousi, S.; Palla, E.; Katsiari, M.; Roussou, Z.; Maguina, A.; Platsouka, E.D. Molecular identification of tigecycline- and colistin-resistant carbapenemase-producing *Acinetobacter baumannii* from a Greek hospital from 2011 to 2013. *J. Med. Microbiol.* **2015**, *64*, 993–997. [CrossRef] [PubMed]

6. Agodi, A.; Voulgari, E.; Barchitta, M.; Quattrocchi, A.; Bellocchi, P.; Poulou, A.; Santangelo, C.; Castiglione, G.; Giaquinta, L.; Romeo, M.A.; et al. Spread of a carbapenem- and colistin-resistant *Acinetobacter baumannii* ST2 clonal strain causing outbreaks in two Sicilian hospitals. *J. Hosp. Infect.* **2014**, *86*, 260–266. [CrossRef] [PubMed]

7. Cai, Y.; Chai, D.; Wang, R.; Liang, B.; Bai, N. Colistin resistance of *Acinetobacter baumannii*: Clinical reports, mechanisms and antimicrobial strategies. *J. Antimicrob. Chemother.* **2012**, *67*, 1607–1615. [CrossRef] [PubMed]

8. Liu, Y.Y.; Wang, Y.; Walsh, T.R.; Yi, L.X.; Zhang, R.; Spencer, J.; Doi, Y.; Tian, G.; Dong, B.; Huang, X.; et al. Emergence of plasmid-mediated colistin resistance mechanism MCR-1 in animals and human beings in China: A microbiological and molecular biological study. *Lancet Infect. Dis.* **2016**, *16*, 161–168. [CrossRef]

9. Zurfuh, K.; Poirel, L.; Nordmann, P.; Nuesch-Inderbinen, M.; Hachler, H.; Stephan, R. Occurrence of the plasmid-borne *mcr-1* colistin resistance gene in extended-spectrum-beta-lactamase-producing Enterobacteriaceae in river water and imported vegetable samples in Switzerland. *Antimicrob. Agents Chemother.* **2016**, *60*, 2594–2595. [CrossRef] [PubMed]

10. Rhouma, M.; Beaudry, F.; Letellier, A. Resistance to colistin: What is the fate for this antibiotic in pig production? *Int. J. Antimicrob. Agents* **2016**, *48*, 119–126. [CrossRef] [PubMed]

11. Xavier, B.B.; Lammens, C.; Ruhal, R.; Kumar-Singh, S.; Butaye, P.; Goossens, H.; Malhotra-Kumar, S. Identification of a novel plasmid-mediated colistin-resistance gene, *mcr-2*, in *Escherichia coli*, Belgium, June 2016. *Euro Surveill.* **2016**, *21*. [CrossRef] [PubMed]

12. Yin, W.; Li, H.; Shen, Y.; Liu, Z.; Wang, S.; Shen, Z.; Zhang, R.; Walsh, T.R.; Shen, J.; Wang, Y. Novel plasmid-mediated colistin resistance gene *mcr-3* in *Escherichia coli*. *MBio* **2017**, *8*, e00543-17. [CrossRef] [PubMed]

13. Carattoli, A.; Villa, L.; Feudi, C.; Curcio, L.; Orsini, S.; Luppi, A.; Pezzotti, G.; Magistrali, C.F. Novel plasmid-mediated colistin resistance *mcr-4* gene in *Salmonella* and *Escherichia coli*, Italy 2013, Spain and Belgium, 2015 to 2016. *Euro Surveill.* **2017**, *22*, 30589. [CrossRef] [PubMed]

14. Borowiak, M.; Fischer, J.; Hammerl, J.A.; Hendriksen, R.S.; Szabo, I.; Malorny, B. Identification of a novel transposon-associated phosphoethanolamine transferase gene, *mcr-5*, conferring colistin resistance in d-tartrate fermenting *Salmonella enterica* subsp. *enterica* serovar Paratyphi B. *J. Antimicrob. Chemother.* **2017**. [CrossRef] [PubMed]

15. Poirel, L.; Jayol, A.; Nordmann, P. Polymyxins: Antibacterial activity, susceptibility testing, and resistance mechanisms encoded by plasmids or chromosomes. *Clin. Microbiol. Rev.* **2017**, *30*, 557–596. [CrossRef] [PubMed]

16. Srinivas, P.; Rivard, K. Polymyxin resistance in Gram-negative pathogens. *Curr. Infect. Dis. Rep.* **2017**, *19*, 38. [CrossRef] [PubMed]

17. Weber, B.S.; Harding, C.M.; Feldman, M.F. Pathogenic *Acinetobacter*: From the cell surface to infinity and beyond. *J. Bacteriol.* **2015**, *198*, 880–887. [CrossRef] [PubMed]

18. Kroger, C.; Kary, S.C.; Schauer, K.; Cameron, A.D. Genetic regulation of virulence and antibiotic resistance in *Acinetobacter baumannii*. *Genes (Basel)* **2016**, *8*, 12. [CrossRef] [PubMed]

19. Velkov, T.; Thompson, P.E.; Nation, R.L.; Li, J. Structure-activity relationships of polymyxin antibiotics. *J. Med. Chem.* **2010**, *53*, 1898–1916. [CrossRef] [PubMed]

20. Hancock, R.E.; Scott, M.G. The role of antimicrobial peptides in animal defenses. *Proc. Natl. Acad. Sci. USA* **2000**, *97*, 8856–8861. [CrossRef] [PubMed]

21. Baeuerlein, A.; Ackermann, S.; Parlesak, A. Transepithelial activation of human leukocytes by probiotics and commensal bacteria: Role of Enterobacteriaceae-type endotoxin. *Microbiol. Immunol.* **2009**, *53*, 241–250. [CrossRef] [PubMed]

22. Li, J.; Nation, R.L.; Milne, R.W.; Turnidge, J.D.; Coulthard, K. Evaluation of colistin as an agent against multi-resistant Gram-negative bacteria. *Int. J. Antimicrob. Agents* **2005**, *25*, 11–25. [CrossRef] [PubMed]

23. Deris, Z.Z.; Akter, J.; Sivanesan, S.; Roberts, K.D.; Thompson, P.E.; Nation, R.L.; Li, J.; Velkov, T. A secondary mode of action of polymyxins against Gram-negative bacteria involves the inhibition of NADH-quinone oxidoreductase activity. *J. Antibiot. (Tokyo)* **2014**, *67*, 147–151. [CrossRef] [PubMed]

24. Lesho, E.; Yoon, E.J.; McGann, P.; Snesrud, E.; Kwak, Y.; Milillo, M.; Onmus-Leone, F.; Preston, L.; St Clair, K.; Nikolich, M.; et al. Emergence of colistin-resistance in extremely drug-resistant *Acinetobacter baumannii* containing a novel *pmrCAB* operon during colistin therapy of wound infections. *J. Infect. Dis.* **2013**, *208*, 1142–1151. [CrossRef] [PubMed]

25. Rolain, J.M.; Diene, S.M.; Kempf, M.; Gimenez, G.; Robert, C.; Raoult, D. Real-time sequencing to decipher the molecular mechanism of resistance of a clinical pan-drug-resistant *Acinetobacter baumannii* isolate from Marseille, France. *Antimicrob. Agents Chemother.* **2013**, *57*, 592–596. [CrossRef] [PubMed]

26. Snitkin, E.S.; Zelazny, A.M.; Gupta, J.; Program, N.C.S.; Palmore, T.N.; Murray, P.R.; Segre, J.A. Genomic insights into the fate of colistin resistance and *Acinetobacter baumannii* during patient treatment. *Genome Res.* **2013**, *23*, 1155–1162. [CrossRef] [PubMed]

27. Adams, M.D.; Nickel, G.C.; Bajaksouzian, S.; Lavender, H.; Murthy, A.R.; Jacobs, M.R.; Bonomo, R.A. Resistance to colistin in *Acinetobacter baumannii* associated with mutations in the PmrAB two-component system. *Antimicrob. Agents Chemother.* **2009**, *53*, 3628–3634. [CrossRef] [PubMed]

28. Arroyo, L.A.; Herrera, C.M.; Fernandez, L.; Hankins, J.V.; Trent, M.S.; Hancock, R.E. The PmrCAB operon mediates polymyxin resistance in *Acinetobacter baumannii* ATCC 17978 and clinical isolates through phosphoethanolamine modification of lipid A. *Antimicrob. Agents Chemother.* **2011**, *55*, 3743–3751. [CrossRef] [PubMed]

29. Beceiro, A.; Llobet, E.; Aranda, J.; Bengoechea, J.A.; Doumith, M.; Hornsey, M.; Dhanji, H.; Chart, H.; Bou, G.; Livermore, D.M.; et al. Phosphoethanolamine modification of lipid A in colistin-resistant variants of *Acinetobacter baumannii* mediated by the PmrAB two-component regulatory system. *Antimicrob. Agents Chemother.* **2011**, *55*, 3370–3379. [CrossRef] [PubMed]

30. Park, Y.K.; Choi, J.Y.; Shin, D.; Ko, K.S. Correlation between overexpression and amino acid substitution of the PmrAB locus and colistin resistance in *Acinetobacter baumannii*. *Int. J. Antimicrob. Agents* **2011**, *37*, 525–530. [CrossRef] [PubMed]

31. Pelletier, M.R.; Casella, L.G.; Jones, J.W.; Adams, M.D.; Zurawski, D.V.; Hazlett, K.R.; Doi, Y.; Ernst, R.K. Unique structural modifications are present in the lipopolysaccharide from colistin-resistant strains of *Acinetobacter baumannii*. *Antimicrob. Agents Chemother.* **2013**, *57*, 4831–4840. [CrossRef] [PubMed]

32. Boll, J.M.; Tucker, A.T.; Klein, D.R.; Beltran, A.M.; Brodbelt, J.S.; Davies, B.W.; Trent, M.S. Reinforcing lipid A acylation on the cell surface of *Acinetobacter baumannii* promotes cationic antimicrobial peptide resistance and desiccation survival. *MBio* **2015**, *6*, e00478-15. [CrossRef] [PubMed]

33. Moffatt, J.H.; Harper, M.; Adler, B.; Nation, R.L.; Li, J.; Boyce, J.D. Insertion sequence ISAba11 is involved in colistin resistance and loss of lipopolysaccharide in *Acinetobacter baumannii*. *Antimicrob. Agents Chemother.* **2011**, *55*, 3022–3024. [CrossRef] [PubMed]

34. Moffatt, J.H.; Harper, M.; Harrison, P.; Hale, J.D.; Vinogradov, E.; Seemann, T.; Henry, R.; Crane, B.; St Michael, F.; Cox, A.D.; et al. Colistin resistance in *Acinetobacter baumannii* is mediated by complete loss of lipopolysaccharide production. *Antimicrob. Agents Chemother.* **2010**, *54*, 4971–4977. [CrossRef] [PubMed]

35. Hood, M.I.; Becker, K.W.; Roux, C.M.; Dunman, P.M.; Skaar, E.P. Genetic determinants of intrinsic colistin tolerance in *Acinetobacter baumannii*. *Infect. Immun.* **2013**, *81*, 542–551. [CrossRef] [PubMed]

36. Lean, S.S.; Suhaili, Z.; Ismail, S.; Rahman, N.I.; Othman, N.; Abdullah, F.H.; Jusoh, Z.; Yeo, C.C.; Thong, K.L. Prevalence and genetic characterization of carbapenem- and polymyxin-resistant *Acinetobacter baumannii* isolated from a tertiary hospital in Terengganu, Malaysia. *ISRN Microbiol.* **2014**, *2014*, 953417. [CrossRef] [PubMed]

37. Bojkovic, J.; Richie, D.L.; Six, D.A.; Rath, C.M.; Sawyer, W.S.; Hu, Q.; Dean, C.R. Characterization of an *Acinetobacter baumannii* lptD deletion strain: Permeability defects and response to inhibition of lipopolysaccharide and fatty acid biosynthesis. *J. Bacteriol.* **2015**, *198*, 731–741. [CrossRef] [PubMed]

38. Moffatt, J.H.; Harper, M.; Mansell, A.; Crane, B.; Fitzsimons, T.C.; Nation, R.L.; Li, J.; Adler, B.; Boyce, J.D. Lipopolysaccharide-deficient *Acinetobacter baumannii* shows altered signaling through host Toll-like receptors and increased susceptibility to the host antimicrobial peptide LL-37. *Infect. Immun.* **2013**, *81*, 684–689. [CrossRef] [PubMed]

39. Maifiah, M.H.; Cheah, S.E.; Johnson, M.D.; Han, M.L.; Boyce, J.D.; Thamlikitkul, V.; Forrest, A.; Kaye, K.S.; Hertzog, P.; Purcell, A.W.; et al. Global metabolic analyses identify key differences in metabolite levels between polymyxin-susceptible and polymyxin-resistant *Acinetobacter baumannii*. *Sci. Rep.* **2016**, *6*, 22287. [CrossRef] [PubMed]

40. Malinverni, J.C.; Silhavy, T.J. An ABC transport system that maintains lipid asymmetry in the Gram-negative outer membrane. *Proc. Natl. Acad. Sci. USA* **2009**, *106*, 8009–8014. [CrossRef] [PubMed]

41. Audet, A.; Nantel, G.; Proulx, P. Phospholipase A activity in growing *Escherichia coli* cells. *Biochim. Biophys. Acta* **1974**, *348*, 334–343. [CrossRef]

42. Thi Khanh Nhu, N.; Riordan, D.W.; Do Hoang Nhu, T.; Thanh, D.P.; Thwaites, G.; Huong Lan, N.P.; Wren, B.W.; Baker, S.; Stabler, R.A. The induction and identification of novel colistin resistance mutations in *Acinetobacter baumannii* and their implications. *Sci. Rep.* **2016**, *6*, 28291. [CrossRef] [PubMed]

43. Hood, M.I.; Jacobs, A.C.; Sayood, K.; Dunman, P.M.; Skaar, E.P. *Acinetobacter baumannii* increases tolerance to antibiotics in response to monovalent cations. *Antimicrob. Agents Chemother.* **2010**, *54*, 1029–1041. [CrossRef] [PubMed]

44. Ni, W.; Li, Y.; Guan, J.; Zhao, J.; Cui, J.; Wang, R.; Liu, Y. Effects of efflux pump inhibitors on colistin resistance in multidrug-resistant Gram-negative bacteria. *Antimicrob. Agents Chemother.* **2016**, *60*, 3215–3218. [CrossRef] [PubMed]

45. Andersson, D.I. Persistence of antibiotic resistant bacteria. *Curr. Opin. Microbiol.* **2003**, *6*, 452–456. [CrossRef] [PubMed]

46. Mu, X.; Wang, N.; Li, X.; Shi, K.; Zhou, Z.; Yu, Y.; Hua, X. The effect of colistin resistance-associated mutations on the fitness of *Acinetobacter baumannii*. *Front. Microbiol.* **2016**, *7*, 1715. [CrossRef] [PubMed]

47. Geisinger, E.; Isberg, R.R. Interplay between antibiotic resistance and virulence during disease promoted by multidrug-resistant bacteria. *J. Infect. Dis.* **2017**, *215*, S9–S17. [CrossRef] [PubMed]

48. Beceiro, A.; Tomas, M.; Bou, G. Antimicrobial resistance and virulence: A successful or deleterious association in the bacterial world? *Clin. Microbiol. Rev.* **2013**, *26*, 185–230. [CrossRef] [PubMed]

49. McConnell, M.J.; Actis, L.; Pachon, J. *Acinetobacter baumannii*: Human infections, factors contributing to pathogenesis and animal models. *FEMS Microbiol. Rev.* **2013**, *37*, 130–155. [CrossRef] [PubMed]

50. Antunes, L.C.; Visca, P.; Towner, K.J. *Acinetobacter baumannii*: Evolution of a global pathogen. *Pathog. Dis.* **2014**, *71*, 292–301. [CrossRef] [PubMed]

51. Rolain, J.M.; Roch, A.; Castanier, M.; Papazian, L.; Raoult, D. *Acinetobacter baumannii* resistant to colistin with impaired virulence: A case report from France. *J. Infect. Dis.* **2011**, *204*, 1146–1147. [CrossRef] [PubMed]

52. Hraiech, S.; Roch, A.; Lepidi, H.; Atieh, T.; Audoly, G.; Rolain, J.M.; Raoult, D.; Brunel, J.M.; Papazian, L.; Bregeon, F. Impaired virulence and fitness of a colistin-resistant clinical isolate of *Acinetobacter baumannii* in a rat model of pneumonia. *Antimicrob. Agents Chemother.* **2013**, *57*, 5120–5121. [CrossRef] [PubMed]

53. Pournaras, S.; Poulou, A.; Dafopoulou, K.; Chabane, Y.N.; Kristo, I.; Makris, D.; Hardouin, J.; Cosette, P.; Tsakris, A.; De, E. Growth retardation, reduced invasiveness, and impaired colistin-mediated cell death associated with colistin resistance development in *Acinetobacter baumannii*. *Antimicrob. Agents Chemother.* **2014**, *58*, 828–832. [CrossRef] [PubMed]

54. Lopez-Rojas, R.; Jimenez-Mejias, M.E.; Lepe, J.A.; Pachon, J. *Acinetobacter baumannii* resistant to colistin alters its antibiotic resistance profile: A case report from Spain. *J. Infect. Dis.* **2011**, *204*, 1147–1148. [CrossRef] [PubMed]

55. Lopez-Rojas, R.; McConnell, M.J.; Jimenez-Mejias, M.E.; Dominguez-Herrera, J.; Fernandez-Cuenca, F.; Pachon, J. Colistin resistance in a clinical *Acinetobacter baumannii* strain appearing after colistin treatment: Effect on virulence and bacterial fitness. *Antimicrob. Agents Chemother.* **2013**, *57*, 4587–4589. [CrossRef] [PubMed]

56. Eveillard, M.; Soltner, C.; Kempf, M.; Saint-Andre, J.P.; Lemarie, C.; Randrianarivelo, C.; Seifert, H.; Wolff, M.; Joly-Guillou, M.L. The virulence variability of different *Acinetobacter baumannii* strains in experimental pneumonia. *J. Infect.* **2010**, *60*, 154–161. [CrossRef] [PubMed]

57. Durante-Mangoni, E.; Del Franco, M.; Andini, R.; Bernardo, M.; Giannouli, M.; Zarrilli, R. Emergence of colistin resistance without loss of fitness and virulence after prolonged colistin administration in a patient with extensively drug-resistant *Acinetobacter baumannii*. *Diagn. Microbiol. Infect. Dis.* **2015**, *82*, 222–226. [CrossRef] [PubMed]

58. Dahdouh, E.; Gomez-Gil, R.; Sanz, S.; Gonzalez-Zorn, B.; Daoud, Z.; Mingorance, J.; Suarez, M. A novel mutation in *pmrB* mediates colistin resistance during therapy of *Acinetobacter baumannii*. *Int. J. Antimicrob. Agents* **2017**, *49*, 727–733. [CrossRef] [PubMed]

59. Dafopoulou, K.; Xavier, B.B.; Hotterbeekx, A.; Janssens, L.; Lammens, C.; De, E.; Goossens, H.; Tsakris, A.; Malhotra-Kumar, S.; Pournaras, S. Colistin-resistant *Acinetobacter baumannii* clinical strains with deficient biofilm formation. *Antimicrob. Agents Chemother.* **2016**, *60*, 1892–1895. [CrossRef] [PubMed]

60. Wand, M.E.; Bock, L.J.; Bonney, L.C.; Sutton, J.M. Retention of virulence following adaptation to colistin in *Acinetobacter baumannii* reflects the mechanism of resistance. *J. Antimicrob. Chemother.* **2015**, *70*, 2209–2216. [CrossRef] [PubMed]

61. Fernandez-Reyes, M.; Rodriguez-Falcon, M.; Chiva, C.; Pachon, J.; Andreu, D.; Rivas, L. The cost of resistance to colistin in *Acinetobacter baumannii*: A proteomic perspective. *Proteomics* **2009**, *9*, 1632–1645. [CrossRef] [PubMed]

62. Lopez-Rojas, R.; Dominguez-Herrera, J.; McConnell, M.J.; Docobo-Perez, F.; Smani, Y.; Fernandez-Reyes, M.; Rivas, L.; Pachon, J. Impaired virulence and In Vivo fitness of colistin-resistant *Acinetobacter baumannii*. *J. Infect. Dis.* **2011**, *203*, 545–548. [CrossRef] [PubMed]

63. Lopez-Rojas, R.; Garcia-Quintanilla, M.; Labrador-Herrera, G.; Pachon, J.; McConnell, M.J. Impaired growth under iron-limiting conditions associated with the acquisition of colistin resistance in *Acinetobacter baumannii*. *Int. J. Antimicrob. Agents* **2016**, *47*, 473–477. [CrossRef] [PubMed]

64. Valencia, R.; Arroyo, L.A.; Conde, M.; Aldana, J.M.; Torres, M.J.; Fernandez-Cuenca, F.; Garnacho-Montero, J.; Cisneros, J.M.; Ortiz, C.; Pachon, J.; et al. Nosocomial outbreak of infection with pan-drug-resistant *Acinetobacter baumannii* in a tertiary care university hospital. *Infect. Control Hosp. Epidemiol.* **2009**, *30*, 257–263. [CrossRef] [PubMed]

65. Beceiro, A.; Moreno, A.; Fernandez, N.; Vallejo, J.A.; Aranda, J.; Adler, B.; Harper, M.; Boyce, J.D.; Bou, G. Biological cost of different mechanisms of colistin resistance and their impact on virulence in *Acinetobacter baumannii*. *Antimicrob. Agents Chemother.* **2014**, *58*, 518–526. [CrossRef] [PubMed]

66. Jones, C.L.; Singh, S.S.; Alamneh, Y.; Casella, L.G.; Ernst, R.K.; Lesho, E.P.; Waterman, P.E.; Zurawski, D.V. In Vivo fitness adaptations of colistin-resistant *Acinetobacter baumannii* isolates to oxidative stress. *Antimicrob. Agents Chemother.* **2017**, *61*, e00598-16. [CrossRef] [PubMed]

67. Durante-Mangoni, E.; Zarrilli, R. Global spread of drug-resistant *Acinetobacter baumannii*: Molecular epidemiology and management of antimicrobial resistance. *Future Microbiol.* **2011**, *6*, 407–422. [CrossRef] [PubMed]

68. Oikonomou, O.; Sarrou, S.; Papagiannitsis, C.C.; Georgiadou, S.; Mantzarlis, K.; Zakynthinos, E.; Dalekos, G.N.; Petinaki, E. Rapid dissemination of colistin and carbapenem resistant *Acinetobacter baumannii* in Central Greece: Mechanisms of resistance, molecular identification and epidemiological data. *BMC Infect. Dis.* **2015**, *15*, 559. [CrossRef] [PubMed]

69. Li, J.; Nation, R.L.; Owen, R.J.; Wong, S.; Spelman, D.; Franklin, C. Antibiograms of multidrug-resistant clinical *Acinetobacter baumannii*: Promising therapeutic options for treatment of infection with colistin-resistant strains. *Clin. Infect. Dis.* **2007**, *45*, 594–598. [CrossRef] [PubMed]

70. Mendes, R.E.; Fritsche, T.R.; Sader, H.S.; Jones, R.N. Increased antimicrobial susceptibility profiles among polymyxin-resistant *Acinetobacter baumannii* clinical isolates. *Clin. Infect. Dis.* **2008**, *46*, 1324–1326. [CrossRef] [PubMed]

Permissions

All chapters in this book were first published in ANTIBIOTICS, by MDPI; hereby published with permission under the Creative Commons Attribution License or equivalent. Every chapter published in this book has been scrutinized by our experts. Their significance has been extensively debated. The topics covered herein carry significant findings which will fuel the growth of the discipline. They may even be implemented as practical applications or may be referred to as a beginning point for another development.

The contributors of this book come from diverse backgrounds, making this book a truly international effort. This book will bring forth new frontiers with its revolutionizing research information and detailed analysis of the nascent developments around the world.

We would like to thank all the contributing authors for lending their expertise to make the book truly unique.

They have played a crucial role in the development of this book. Without their invaluable contributions this book wouldn't have been possible. They have made vital efforts to compile up to date information on the varied aspects of this subject to make this book a valuable addition to the collection of many professionals and students.

This book was conceptualized with the vision of imparting up-to-date information and advanced data in this field. To ensure the same, a matchless editorial board was set up. Every individual on the board went through rigorous rounds of assessment to prove their worth. After which they invested a large part of their time researching and compiling the most relevant data for our readers.

The editorial board has been involved in producing this book since its inception. They have spent rigorous hours researching and exploring the diverse topics which have resulted in the successful publishing of this book. They have passed on their knowledge of decades through this book. To expedite this challenging task, the publisher supported the team at every step. A small team of assistant editors was also appointed to further simplify the editing procedure and attain best results for the readers.

Apart from the editorial board, the designing team has also invested a significant amount of their time in understanding the subject and creating the most relevant covers. They scrutinized every image to scout for the most suitable representation of the subject and create an appropriate cover for the book.

The publishing team has been an ardent support to the editorial, designing and production team. Their endless efforts to recruit the best for this project, has resulted in the accomplishment of this book. They are a veteran in the field of academics and their pool of knowledge is as vast as their experience in printing. Their expertise and guidance has proved useful at every step. Their uncompromising quality standards have made this book an exceptional effort. Their encouragement from time to time has been an inspiration for everyone.

The publisher and the editorial board hope that this book will prove to be a valuable piece of knowledge for researchers, students, practitioners and scholars across the globe.

List of Contributors

Ellen Berni, Laura A. Scott, Sara Jenkins-Jones and Christopher Ll. Morgan
Global Epidemiology and Medical Statistics, Pharmatelligence, Cardiff CF14 3QX, UK

Craig J. Currie
Global Epidemiology and Medical Statistics, Pharmatelligence, Cardiff CF14 3QX, UK
Cochrane Institute of Primary Care and Public Health, Cardiff University, The Pharma Research Centre, Abton House, Wedal Road, Cardiff CF14 3QX, UK

Hanka De Voogd and Monica S. Rocha
Mylan Established Pharmaceuticals Division, Weesp 1381 CP, The Netherlands

Chris C. Butler
Nuffield Department of Primary Care Health Sciences, University of Oxford, Oxford OX2 6GG, UK

Yōko Takahashi and Takuji Nakashima
Kitasato Institute for Life Sciences, Kitasato University, 5-9-1 Shirokane, Minato-ku, Tokyo 108-8641, Japan

Ashraf M. A. Abdalla and Abdelazim Y. Abdelgadir
Department of Forest Products and Industries, Faculty of Forestry, University of Khartoum, Khartoum 11111, Sudan

Enass Y. A. Salih
Department of Forest Products and Industries, Faculty of Forestry, University of Khartoum, Khartoum 11111, Sudan
Faculty of Pharmacy, Division of Pharmaceutical Biosciences, University of Helsinki, FIN-00014 Helsinki, Finland
Viikki Tropical Resources Institute (VITRI), Department of Forest Sciences, University of Helsinki, FIN-00014 Helsinki, Finland

Mustafa K. M. Fahmi
Department of Forest Products and Industries, Faculty of Forestry, University of Khartoum, Khartoum 11111, Sudan
Viikki Tropical Resources Institute (VITRI), Department of Forest Sciences, University of Helsinki, FIN-00014 Helsinki, Finland

Hiba A. Ali
Commission for Biotechnology and Genetic Engineering, National Centre for Research, Khartoum, Sudan

Pia Fyhrquist
Faculty of Pharmacy, Division of Pharmaceutical Biosciences, University of Helsinki, FIN-00014 Helsinki, Finland

Markku Kanninen, Marketta Sipi and Olavi Luukkanen
Viikki Tropical Resources Institute (VITRI), Department of Forest Sciences, University of Helsinki, FIN-00014 Helsinki, Finland

Mai H. Elamin
Department of Phytochemistry, Faculty of Pharmacy, University of Sciences and Technology, Omdurman, Sudan

Ulugbek A. Abdufattaev
The Republican Specialized Center of Urology, 100109 Tashkent, Uzbekistan

Jakhongir F. Alidjanov
The Republican Specialized Center of Urology, 100109 Tashkent, Uzbekistan
Clinic of Urology, Paediatric Urology and Andrology, Justus-Liebig-University, 35392 Giessen, Germany

Adrian Pilatz and Florian M. E.Wagenlehner
Clinic of Urology, Paediatric Urology and Andrology, Justus-Liebig-University, 35392 Giessen, Germany

Kurt G. Naber
Department of Urology, School of Medicine, Technical University of Munich, D-80333 Munich, Germany

Sidney Hayes, Karthic Rajamanickam and Connie Hayes
Department of Microbiology and Immunology, College of Medicine, University of Saskatchewan, Saskatoon, SK S7N 5E5, Canada

Yao Liu and Eefjan Breukink
Department of Membrane Biochemistry and Biophysics, Utrecht University, Utrecht 3584 CH, The Netherlands

Gabriela Lopes Fernandes and Debora Barros Barbosa
Department of Dental Materials and Prosthodontics, School of Dentistry, Araçatuba, São Paulo State University (UNESP), Araçatuba 16015-050, São Paulo, Brazil

Renan Aparecido Fernandes
Department of Dental Materials and Prosthodontics, School of Dentistry, Araçatuba, São Paulo State University (UNESP), Araçatuba 16015-050, São Paulo, Brazil

Department of Dentistry, University Center of Adamantina (UNIFAI), Adamantina 17800-000, São Paulo, Brazil

Alberto Carlos Botazzo Delbem, Jackeline Gallo do Amaral and José Antonio Santos Souza
Department of Pediatric Dentistry and Public Health, School of Dentistry, Araçatuba, São Paulo State University (UNESP), Araçatuba 16015-050, São Paulo, Brazil

Francisco Nunes de Souza Neto and Emerson Rodrigues Camargo
Department of Chemistry, Federal University of São Carlos, São Carlos 13565-905, São Paulo, Brazil

Luiz Fernando Gorup
Department of Chemistry, Federal University of São Carlos, São Carlos 13565-905, São Paulo, Brazil
FACET — Department of Chemistry, Federal University of Grande Dourados, Dourados 79804-970, Mato Grosso do Sul, Brazil

Douglas Roberto Monteiro
Graduate Program in Dentistry (GPD — Master´s Degree), University of Western São Paulo (UNOESTE), Presidente Prudente 19050-920, São Paulo, Brazil

Alessandra Marçal Agostinho Hunt
Department of Microbiology and Molecular Genetics, Michigan State University, East Lansing, MI 48823, USA

Catarina Moreirinha, Carla Pereira and Adelaide Almeida
Departament of Biology and CESAM, Campus Universitário de Santiago, Universidade de Aveiro, 3810-193 Aveiro, Portugal

Nádia Osório and Sara Simões
Escola Superior de Tecnologia da Saúde, Rua 5 de Outubro, SM Bispo. Instituto Politécnico de Coimbra, Apartado 7006, 3046-854 Coimbra, Portugal

Ivonne Delgadillo
Departament of Chemistry, QOPNA, University of Aveiro, Campus Universitário de Santiago, 3810-193 Aveiro, Portugal

Jie Feng, Wanliang Shi, Genevieve M. Tauxe, Conor J. McMeniman and Ying Zhang
Department of Molecular Microbiology and Immunology, Bloomberg School of Public Health, Johns Hopkins University, Baltimore, MD 21205, USA

Judith Miklossy
International Alzheimer Research Centre, Prevention Alzheimer International Foundation, Martigny-Croix CP 16 1921, Switzerland

Soumya Ghosh, Robyn McArthur, Zhi Chao Guo, Rory McKerchar, Kingsley Donkor and Naowarat Cheeptham
Department of Biological Sciences, Thompson Rivers University, Kamloops, BC V2C 0C8, Canada

Jianping Xu
Department of Biology, McMaster University, Hamilton, ON L8S 4K1, Canada

Jiage Feng
Department of Chemistry, University of Adelaide, North Tce, Adelaide, SA 5005, Australia

Ashleigh S. Paparella, Grant W. Booker and Steven W. Polyak
School of Biological Sciences, University of Adelaide, North Tce, Adelaide, SA 5005, Australia

Andrew D. Abell
School of Biological Sciences, University of Adelaide, North Tce, Adelaide, SA 5005, Australia
Centre for Nanoscale BioPhotonics (CNBP), University of Adelaide, Adelaide, SA 5005, Australia

Aida Duarte
Microbiology and Immunology Department, Interdisciplinary Research Centre Egas Moniz (CiiEM), Faculty of Pharmacy, Universidade de Lisboa, 1649-003 Lisboa, Portugal

Cátia Caneiras
Microbiology and Immunology Department, Interdisciplinary Research Centre Egas Moniz (CiiEM), Faculty of Pharmacy, Universidade de Lisboa, 1649-003 Lisboa, Portugal
Institute of Environmental Health (ISAMB), Faculty of Medicine, Universidade de Lisboa, 1649-028 Lisboa, Portugal

Filipa Calisto
Microbiology and Immunology Department, Interdisciplinary Research Centre Egas Moniz (CiiEM), Faculty of Pharmacy, Universidade de Lisboa, 1649-003 Lisboa, Portugal
Instituto de Tecnologia Química e Biológica António Xavier, Universidade Nova de Lisboa, 2780-157 Oeiras, Portugal

Gabriela Jorge da Silva
Faculty of Pharmacy, Universidade de Coimbra, Polo das Ciências da Saúde, Azinhaga de Santa Comba, 3000-548 Coimbra, Portugal

Luis Lito
Laboratory of Microbiology, Centro Hospitalar Lisboa Norte, 1649-035 Lisboa, Portugal

José Melo-Cristino
Laboratory of Microbiology, Centro Hospitalar Lisboa Norte, 1649-035 Lisboa, Portugal
Institute of Microbiology, Institute of Molecular Medicine, Faculty of Medicine, Universidade de Lisboa, 1649-028 Lisboa, Portugal

Nadine Schallopp, Sarah Milbredt, Theodor Sperlea, Franziska S. Kemter, Matthias Bruhn and TorstenWaldminghaus
LOEWE Center for Synthetic Microbiology-SYNMIKRO, Philipps-Universität Marburg, Marburg 35032, Germany

Daniel Schindler
LOEWE Center for Synthetic Microbiology-SYNMIKRO, Philipps-Universität Marburg, Marburg 35032, Germany
School of Chemistry, Manchester Institute of Biotechnology, University of Manchester, Manchester M1 7DN, UK

Erika L. Cyphert and Horst A. von Recum
Department of Biomedical Engineering, CaseWestern Reserve University, 10900 Euclid Avenue, Cleveland, OH 44106, USA

Jaqueline D. Wallat and Jonathan K. Pokorski
Department of Macromolecular Science and Engineering, CaseWestern Reserve University, 2100 Adelbert Road, Cleveland, OH 44106, USA

Ángel Manteca and Paula Yagüe
Área de Microbiología, Departamento de Biología Funcional IUOPA, Facultad de Medicina, Universidad de Oviedo, 33006 Oviedo, Spain

Gabriela Jorge Da Silva and Sara Domingues
Faculty of Pharmacy, University of Coimbra, 3000-548 Coimbra, Portugal
Centre for Neurosciences and Cell Biology, University of Coimbra, 3000-548 Coimbra, Portugal

Index

www.ingramcontent.com/pod-product-compliance
Lightning Source LLC
Chambersburg PA
CBHW080515200326
41458CB00012B/4215